Second Edition

Forensic Toxicology

A Comparative Approach

As per the latest
CBME Guidelines |
Competency Based Undergraduate Curriculum
for the Indian Medical Graduate

- **For MBBS, Postgraduate Students of Forensic Medicine and Toxicology, and BPMT Students**
- **For Students Preparing for NEET-PG and other Entrance Examinations**
- **Reference Guide for Clinicians and Medical Officers Dealing in Forensic-Toxicological Emergencies**

Second Edition

Forensic
Toxicology

A Comparative Approach

*As per the latest
CBME Guidelines |
Competency Based Undergraduate Curriculum
for the Indian Medical Graduate*

- For MBBS, Postgraduate Students of Forensic Medicine and Toxicology, and BPMT Students
- For Students Preparing for NEET-PG and other Entrance Examinations
- Reference Guide for Clinicians and Medical Officers Dealing in Forensic-Toxicological Emergencies

Vipul Ambade MBBS, MD, LLB

Professor and Head
Department of Forensic Medicine
Government Medical College
Gondia, Maharashtra

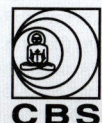

CBS

CBS Publishers & Distributors Pvt Ltd

New Delhi • Bengaluru • Chennai • Kochi • Kolkata • Lucknow • Mumbai
Hyderabad • Jharkhand • Nagpur • Patna • Pune • Uttarakhand

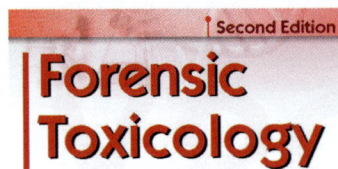

Second Edition

Forensic Toxicology

A Comparative Approach

ISBN: 978-93-90709-26-7

Second Edition: 2022

First Edition: 2016

Published by Satish Kumar Jain and produced by Varun Jain for

CBS Publishers & Distributors Pvt Ltd

4819/XI Prahlad Street, 24 Ansari Road, Daryaganj, New Delhi 110 002, India
Ph: 011-23289259, 23266861, 23266867   Website: www.cbspd.com
Fax: 011-23243014   e-mail: delhi@cbspd.com; cbspubs@airtelmail.in
Corporate Office: 204 FIE, Industrial Area, Patparganj, Delhi 110 092
Ph: 011-4934 4934   Fax: 011-4934 4935   e-mail: publishing@cbspd.com; publicity@cbspd.com

Branches

- **Bengaluru:** Seema House 2975, 17th Cross, K.R. Road, Banasankari 2nd Stage, Bengaluru 560 070, Karnataka, India
  Ph: +91-80-26771678/79   Fax: +91-80-26771680   e-mail: bangalore@cbspd.com
- **Chennai:** 7, Subbaraya Street, Shenoy Nagar, Chennai 600 030, Tamil Nadu, India
  Ph: +91-44-26680620, 26681266   Fax: +91-44-42032115   e-mail: chennai@cbspd.com
- **Kochi:** 42/1325, 1326, Power House Road, Opp. KSEB, Power House, Ernakulam 682018, Kochi, Kerala , India
  Ph: +91-484-4059061-65   Fax: +91-484-4059065   e-mail: kochi@cbspd.com
- **Kolkata:** 147, Hind Ceramics Compound, 1st Floor, Nilgunj Road, Belghoria, Kolkata-700056, West Bengal, India
  Ph: +91-9096713055/7798394118, 9836841399   e-mail: kolkata@cbspd.com
- **Lucknow:** Basement, Khushnuma Complex, 7, Meerabai Marg (Behind Jawahar Bhawan), Lucknow 226001 (UP), India
  Ph: 0522-4000032   e-mail: tiwari.lucknow@cbspd.com
- **Mumbai:** PWD Shed, Gala No. 25/26, Ramchandra Bhatt Marg, Next to JJ Hospital, Gate No. 2 Opp. Union Bank of India, Noorbaug, Mumbai 400009, Maharashtra, India
  Ph: +91-22-66661880/89   e-mail: mumbai@cbspd.com

Representatives

- **Hyderabad** 0-9885175004 • **Jharkhand** 0-9811541605 • **Nagpur** 0-9421945513
- **Patna**   0-9334159340 • **Pune** 0-9623451994 • **Uttarakhand** 0-9716462459

Printed at HT Media Ltd, Greater Noida, UP, India

to

---

my parents
Late Shri Namdeorao Ambade
and
Smt Chandraprabha Ambade

Preface to the Second Edition

I am deeply overwhelmed after completing the compilation of the material of the second edition of the book *Forensic Toxicology: A Comparative Approach*. Since publishing the first edition, students, readers, and faculty forum have shared their views, comments and suggestions, particularly regarding the references. When I started to work on the second edition I thought it would be a breeze to add modification, recent advances and references, compared to the Herculean task of creating and publishing the first edition. However, once the work commenced, I realized that this revision would require even greater effort than the first edition; and the prevailing COVID-19 pandemic added further hurdles in it.

The most obvious change in the second edition is the inclusion of the references in the running literature in superscript and at the end of each chapter. The treatment pertaining to poisoning is often overlooked in forensic texts and not considered in clinical practice. Management of poisoning has been upgraded to the latest trends to be useful in clinical practice for the physician. The bedside/color test for the detection of different types of poisoning has been greatly updated. Specific Learning Objectives (SLOs) for each chapter as per the competency based learning recommended by the Medical Council of India for medical graduates have been incorporated. Important questions and MCQs are included in this edition to help students prepare for theory as well as practical examinations.

Vipul Ambade
vipulambade@rediffmail.com

Acknowledgments

Since the release of the first edition in 37th Annual Conference of Indian Academy of Forensic Medicine held at BJ Medical College, Ahmedabad, Gujarat, on 17th January, 2016, many students, readers and faculty forums have shared their views, comments and suggestions. To all of them, including in particular the following, my deepest sincere thanks: Dr Chetan Jani, Dr Kalidas Chavan, Dr Numan Hussaini, Dr Rajesh Bardale, Dr Harshwardhan Khartade, Dr Ravindra Deokar, Dr Ulhas Gonnade, Dr Shailendra Dhawne, Dr Jaideo Borkar, Dr Ajit Malani, Dr Manish Tiwari, Dr Ajay Taware, Dr Amol Shinde, Dr Naresh Zanzad, Dr SK Singhal, Dr Ajit Pathak, Dr Mohan Pawar, Dr Pawan Sable, Dr Swapnil Akhade, Dr Pawan Tekade, Dr Sharad Kuchewar, Dr Sachin Gadge, Dr Ravi Meshram, Dr Arun Jaiswani, Dr Ashok Najan, Dr Dayanand Kolpe, Dr Amol Maiyyar, Dr Arti Narde, Dr Shailesh Wakde, Dr Ajay Shendarkar, Dr Praveen Jadhav, Dr Pratik Gilbe, Dr Indrajeet Khandekar and many more with special thanks to Dr Manu Sharma for his overall technical support during the correction of revised edition of this book.

I would also like to acknowledge the unquestionable support of CBS Publishers & Distributors and Mr YN Arjuna (Senior Vice President—Publishing, Editorial and Publicity) along with his entire team for excellent formatting of this book.

Lastly, I am thankful to my wife Dr Hemlata, lovely daughters Vidhi and Aarohi, and my relatives and friends for helping me accomplish the task and extend their support even during the prevailing COVID-19 pandemic.

Vipul Ambade

Preface to the First Edition

It is a great pleasure that I am presenting the book *Forensic Toxicology: A Comparative Approach*. Taking into consideration that toxicology is very vast and difficult to remember, this book is presented in a simple and lucid language. The most important distinguishing feature of this book is that the different poisons of a group are discussed in a comparative point-wise manner in a tabular form for better understanding, learning and easy comparison. Apart from the numerous tabular charts, more than 180 photographs and figures related to poison/autopsy findings are included in this book. A separate chapter on preservation of viscera and other materials containing guidelines for collection, preservation and dispatch; and a new chapter on biological and chemical warfare are also included. Latest trends in the management of poisoning cases have been tried to cover in the book.

While preparing this book, I have gone through various textbooks and journals, and I am indebted to these authors. This book is primarily designed for undergraduate students and I hope it will make toxicology easier for students to learn and study. It will surely help the postgraduate students in preparing for examination and prove useful to the medical officers/practitioners while dealing the case of poisoning. I would definitely welcome the valuable suggestion and healthy criticism, which will be of immense help for future improvement of this book.

Vipul Ambade
vipulambade@rediffmail.com

Acknowledgments

I began my career in forensic medicine about 20 years back under the guidance of my teacher Dr AC Mohanty, a man with great vision and tremendous knowledge. While working with him, he not only made me realize the importance of the subject but also changed my outlook towards the dead victim. I gratefully acknowledge him for his guidance and influence which made me to persist my career in forensic.

It is with a great pleasure and deep sense of gratitude that I acknowledge my debt to my respected teacher Dr AP Dongre (Ex-Dean, Government Medical College, Yeotmal) for his affectionate guidance and constant support.

I am indebted to my revered teacher Dr AN Keoliya (Dean, Government Medical College, Gondia) for fostering me while learning and exploring my potential for different administrative and non-administrative work.

I am obliged to Dr Abhimanyu Niswade (Dean, Government Medical College, Nagpur) for allowing to embrace this work in the institution.

I am very grateful to my senior colleagues during postgraduation, Dr Ashesh Wankhede (Professor and Head, Forensic Medicine, Government Medical College, Jagdalpur, Chhattisgarh), Dr Anil Batra (Professor and Head, Forensic Medicine, Government Medical College, Akola) and Dr Kailash Zine (Professor and Head, Forensic Medicine, Government Medical College, Aurangabad) for being the first teachers who taught me medicolegal work.

I am also thankful to my classmates Dr Prakash Mohite (Professor and Head, Forensic Medicine, Medical College, Sawangi) and Dr Manish Shrigiriwar (OSD, Super-speciality Hospital, Nagpur) for their constant encouragement and unremitting help.

I respectfully thanks to Dr PG Dixit, Professor and Head, Forensic Medicine, Government Medical College, Nagpur, for permitting to carry out this work in the department.

I am respectfully thankful to Dr LK Bade, Dr HT Katade, Dr SS Gupta, Dr RK Singh (Raipur), Dr BH Tirpude (Sevagram), Dr SD Nanandkar, Dr SC Mohite, Dr Harish Pathak (Mumbai), Dr VR Agrawal (Pune), Dr HV Godbole, Dr RN Kagne (Pondicherry) for their guidance and blessing.

I am grateful to my friend Dr Linesh Khobragade (Consultant Pharmacologist, Sarjah), Dr Satin Meshram and Dr Nilesh Tumram (Department of Forensic Medicine, Government Medical College, Nagpur) without whom this endeavor would not have been possible.

I am thankful to Vinia Ambade (BE, Pune), Dr Raj Bhagwatkar (BDS, Nagpur), Dr Avinash Turankar (Department of Pharmacology, Nagpur) and Dr Pravin Shingade (Department of Medicine, Nagpur) for their help while preparing and editing the manuscript.

I am also thankful to Dr Hemant Kukde (Mumbai), Dr Nitin Barmate (Raipur), Shri Pramod Mandekar, Mr Sudesh Rathod (Yeotmal), Shri Gurudyal Pathak, Shri Ghodmare (Nagpur), Mr Arun Gujar (Pune), Mr Shantnu Sarkar and Mr Rajesh Shrivas (Nagpur) for their kind help.

Finally, I express my sincere gratitude and acknowledgment to my wife Dr Hemlata and lovely daughters Vidhi and Aarohi in accomplishing the task.

Vipul Ambade

Contents

Competencies

Number	Competency: The student shoud be able to

Topic: Forensic Pathology

FM2.14 Describe and discuss examination of clothing, preservation of viscera on postmortem examination for chemical analysis and other medico-legal purposes, postmortem artefacts

FM2.19 Investigation of anaesthetic, operative deaths: Describe and discuss special protocols for conduction of autopsy and for collection, preservation and dispatch of related material evidences

FM2.35 Demonstrate professionalism while conducting autopsy in medicolegal situations, interpretation of findings and making inference/opinion, collection preservation and dispatch of biological or trace evidences

Topic: Forensic Laboratory Investigation in Medico-legal Practice

FM6.1 Describe different types of specimen and tissues to be collected both in the living and dead: Body fluids (blood, urine, semen, faeces, saliva), skin, nails, tooth pulp, vaginal smear, viscera, skull, specimen for histo-pathological examination, blood grouping, HLA typing and DNA fingerprinting. Describe Locard's Exchange Principle

FM6.2 Describe the methods of sample collection, preservation, labelling, dispatch, and interpretation of reports

FM6.3 Demonstrate professionalism while sending the biological or trace evidences to Forensic Science laboratory, specifying the required tests to be carried out, objectives of preservation of evidences sent for examination, personal discussions on interpretation of findings

FM7.1 Enumerate the indications and describe the principles and appropriate use for: DNA profiling, Facial Reconstruction, Polygraph (Lie Detector), Narcoanalysis, Brain Mapping, Digital autopsy, Virtual Autopsy, Imaging technologies

Topic: Toxicology: General Toxicology

FM8.1 Describe the history of Toxicology

FM8.2 Define the terms Toxicology, Forensic Toxicology, Clinical Toxicology and poison

FM8.3 Describe the various types of poisons and diagnosis of poisoning in living and dead

FM8.4 Describe the Laws in relations to poisons including NDPS Act, Medico-legal aspects of poisons

FM8.5 Describe Medico-legal autopsy in cases of poisoning including preservation and dispatch of viscera for chemical analysis

FM8.6 Describe the general symptoms, principles of diagnosis and management of common poisons encountered in India

FM8.7 Describe simple bedside clinic tests to detect poison/drug in patient's body fluids

FM8.8 Describe basic methodologies in treatment of poisoning: Decontamination, supportive therapy, antidote therapy, procedures of enhanced elimination

FM8.9 Describe the procedure of intimation of suspicious cases or actual cases of foul play to the police, maintenance of records, preservation and despatch of relevant samples for laboratory analysis.

FM8.10   Describe the general principles of Analytical Toxicology and give a brief description of analytical methods available for toxicological analysis: Chromatography—Thin Layer Chromatography, Gas Chromatography, Liquid Chromatography and Atomic Absorption Spectroscopy

Topic: Toxicology: Chemical Toxicology

FM9.1   Describe General Principles and basic methodologies in treatment of poisoning: Decontamination, supportive therapy, antidote therapy, procedures of enhanced elimination with regard to: Caustics Inorganic—sulphuric, nitric, and hydrochloric acids; Organic—Carboloic Acid (phenol), Oxalic and acetylsalicylic acids

FM9.2   Describe General Principles and basic methodologies in treatment of poisoning: Decontamination, supportive therapy, antidote therapy, procedures of enhanced elimination with regard to Phosphorus, Iodine, Barium

FM9.3   Describe General Principles and basic methodologies in treatment of poisoning: Decontamination, supportive therapy, antidote therapy, procedures of enhanced elimination with regard to arsenic, lead, mercury, copper, iron, cadmium and thallium

FM9.4   Describe General Principles and basic methodologies in treatment of poisoning: Decontamination, supportive therapy, antidote therapy, procedures of enhanced elimination with regard to ethanol, methanol, ethylene glycol

FM9.5   Describe General Principles and basic methodologies in treatment of poisoning: Decontamination, supportive therapy, antidote therapy, procedures of enhanced elimination with regard to Organophosphates, Carbamates, Organochlorines, Pyrethroids, Paraquat, Aluminium and Zinc phosphide

FM9.6   Describe General Principles and basic methodologies in treatment of poisoning: Decontamination, supportive therapy, antidote therapy, procedures of enhanced elimination with regard to ammonia, carbon monoxide, hydrogen cyanide and derivatives, methyl isocyanate, tear (riot control) gases

Topic: Toxicology : Pharmaceutical Toxicology

FM10.1   Describe General Principles and basic methodologies in treatment of poisoning: Decontamination, supportive therapy, antidote therapy, procedures of enhanced elimination with regard to: (a) Antipyretics: Paracetamol, Salicylatess (b) Anti-Infective, (Common antibiotics—an overview), (c) Neuropsychotoxicology: Barbiturates, benzodiazepins; phenytoin, lithium, haloperidol, neuroleptics, tricyclics, (d) Narcotic Analgesics, Anaesthetics, and Muscle Relaxants, (e) Cardiovascular Toxicology Cardiotoxic plants—oleander, odollam, aconite, digitalis, (f) Gastrointestinal and Endocrinal Drugs—Insulin

Topic: Toxicology: Biotoxicology

FM11.1   Describe features and management of Snake bite, scorpion sting, bee and wasp sting and spider bite

Topic: Toxicology: Sociomedical Toxicology

FM12.1   Describe features and management of abuse/poisoning with following chemicals: Tobacco, cannabis, amphetamines, cocaine, hallucinogens, designer drugs and solvent

Topic: Toxicology: Environmental Toxicology

FM13.1   Describe toxic pollution of environment, its medico-legal aspects & toxic hazards of occupation and industry

FM13.2   Describe medico-legal aspects of poisoning in Workman's Compensation Act

Topic: Skills in Toxicology

FM14.2   Demonstrate the correct technique of clinical examination in a suspected case of poisoning and prepare medico-legal report in a simulated/supervised environment

FM14.3   Assist and demonstrate the proper technique in collecting, preserving and dispatch of the exhibits in a suspected case of poisoning, along with clinical examination

FM14.16 To examine and prepare medico-legal report of drunk person in a simulated/supervised environment

FM14.17 To identify and draw medico-legal inference from common poisons: Datura, castor, cannabis, opium, aconite copper sulphate, pesticides compounds, marking nut, oleander, Nux vomica, abrus seeds, Snakes, capsicum, calotropis, lead compounds and tobacco.

Integration Topics

PH1.22 Describe drugs of abuse (dependence, addiction, stimulants, depressants, psychedelics, drugs used for criminal offences)

PH5.7 Demonstrate an understanding of the legal and ethical aspects of prescribing drugs

IM20.1 Enumerate the poisonous snakes of your area and describe the distinguishing marks of each

IM20.2 Describe, demonstrate in a volunteer or a mannequin and educate (to other health care workers/patients) the correct initial management of patient with a snake bite in the field

IM20.3 Describe the initial approach to the stabilisation of the patient who presents with snake bite

IM20.4 Elicit and document and present an appropriate history, the circumstance, time, kind of snake, evolution of symptoms in a patient with snake bite

IM21.2 Enumerate the common plant poisons seen in your area and describe their toxicology, clinical features, prognosis and specific approach to detoxification

IM21.3 Enumerate the common corrosives used in your area and describe their toxicology, clinical features, prognosis and approach to therapy

IM21.4 Enumerate the commonly observed drug overdose in your area and describe their toxicology, clinical features, prognosis and approach to therapy

IM21.5 Observe and describe the functions and role of a poison center in suspected poisoning

IM21.6 Describe the medico-legal aspects of suspected suicidal or homicidal poisoning and demonstrate the correct procedure to write a medico legal report on a suspected poisoning

IM21.7 Counsel family members of a patient with suspected poisoning about the clinical and medico legal aspects with empathy

IM21.8 Enumerate the indications for psychiatric consultation and describe the precautions to be taken in a patient with suspected suicidal ideation/gesture

Reference

Medical Council of India, Competency Based Undergraduate Curriculum for the Indian Medical Graduate. Volume-1 (2018). UG-Curriculum-Vol-I.pdf (nmc.org.in)

General Toxicology

Toxicology is derived from the combination of two words 'toxic' from Greek toxikon meaning arrow poison and 'logy' meaning study.[1,2] The history of poison is as old as human existence. Even in mythological story like Mahabharata, the Pandavas son Bhim was poisoned by Duryodhana.

Toxicology is defined as the branch of science which deals with the poisons in all its aspect. Thus, it is the study of poison deals with its source, properties, absorption, fate, action, fatal dose and fatal period, signs and symptoms, laboratory investigation, diagnosis, treatment, postmortem findings and medicolegal aspect of different poisoning cases. Mathieu Orfila is considered as the Father of Modern Toxicology, who has given the subject its first formal treatment in his Traité des poison in 1813.[3]

Forensic toxicology	*Clinical toxicology*
It deals with medicolegal aspects of poisoning, including causes and circumstances of death.	It deals with mechanism of action, clinical manifestations, laboratory investigation, diagnosis and treatment of a poison.
Poison	*Drugs*
• Poison is a substance which when ingested, injected, inhaled, applied or administered causes disease, ill health or death of a person. • It is used to curtail the life or to minimize the life or to get rid of life. • When the substance is given with the **intention of causing harm** or death, it is considered as **poison**.	• Whereas, drug is any substance used in the diagnosis, treatment, investigation, and prevention and modification of disease. • It is used to sustain or to prolong life or to get relief. • When a substance is given with the **intention of sustaining life**, it is considered as a **drug**, irrespective of the dose.

Legal difference
There is no legal definition of poison. Legally the poison and drug are differentiated on the **basis of the intention** with which that substance is given.

Medical difference
The difference between the poison and the drug is of **dose with which that substance is given**. Since a drug in therapeutic dose or lesser dose produces desirable or beneficial effect but the same drug when given in higher dose produces deleterious effect and acts as a poison, e.g. digitalis, barbiturates, diazepam, etc.

All drugs are poison when taken in **excess dose** and with **intention** to cause harm. But all poisons are not drugs even when taken in low dose.

CLASSIFICATION OF POISONS

Poisons can be classified according to the
1. Action of poison
2. Nature of poison
3. Source of poison

ACTION OF POISON

Poisons are classified into 2 groups: (a) Local and (b) Systemic (Table 1.1).

NATURE OF POISON

For the medicolegal purpose, poisons are classified as:

1. Homicidal Poisoning

There is no ideal homicidal poison. However, thallium and fluoride (present in rodenticides) are near to ideal homicidal poisons.[4] The commonly used poisons for homicidal purpose are arsenic, aconite, strychnine, snake venom, opium (Table 1.2).

Table 1.1: Classification of poison on the basis of action

A. Local	B. Systemic
1. Corrosives **a. Acids:** i. Inorganic: *Sulfuric acid, hydrochloric acid, nitric acid* ii. Organic: *Acetic acid, oxalic acid, carbolic acid* **b. Alkalies:** i. *Hydroxide of sodium, potassium and ammonium* ii. *Carbonates of sodium, potassium and ammonium* **c. Metallic:** *Mercuric chlorides* **2. Irritants** **a. Mechanical:** i. Glass pieces or powder ii. Hairs and fibers iii. Metallic chips, nails, pins iv. Diamond dust or powder **b. Chemical:** i. Inorganic **Non-metals:** *Phosphorus, iodine, fluorine, chlorine, bromine* **Metals:** *Arsenic, lead, mercury, copper, iron, zinc, thallium* ii. Organic: Agricultural poisoning like Insecticidal: *Organophosphorus, organochlorine, carbamate, pyrethroids* Rodenticidal Fungicidal Herbicidal **c. Vegetables:** *Abrus precatorius, Ricinus communis, Croton tiglium, Semicarpus anacardium, Calotropis, Plumbago rosea, Capsicum* **d. Animals:** *Snakes, scorpions, bees, wasps, spiders, cantharides, and poisonous fish*	**1. Cardiac poisons:** *Cyanide, aconite, digitalis, tobacco, Cerbera thevetia, Nerium odorum* **2. Respiratory poisons** (asphyxiant gases), e.g. *CO, CO_2, SO_2, H_2S, NH_3, phosphine (PH_3), war gases and sewer gases* **3. Hepatotoxic poisons:** *Phosphorus, chloroform, trichloroethane, carbon tetrachloride.* **4. Nephrotoxic poisons:** *Mercury, carbolic, oxalic, snake poison* **5. Miscellaneous:** *Food poison, drug abuse* **6. Neurotics** **a. Cerebral:** i. Somniferous: Opium and its alkaloids like *morphine, codeine, thebaine, papaverine, noscapine, and narcine* ii. Inebriants: Alcohols—*ethyl and methyl alcohol* Anaesthetic agents: *Ether, chloroform, nitrous oxide.* Coal tar derivatives, e.g. *naphthalene* iii. Deliriants: *Datura, cannabis, cocaine* iv. Depressant (sedatives and hypnotics): *Barbiturates, benzodiazepam, chloral hydrate, paraldehyde* v. Stimulants: *Amphetamines, camphor, caffeine, cocaine* vi. Hallucinogens: *LSD (lysergic acid diethylamide), mescaline (peyote)* **b. Spinal:** i. Excitants: *Strychnos nux-vomica* ii. Depressants: *Lathyrus sativus (khesari daal), gelsemium (jasmine).* **c. Peripheral:** *Conium, curare*

2. Suicidal Poisoning

There is no ideal suicidal poison. However, opium and barbiturates are near to ideal suicidal poisons.[4] The commonly used poisons for suicidal purpose are insecticides, rodenticides, cyanides, carbolic acid, barbiturates, diazepam, opium (Table 1.2).

3. Accidental Poisoning

Accidental poisoning can occur due to any poison but commonly occurs due to insecticides, snakebite, and gas leakage from industries. It occurs due to:

a. Mistaken with other materials
b. Carelessness in storing poisons
c. Quack remedies
d. While working or exposure in industry, in agricultural fields or in laboratory
e. Snakes, scorpions or insects bites
f. Leakage of gas from industries
g. Accidental consumption of poison by children
h. Food poisoning
i. Drug overdose or misuse or addiction

4. Other Types of Poisoning on the basis of its Nature (Table 1.3)

Table 1.2: Characteristics of an ideal homicidal and suicidal poison

Ideal homicidal poison	Ideal suicidal poison
1. Cheap	Cheap
2. Easily available	Easily available
3. Highly toxic	Highly toxic
4. Odorless, colorless, tasteless	Tasteless, odorless, colorless/pleasant
5. Capable of being easily given with food or drinks	Capable of being easily taken with food or drinks
6. Produces features that resemble natural disease to avoid suspicion	Should lead to painless death
7. No antidote available	Not necessary
8. Completely metabolised so that it is not detected on TA/PM examination	Not necessary

Table 1.3: Classification of poison on the basis of its nature

Nature of poison	Description	Examples
1. Homicidal:	These are the poisons used for killing other	Arsenic, aconite, lead, strychnine, etc.
2. Suicidal:	These are the poisons used to commit suicide	Insecticides, cyanides, carbolic, barbiturates, etc.
3. Accidental:	These are the poisons which cause poisoning due to accidental circumstances	Insecticides, snakebites, food poisoning, gas leakage, etc.
4. Abortifacients:	These are the poisons used for inducing criminal abortion	Arsenic, lead, ergot, quinine, Calotropis, Plumbago, Nerium, *Cerbera thevetia*, aconite, strychnine, etc.
5. Aphrodisiac agents:	These are the poisons which increase the sexual desire	Alcohol, Datura, cocaine, Cannabis preparations
6. Arrow poisons:	These are the poisons commonly applied on the arrow head/tip	Strychnine, Curare, aconite, Abrus, Calotropis, Plumbago and snake venom
7. Cattle poisons:	These are the poisons used for killing cattle	Strychnine, Curare, aconite, Abrus, Calotropis, Plumbago, Nerium, *Cerbera thevetia*
8. Stupefying poisons:	These are the poisons which alter the consciousness of the person and are commonly given for purpose of rape, robbery, dacoity and theft	Datura, cocaine, Cannabis preparations, alcohol
9. Malingering purpose:	These are the poisons used for malingering purpose to avoid duty or to make false charges against enemy	*Semicarpus anacardium*—branding; Abrus—conjunctivitis
10. Vitriolage:	Agents used to cause bodily injury	Corrosives

SOURCE OF POISON

Depending upon the source, poisons are classified as shown in Table 1.4.

Table 1.4: Source of poison with its examples

Source	Examples
1. Domestic/ household	Detergents, disinfectants, phenols, kerosene, etc.
2. Agricultural	Organophosphorus, organochlorine, carbamates
3. Vegetables	All vegetable irritants, Datura, Cannabis, etc.
4. Animals	Snakes venoms, insect bite
5. Medicinal source	Wrong medication, over medication and abuse barbiturate, diazepam, opium, etc.
6. Industrial source	Factories where poisons are produced as by-products, e.g. carbide, methyl isocyanate, phosphine, carbon monoxide, cyanides, etc.
7. Commercial source	From storehouse, selling shops, etc. e.g. alcohols, opium, cocaine, etc.
8. Food and drink	Preservatives of foodgrains, additives like coloring and odoring agents, and food poisoning itself
9. Miscellaneous	Sewer gases

PROPERTIES

Color, odor, taste, solubility, form, etc. in relation to particular poison is described in particular chapter.

ABSORPTION

The absorption of poison/drug may be direct or indirect through mucous membrane or skin.

Direct: Through parenteral routes.

Mucous membranes (MM): Sublingual, inhalation, oral and other orifices.

Skin: Example phosphorus, phenol, insecticidal poison.

Routes of Administration

1. Oral
2. Parenteral/injection—SC, IM, IV, intra-dermal, intra-arterial, etc.
3. Inhalation
4. Sublingual
5. Other natural orifices (e.g. nasal, rectal, vaginal, urethral, etc.).
6. Contact poisoning, i.e. through skin or wounds, or ulcers
7. Through pellets (chemical or bacterial poison pellets fired with airgun).

FATE OF POISON

1. Eliminated as such by defecation or vomitus.
2. Neutralized or inactivated in GIT.
3. Metabolized or detoxified in the body.
4. Eliminated after absorption by urine, breath, bile, milk, sweat, saliva, tear, etc.
5. Gets deposited in some organs or tissue. Heavy metals and radioactive substances stored in epidermis, hair, nails and bones and organophosphorus compounds in fat.

ACTION OF POISON

The poison may be:

1. **Local action:** The poison exerts its effect at the site of contact, e.g. corrosive burns with strong acids, dilatation of pupil with atropine, tingling and numbness sensation with aconite.
2. **Systemic action:** The poison acts on a particular organ/part of the body after absorption of the poison to produce systemic action, e.g. strychnine acts on spinal cord, digitalis acts on heart, curare acts on peripheral nerves, opium/barbiturates acts on CNS.
3. **Combined action:** Some poisons have both local as well as systemic action after its absorption, e.g. carbolic acid, phosphorus, snake venom.

Poison	Local action	Systemic action
Oxalic/carbolic	Corrosive	Renal and CNS toxicity
Phosphorus	On GIT	Liver and CNS toxicity
Snake venom	At the site of bite	Also present

4. General action: The action of poison is not restricted to particular organ but involved multiple system, e.g. metallic poison, insecticidal poison.

FACTORS AFFECTING THE ACTION OF POISONS

1. **Dose:** The action of the poison is directly proportional to its dose. Higher the dose, more will be the fatality and lesser the dose, less will be the fatality with the following exceptions:[4]

   a. Idiosyncrasy: It is the abnormal response of a drug or hypersensitivity due to inborn peculiarities leading to reaction/death even in a small dose of a drug, e.g. quinine, aspirin, morphine, etc.

   b. Allergy: It is the hypersensitivity acquired as a result of previous exposure due to the formation of antibodies, e.g. penicillin, NSAID, anti-snake venom.

   c. Tolerance: It is the capacity of the body to sustain the action of certain drugs or agents without any immediate harm, e.g. alcohol, opium, tobacco, cannabis, etc. The repeated and chronic use of these agents results in addiction and drug dependence.

   d. Synergism: The final response due to combination of substances is more than the sum of their individual action, e.g. alcohol with cocaine or barbiturates or with antidepressants, anticonvulsants, tranquilizers and antihistaminic.

   e. Cumulative poisons: Some poisons are not readily excreted from the body and are retained or tend to accumulate in the body and may not cause any toxic effect when ingested/enter the body in a low dose, e.g. lead, arsenic, digitalis, carbon monoxide (CO), strychnine, and barbiturates.

2. **Form of poison**

   a. Physical form: The poison in gaseous/vapor form is more poisonous than liquids, and liquids are more toxic than solids. The solid poison which is in fine powder form is more poisonous than coarse form.

   [Gases/vapors > liquid > solid (fine > coarse)]

   b. Chemical form: Pure arsenic and mercury are not poisonous while their compounds are highly poisonous.

   Similarly, some compound of an individual metal is not toxic and other compound of the same metal is deadly toxic, e.g. barium sulfate is non-toxic and used in barium meal in radiological investigation; whereas barium sulfide is highly toxic.

   c. Concentrated form: Normally more the concentration, more will be the absorption and more its toxicity. But the dilute solution of oxalic acid is more rapidly absorbed and is much more fatal.[5]

3. **Condition of stomach[5]:** It delays or facilitates the absorption of poison and it depends on:

   a. Empty stomach—absorbs poison rapidly.

   b. Food contents in stomach:
   - Presence of food in the stomach acts as diluents.
   - Fatty food delays the absorption process of poisoning except phosphorus.

   c. Abnormal conditions of the stomach also lead to delay in the absorption of poison.
   - Pyloric stenosis which delays the emptying of food.
   - Gastrojejunostomy causes repeated backward flow of gastric contents.

   d. Achlorhydric subjects—the salts of cyanides is ineffective due to lack of hydrochloric acid (HCl) in the stomach which is required for their conversion to hydrogen cyanide before absorption.

4. **Routes of administration of poison**

   a. Route: Rate of absorption depends upon the route of administration. Through some routes, poisons are absorbed very rapidly and exert their action promptly. The rate of absorption is fastest through inhalation routes. This is followed by IV, IM and other parenteral routes as compared to oral and direct skin contact. Injured or ulcerated skin absorbs poison quicker than intact skin. The absorption is more rapid in oral route than rectal route.

b. **Different route:** The action of poisons is different when they are introduced through different routes, e.g.
  - Snake venom is effective only when injected and harmless when taken orally.
  - Cocaine: On ingestion acts as deliriants, on injection it acts as local anesthetic.
  - Curare: On ingestion is inert, on injection it is highly toxic.

5. **General condition of the body**
  a. **Age:** Some poisons are better tolerated in some ages and badly in other ages. Opium is better tolerated by elderly and atropine is better tolerated by children.
  b. **Physique and health:** Well-built person with good physique and health will tolerate poison better than weak and lean subject.
  c. **Presence of any disease:** Usually, in disease conditions the effect of poison is more.
    - In liver pathology, Morphine is more poisonous.
    - In renal damage, Mercury is more poisonous.
    - In head injury or raised ICP, Morphine is more dangerous/lethal.
    - However, some poisons are well-tolerated during disease conditions like:
      – Sedatives and tranquilizers in Manic and deliriant patients
      – Digitalis in heart failure.
      – Strychnine in paralysis.
      – Cyanide in achlorhydria.
  d. **Sleep:** Absorption is less during sleep due to slow metabolism and hence has slow action but depressant drugs may cause more harm during sleep.

  e. **Exercise:** It decreases the action of drug as more blood is drawn to the muscle, e.g. alcohol.

DIAGNOSIS OF POISONING

The diagnosis of poisoning is not always possible due to various reasons.

1. Usually patient is not in a position to narrate the story or to give the history.
2. Sometimes in spite of knowing the nature of poisoning consumed by the patient, the relatives do not come forward due to fear of being involved in police investigation.
3. Also due to ignorance of the importance of giving proper history of poisoning to the doctor, the physician's task becomes more difficult as none is willing to give correct history to avoid police investigation.
4. Unlike in other clinical conditions arising out of natural disease, there are very few **toxic syndrome or toxidrome**[6] (refer to a group of clinical features that are consistently encountered in relation to a specific toxin) characterized by typical signs and symptoms.

In Living Subject

1. History of the case as stated by patient, relatives or friends:
   It includes time of onset, symptoms, progress, in relation to food/drink and condition of others who took the same, possible source of poison, any past history of poisoning, history of depression and about the properties of the poisonous material like smell, taste, color, consistency, etc.
2. Signs and symptoms of the patient
3. Detailed physical examination
4. Laboratory investigation of vomitus, blood, etc. or any material brought by the relatives. The toxicological analysis (TA) of gastric lavage fluid, blood, urine, stools and vomitus confirms the nature of the poison. The detection of the poison in suspected food, fluid or utensils help as corroborative evidence.

In Dead Subject

1. History as provided by police or relatives should be taken in the same line as in case of living victims. In addition, history should also contain:
   i. Period of survival after poisoning and their symptoms.
   ii. Details of treatment if given.
2. Postmortem examination of a body
   a. External examination (*see* page 13):
      i. Clothes examined for vomitus stain with its color and smell.
      ii. Body for any injection marks.
      iii. Mouth and nostrils for presence of froth—in insecticidal poisons, morphine, barbiturates, strychnine and cyanides.
      iv. PM lividity for peculiar color—in carbon monoxide (cherry red), hydrogen sulphide (bluish green), cyanides (pink) and opium (black lividity).
      v. Skin for different colors—in acute copper and phosphorous poisoning (yellow due to jaundice) and asphyxiants poisoning (bluish due to cyanosis).
      vi. Gums and teeth for color changes, particularly in metallic poisons like copper, mercury, lead (bluish color).
   b. Internal examination (*see* page 14):
      i. Organs/viscera should be examined for any congestion and edema.
      ii. Stomach should be examined for color and smell of its content along with submucosal hemorrhage, softening, congestion and perforations of its wall. In poisoning, these changes are more marked at greater curvature of stomach.[4]
      iii. Small intestine should also be examined for the above changes, particularly in the duodenum and jejunum.
3. Preservation of viscera and other materials for laboratory investigation like TA.
4. Moral and circumstantial evidence in suicidal and homicidal poisoning.
   i. In suicidal poisoning, it includes suicidal note, cause of suicide with evidence of ingestion/purchase of poison. The container of the poison may be found near the dead body or victim.
   ii. In homicidal poison, it includes history of quarrel or other cause/motive of homicide with evidence of ingestion/injection/purchase of poison. The relatives are very eager to dispose of the dead body.

TREATMENT OF POISONING

If the specific nature of the poison is not known, then it should be treated on the lines of general principles of treatment of poisoning which are as follows:

1. Removal of patient from the source of exposure
2. Removal of unabsorbed poison
3. Dilution of unabsorbed poison
4. Elimination of absorbed poison
5. Specific antidote
6. Symptomatic treatment

However, **Stabilization and Evaluation** of the patient should be done before starting the actual treatment like decontamination (removal of unabsorbed poison), poison elimination (by means of diuresis, dialysis) and specific antidote administration.[6] *Stabilization* refers to correction of life-threatening problems like airway, breathing, circulation and CNS depression. *Evaluation* includes complete assessment/examination and diagnosis/laboratory investigation of the patient of poisoning. *Moreover, most poisoned patients can be treated successfully without any contribution from the laboratory other than routine clinical biochemistry and hematology investigations.*

1. Removal of Patient from the Source of Exposure

- In gaseous/volatile poison—remove patient from the source or environment.
- In insecticidal poison—removal of clothes.
- In corrosives poison—removal of soiled clothes.

2. Removal of Unabsorbed Poison

It depends upon the route of administration of poison.

a. In case of **contact poisoning** to skin/injuries:
- Removal of clothes.
- Wash the area with lukewarm water or soap.
- Application of local anesthetic agents.

b. In case of **intravaginal or other natural orifices:**
- Vaginal douching or irrigation with plain water.

c. **Inhaled poison:**
- Removal of patient from source.
- Ensure clear airway and respiration.

d. **Injected poison** (e.g. snakebite, arrow poison):

The spread of injected poison is restricted by:
- Application of ligature/tourniquette proximal to the site of bite.
- Application of ice packs.
- Antidote infiltration after washing of the site of bite.

e. **Ingested poison:**

The ingested poison is removed by:
- Emesis/induction of vomiting.
- Gastric lavage/stomach wash.
- Purgatives and colonic lavage by means of sodium/magnesium sulfate or dulcolax, etc.

Emesis

Emesis means induction of vomiting. It is better than stomach wash within 4–6 hours of ingestion of poisoning. It is absolutely contraindicated in all corrosive poisoning **except carbolic acid**. In rest of the condition, it is relatively contraindicated (Table 1.5).

Table 1.5: Contraindications of emesis[7] [5CVP-M]

Conditions	Reasons for contraindication
a. Corrosive poisoning[7]	Perforation of the stomach
b. CNS stimulant drugs poisoning[7]	Convulsions may be precipitated
c. Kerosene/volatile poisoning	Chances of aspiration/inhalation of fumes
d. Morphine poisoning[7]	May fail to act
e. Coma[7]	Aspiration
f. Children	Aspiration
g. Pregnancy	Abortion
h. Cardiorespiratory diseases	Heart failure may be precipitated

Methods of Emesis

Vomiting can be induced by different methods as shown in Table 1.6.

Table 1.6: Method of induction of vomiting

a. Mechanical irritation of throat	Finger—stimulating the posterior wall of pharynx
b. Plain lukewarm water	Good amount of water
c. Common salt	1 TSF in one glass of water
d. Mustard powder	1 TSF in one glass of water
e. Copper sulfate	Weak solution
f. Ipecacuhana syrup	15–30 ml orally[7]
g. Zinc sulfate	1–2 gm in one glass of water
h. Ammonium carbonate	1–2 gm in one glass of water
i. Apomorphine hydrochloride	6 mg IM/SC[7], is centrally acting potent emetic agent.

Household emetics: These are the emetics available in the house. Top four methods are the examples of household emetics.

Gastric Lavage

Gastric lavage/Stomach wash is the cleaning of the stomach with fluid. The volume of each wash depends on the age group of the person. It is done by means of following gastric lavage tubes:

In age group	GL tube	Volume of each wash
Adults	Stomach tube (Boa's/Ewald's)	200–300 ml
Children	Male urinary rubber catheter	100–200 ml
Infants	Ryle's tube	<100 ml

Indications of Stomach Wash

1. Stomach wash is indicated within 4–6 hours of ingestion of any poison. However, it should be done even if the patient is brought after 6 hours of ingestion of poison. It is absolutely contraindicated in corrosive poison except carbolic acid poisoning (Table 1.7).
2. It is also useful in unconscious and depressed condition of the patient after ingestion of poison as the gastric emptying time is delayed.[4]
3. In **injected morphine poisoning** due to its property of re-secretion in the stomach.

Table 1.7: Contraindications of gastric lavage

a. Corrosives	Except carbolic acid
b. Convulsions	Anesthetize or sedate the patient first
c. Coma/petroleum	Do cuffed intubation in such cases
d. Children	Use Ryle's tube or rubber catheter
e. Esophageal varices	Lead to massive hemorrhage

Stomach Tube (Boa's or Ewald's Tube)

Stomach tube is a rubber tube having 1.5 meter length and about 1.5 cm diameter. It is inserted at its lower rounded end through the mouth and has following parts:

a. **Lower rounded perforated end:** It is rounded to prevent damage to the GIT during insertion.

b. **Mouth gag:** It is made up of wooden and have central aperture for the insertion of stomach tube. One end of the gag is pointed to open the clenched teeth.

c. **Rubber tube markings:** It is marked at 40 cm, 50 cm and 60 cm.

d. **Suction bulb:** It is used to force open the perforated lower end when blocked and to take out the stomach fluid.

e. **Funnel end:** It is funnel shaped to pour fluid in the stomach for washing.

Procedure for Stomach Wash

The mouth gag is placed between upper and lower anterior teeth with the patient being on his/her left lateral side and head lower down. The lower perforated end of the tube is lubricated with glycerin or liquid paraffin and is inserted through the central hole of mouth gag, till the 50 cm marking on rubber tube (Fig. 1.1).

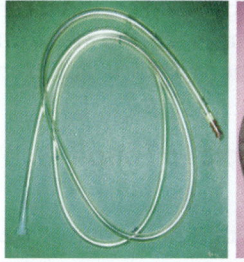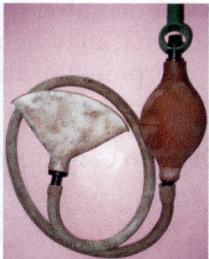

Fig. 1.1: Ryle's tube and stomach tube

The stomach tube may either enter the stomach or respiratory passage.

Stomach tube in respiratory passage	Stomach tube in the stomach
1. Cough starts	1. No cough reflex
2. Air bubbles come out when funnel end of the tube is dipped in water	2. No air bubbles. However, sound of air movement heard when stomach area is auscultated

When confirmed that the tube is in the stomach (as above), then 100–200 ml plain warm water or fresh lukewarm water or normal saline is poured through the funnel end of the tube. The fluid enters the stomach by means of gravity when the funnel end of the tube is held at a higher level than the body. After 1–2 minutes, the fluid from the stomach is removed out either by suction pump or by means of siphon action (when funnel end of the tube is taken lower than the level of body).

This first washing sample by lukewarm water or normal saline is preserved for toxicological analysis. Later on, the washing is done with not >300 ml of either plain water or $KMnO_4$ solution (1 : 1000) or with specific antidote to particular poison. This process of entry and removal of fluid from the stomach is repeated till the color of lavage fluid remains same. At the end, the tube is removed properly to avoid aspiration of fluid to respiratory tract by pinching or bending between the finger.[4]

However, in certain cases, the lavage fluid ($KMnO_4$ solution) is left in the stomach to neutralize the un-removed part of the poison, if any. The fluid ($KMnO_4$ solution, activated charcoal, demulcent) can also be left in certain poison that may be re-secreted in stomach (e.g. morphine) or that remains adherent to gastric mucosa.

3. Dilution of Unabsorbed Poison

It is done by giving:

 a Water to drink that helps in two ways:
  - It reduces the local damaging action
  - It delays the rate of absorption

 b. Bulky bland food, e.g. banana, boiled potato, mashed rice.

 c. Demulcents/fats: It delays the process of absorption and also protects the stomach wall. This method is of **no use in oxalic acid poisoning** (where dilution is contraindicated), and **phosphorus poisoning** (where fats are contraindicated).

4. Elimination of Absorbed Poison

It is done by:

 a. Diuresis (increased urination/forced diuresis) by using fluids and drugs like frusemide or mannitol infusion.

 b. Diaphoresis (increased sweating/perspiration) by applying hot packs and neostigmine or pilocarpine injection.

 c. Dialysis: In case kidney is not functioning (peritoneal or hemodialysis).

 d. Chelating agents: See antidotes

 e. Exchange transfusion: Capable of removing many of the toxins that are not removed by hemodialysis. It is best indicated in cerebral depressant, cardiac poison (digoxin, quinine), organophosphorus, phenol, paraquat, paracetamol, amanitin poisoning.[6]

5. Specific Antidote

Antidote is the substance which counteracts the deleterious effects of the poison without itself being harmful to the body. It is indicated when poison is absorbed from the GIT or shows clinical systemic manifestation of poison (*see* Appendix Table 1).

Types and Uses of Antidotes

  I. **Physical (mechanical) antidotes:** These are the antidotes which **prevent the action of poison mechanically** without destroying or neutralizing the poison. Different physical antidotes with their examples and uses are given in Table 1.8.

 II. **Chemical antidotes:** These are the substances which **chemically react with the poison** and thereby disintegrate or inactivate the poison (Table 1.9).

III. **Pharmacological or physiological antidotes:** These are the substances which have a pharmacologically opposite action as compared to the poison (Table 1.10).

IV. **Universal antidote:** It is so-called because it can be used in all cases of poisoning, especially when the nature of poison is not known. It is the combination of physical and chemical antidotes (Table 1.11). Dose is 15–30 g or 1 TSF in a glass of water.[5,13] It can be repeated 12–24 hourly. It is nowadays obsolete but can be used as first aid measure at home.[12–13]

 V. **Chelating agents:** These are the substances which act on the absorbed metallic poison and form a non-ionized complex with the metal ion freely available in the blood circulation, so that the metal ion is not available for absorption and thereby cannot affect the enzyme system of the body. The commonly used chelating agents are BAL, EDTA, Penicillamine, and Desferrioxamine (Table 1.12).

VI. **Serological/biological antidotes:** These are the substance prepared by injecting the antigen (like snake venom) in the animal blood, so that the sensitized animal serum can be used as an antidote, e.g. antivenom serum.

Table 1.8: Different types of physical antidotes

Physical antidote	Examples	Action/properties	Uses
Demulcent	Oil, ghee, butter, milk, egg albumin (egg white), starch, barley, water, etc.	These substances have soothing action and form a protective layer on the mucosa of stomach so that the poison does not absorb	Corrosive/irritant, except phosphorus
Bulky foods	Banana, mashed potato, boiled rice, vegetables, etc.	These substances engulf the poison and make it unavailable for causing effects and for its absorption	Mechanical irritant
Adsorbent	Activated charcoal (dose: 1 gm/kg body weight[12] in water orally)[6]	It adsorbs the alkaloid poison in their pores so that poison is not available for absorption in stomach	Irritant poison
Diluents	Water, milk, drinks, etc.	It dilutes the poison, thereby delaying the absorption of poison	Corrosive/irritant, except oxalic acid

Table 1.9: Chemical antidotes and their uses

Chemical antidote	Uses (action/forms)
a. Weak non-carbonated alkali[5] (CaO, MgO)	Acid poison (neutralizing the acids)
b. Weak vegetables acid[5] (citric, acetic)	Alkali poison (neutralizing alkali)
c. Copper sulfate	Phosphorus (forms copper phosphide)
d. Egg albumin	Mercury chloride (forms mercuric albuminate)
e. Fresh ferric oxide	Arsenic (forms ferric arsenate)
f. Potassium ferrocyanide	Copper
g. Calcium carbonate	Oxalic acid (forms calcium oxalate)
h. $KMnO_4$	Opium/morphine
i. Sodium thiosulfate	Iodine/cyanide

Table 1.10: Pharmacological antidotes and their uses

Pharmacological antidote	Dose[8-11]	Uses/for
Physostigmine/Neostigmine[8]	0.5–2 mg IV	Datura, atropine
Atropine[8]	2 mg IV repeated every 10 min till dryness of mouth	Organophosphorus (OP)
Ethanol[9]	0.7 ml/kg through nasogastric tube followed by 0.15 ml/kg/hour	Methanol
Naloxone[10]	0.4–0.8 mg IV every 2–3 min (max 10 mg)	Opium/morphine
Lorazepam[11]	4 mg IV, repeated after 10 min if required	Strychnine

Table 1.11: Content of universal antidote

Contents	Obtained from[4]	Parts	Action
Charcoal	Burnt bread/toast	2	Adsorbs poison
MgO	Milk of magnesia	1	Neutralizes acid
Tannin	Strong tea	1	Precipitates metal, alkaloids, and glucosides

Table 1.12: Examples of chelating agents with their dose and uses

Chelating agents	Properties	Dose	Adverse effects	Uses[14]
a. BAL (Dimercaprol)	It is an oily, pungent, viscous liquid developed during World War II as an antidote to the arsenical war gas lewisite. It has 2 SH groups which bind with metal ion present in the blood.[14]	5 mg/kg body weight stat **deep IM** followed by **2–3 mg/kg** 4–8 hourly for first 2 days, followed by 12 hourly (1BD) for next 10 days.[14] If given IV, it causes embolism due to presence of arachis oil in *benzyl benzoate*.	Hypertension, tachycardia, sweating, cramps, headache, anxiety. It is CI in iron and cadmium poisoning; *and in G6PD deficiency*[12]	• Arsenic, mercury poisoning • Bismuth, nickel, gold, antimony. • Adjuvant to copper poisoning and Wilson disease. • Adjuvant to calcium disodium edetate in lead poisoning.

Dimercaptosuccinic acid: It is less toxic and effective orally for lead poisoning.

• As, Hg, Pb poisoning

Chelating agents	Properties	Dose	Adverse effects	Uses[14]
b. Calcium disodium edetate (CaNa$_2$ EDTA)	It has higher affinity for metals like Pb, Zn, Cd, Mn, Cu and some radioactive metals by exchanging with calcium present in it.[14]	**1 gm** in 200–300 ml saline/glucose by **slow IV** drip, BD for 3–5 days. Repeated after 5–7 days[14]	Renal damage with proximal tubular necrosis, acute febrile reaction, anaphylaxis	• Lead poisoning • Cu, Fe, Zn, Mn but not in mercury poisoning.

The disodium salt of ethylene diamine tetraacetic acid (Na$_2$ EDTA) is a potent chelator of calcium, it causes tetany. Dose: 50 mg/kg IV infusion for 2–4 hrs.[14]

• Emergency control of Hypercalcemia

Chelating agents	Properties	Dose	Adverse effects	Uses[14]
c. Penicillamine	It is a degradation product of penicillin. It has stable SH-radicle. It selectively chelates Cu, Hg, Pb and Zn. It is adequately absorbed after oral administration.	**30 mg**/kg body weight, **orally** in 4 divided doses for 7 days.[5] **OR** 0.5–1 g/day orally in divided dose for few days 1 hr before meals [14] **OR** Potassium sulfide 20–40 mg to reduce absorption of dietary copper [14]	Usually non-toxic but may cause thrombo-cytopenia, skin rash, renal problems.	• Copper poisoning • Wilson disease • Alternative to dimercaprol for Hg poisoning • Adjuvant to CaNa$_2$ EDTA in lead poisoning. • Cystinuria and cystine stones
d. Desferri-oxamine	Chemical removal of iron from Ferrioxamine yields desferrioxamine which has very high affinity for iron.[14]	0.5–1 g/day IM, repeated 4–12 hourly till serum iron falls below 300 micro-gram/dl.[14] **OR** 10 g/day orally for unabsorbed iron.[5]	It releases histamine and causes skin lesion. Also causes cramps, abd pain, loose motion, fever.	• Iron poisoning. • Transfusion siderosis in thalassemia patients. (BAL is not given in iron poisoning)

Deferiprone: It is an orally active iron chelator particularly in transfusion siderosis and alternative to iron poisoning. Dose: 50–100 mg/kg daily in 2–4 divided doses.[14]

Household Antidotes

These are the substances which are available usually in the house and can be used as antidotes in case of poisoning (Table 1.13)

Table 1.13: Household antidotes and their uses

Household antidotes	Uses/used as
1. Common salt, mustard powder, plain warm water	Emetic agent
2. Charcoal from burnt toast	Adsorbent
3. Flour suspension	Engulf or even adsorb
4. Banana, potato, boiled rice	Physical antidote
5. Oil, ghee, butter, milk, egg albumin	Demulcent
6. Starch solution	Iodine poisoning
7. Milk of magnesia, tooth paste, wall scrapping	Acid poisoning
8. Vinegar, lemon/orange juice	Alkali poisoning
9. Milk	All ingested poison
10. Strong tea (Tannic acid)	Metallic poison, cocaine, nicotine, strychnine[13]

6. Symptomatic Treatment

A. Safeguarding respiration
   1. Clearing the airways
   2. Endotracheal intubation
   3. Tracheostomy
   4. Oxygen inhalation—6 liters/min
   5. Artificial respiration
B. Maintenance of circulation
   1. Vasoconstriction
   2. Stimulants
   3. Blood transfusion
   4. Noradrenaline drip for peripheral circulatory failure
C. Electrolyte imbalance correction
   1. IV fluids for dehydration/shock
   2. Sodium/potassium for electrolyte imbalance
   3. Other fluids
D. Other supportive treatments like
   1. Atropine for abdominal pain
   2. Diazepam for convulsions/restlessness
   3. Adrenaline, antihistaminic and steroids in anaphylactic reactions
   4. Morphine, pethidine for pain
   5. Glucose for hypoglycemia
E. Maintenance of general condition of the patient
   1. Warm and comfortable condition
   2. Good nursing care
   3. Prophylactic antibiotics
   4. Physiotherapy for rehabilitation
   5. Psychotherapy in an attempted suicide

POSTMORTEM FINDINGS IN SUSPECTED POISONING

The postmortem (PM) findings are different in individual poisoning which are described in respective chapters. However, the characteristic findings in different poisoning are as follows:

External Postmortem Findings

1. Postmortem lividity:

Deep blue color	Asphyxiant/aniline
Cherry-red	CO poisoning
Pink	Cyanide
Brown	Phosphorus
Black	Opium
Green	Hydrogen sulfide

2. Froth from mouth and nose — Opium, barbiturate, Cyanide, strychnine, OP (blood tinged)
3. Detectable smell — Insecticidal poison, volatile poison, opium, cyanide, kerosene, phenol
4. Deep cyanosis — Opium, CO_2, sewer gas,
5. Early rigor mortis — Strychnine, HCN
6. Resist decomposition — Arsenic, datura, formalin
7. Stain near mouth and on hands — Nitric acid, copper sulfate, paints
8. Ulceration on lips and mouth — Corrosives
9. Hemorrhage spots under skin/mucosa — Phosphorus
10. Staining, erosion, ulceration near external genital[5] — Abortifacient agents, corrosives
11. Alopecia, hyperpigmentation, hyperkeratosis[5] — Arsenic
12. Injection marks — Opium/cocaine abuser
13. Punctures marks — Bite marks of snakes, scorpion and insect
14. Constriction of pupil — Morphine, phenol, organophosphorus,
15. Dilatation of pupil — Datura, alcohol

Internal Postmortem Findings

1. Corrosion, ulceration and desquamation of lips, mouth, tongue[5]	Corrosive
2. Soft, swollen, bleached (whitish or yellowish) tongue/mouth[5]	Alkali
3. Chalky white teeth	Sulfuric acid
4. Blue lining on gums/teeth	Lead, mercury (chronic poisoning)
5. Corrosion, ulceration and desquamation of GIT mucosa	Corrosives, irritant
6. MM of upper GIT	
Hard/white	Phenol
Yellow	Nitric acid
Bluish green	Copper sulfate
Green	Ferrous sulfate
Black	Sulfuric acid
Grey/slate color	Mercury chloride
Red velvety	Arsenic
Discolor/staining	Colored salts of arsenic, lead, copper
7. Stomach wall	
Thickened and soft	Corrosive, irritant
Hard wall	Formaldehyde
Hard and leather-like	Carbolic acid
Hemorrhage/ ulcerated	Irritant
Ulceration and sloughing	Corrosive
8. Stomach contents	
Blood	Corrosive, irritant
Bluish	Copper sulfate
Luminous in dark	Phosphorus
Powder/tablets	Drug tab, arsenic, oxalic
Detectable smell	Kerosene, alcohol, insecticides, cyanide, formaldehyde, etc.

9. **Small intestine:** May show irritation, corrosion, ulceration as similar to stomach with presence of poisonous remains.

10. **Large intestine:** May show corrosion, ulcerations in strong acid ingestion. It particularly involves the ascending and transverse colons.

11. **Brain and spinal cord:** Brain may be congested, oedematous in cerebral poison with occasional hemorrhagic points at places in asphyxiant poisons. In spinal poison, spinal cord is congestion and edematous.

12. **Larynx and trachea:** Froth may be present in opium and OP poisoning. It is inflamed and hyperemic in inhalation of irritating gases/acid fumes or aspiration of acids.

13. **Chest cavity:** Smell of volatile poisons, cyanide, opium, etc. can be detected.

14. **Lungs:** It may be voluminous, congested and may show Tardieu's spots in asphyxiant poisons. Cut section gives bloodstained frothy fluid in opium and asphyxiant poison.

15. **Heart:** Subendocardial hemorrhagic spots in poisoning with arsenic, phosphorus, mercuric chloride, etc.

16. **Liver:** Different degenerative changes may be present in poisoning with phosphorus, carbon tetrachloride, chloroform, tetrachloroethylene, etc.

17. **Kidneys:** Swollen, reddish, soft, sometimes greasy in touch with hemorrhage in the calyces and other degenerative changes in poisoning with mercury, oxalic acid, carbolic acid, phosphorus, viper snakebite, etc. In case of oxalic acid poisoning, white oxalate crystals are present in the tubules and the calyces.

18. **Uterus and vagina:** Staining, congestion, hemorrhage, ulceration in attempted abortion by use of local abortifacient agents.

DUTIES OF DOCTOR IN POISONING CASES

1. **Treatment:** The primary duty of a doctor is to treat the patient in any case. If the

nature of poison is unknown, then the patient should be treated on general principle of treatment of poisoning.

2. **History in details of the case:** The information about poison with respect to its type, nature, color, smell, etc. should be recorded along with amount/time of consumption of the poison and motive/reason of poisoning. Details about time of onset and nature of manifestation should also be recorded along with its history of vomiting if any with its nature, smell and color.

3. **Informed to authorities:**
   - The doctor must inform to police in all cases of poisoning irrespective of whether it is suicidal or homicidal or accidental poisoning.
   - If the patient is about to die, then arrange for dying deposition or dying declaration.
   - If the patient dies, police must be informed and the body should be sent for postmortem examination.
   - In case of accidental poisoning due to food/water, public health authorities should also be informed so that precautions can be taken for public health safety.

4. **Maintenance of BHT records:** The record is very important for future reference if required to produce in the court/police. Detailed information of the complaint, condition and treatment of the patient should be included in the record. Details about name, age, sex, address, brought by, consent and identification marks of the patient should also be included in the record. The bed head ticket (BHT) record (case paper of the patient) should be prepared meticulously and updated on daily basis. It should be numbered serially before submitting to record section of the hospital.

5. **Preservation of material for toxicological analysis:** A doctor must preserve all possible evidence of suspected poisoning. He should preserve stomach wash, vomitus, urine, blood and also other suspicious articles and utensils used in poisoning.

POISONING AND LAW

1. If the patient of poisoning is brought dead, then doctor should inform the police and send the body for postmortem examination.
2. The doctor is bound to inform to police in poisoning cases irrespective of whether it is suicidal or homicidal or accidental poisoning. As per Sec 39 of CrPC, it is mandatory for a doctor to inform the police for the commission of homicidal poisoning.
3. The doctor has to preserve all possible material/evidence of suspected poisoning. The doctor is bound to provide all information/documents to the police/court in poisoning cases when asked or summoned. If the doctor causes any evidence to disappear or gives false information with the intention of screening the offender is punishable u/s 201 IPC; and if he intentionally omits to give any information relating to poisoning is punishable u/s 202 IPC. Whoever gives any false evidence in any stage of judicial proceeding is punishable u/s 193 IPC.
4. Indian penal code also describes the punishment specifically related to the poisoning and adulteration to deal offences related to drugs and poison (Table 1.14).

ACTS RELATED TO THE USE OF DRUGS AND POISON

In India, dealing of poisons and drugs are governed by Acts which are as follows:

1. **The Opium Act, 1857:** This Act empowers the Central Government to cultivate poppy plants and manufacture opium in the farms authorized by the Government. This Act was amended in 1878.
2. **The Opium Act, 1878:** This Act prohibits transport, possession and sale of opium. This Act was further amended in 1957.

Table 1.14: Punishment for offence related to drugs and poison

Sec of IPC	Offence	Punishment
272	Adulteration of food or drink intended to sell, so as to make it noxious	Imprisonment of either description for a term which may extend to 6 months and/or fine of up to ₹1000
273	Sale of noxious food or drink	Imprisonment of either description for a term which may extend to 6 months and/or fine of up to ₹1000
274	Adulteration of drugs with any changes in its effect intended to sold or use	Imprisonment of either description for a term which may extend to 6 months and/or fine of up to ₹1000
275	Sale of adulterated drugs	Imprisonment of either description for a term which may extend to 6 months and/or fine of up to ₹1000
276	Sale of drug as a different drug or preparation	Imprisonment of either description for a term which may extend to 6 months and/or fine of up to ₹1000
277	Fouling water of public spring or reservoir	Imprisonment of either description for a term which may extend to 3 months and/or fine of up to ₹500
278	Voluntarily making atmosphere noxious	Fine which may extend to ₹500
284	Negligent conduct with respect to poisonous substance so as to endanger human life or likely to cause hurt or injury	Imprisonment of either description for a term which may extend to 6 months and/or fine of up to ₹1000
326A	Voluntarily causing grievous hurt by use of acid	Imprisonment of either description for a term which may not be less than 10 years but may extend to imprisonment of life and fine
326B	Voluntarily throwing or attempting to throw acid on any part of the body with an intention of causing damage or disfigurement	Imprisonment of either description for a term which may not be less than 5 years but may extend to 7 years and fine
328	Causing hurt by means of poison or any intoxicating agent or drug with intent to commit an offence	Imprisonment of either description for a term which may extend to 10 years and fine

3. **The Poisons Act, 1919:** This Act deals with the regulation of import of poisons and grant of license for the possession and sale of poisons.

4. **The Dangerous Drugs Act, 1930:** This Act regulates the import, export, cultivation, manufacture, possession, sale and use of dangerous drugs of abuse like opium, cannabis and cocaine.

5. **The Drugs Act, 1940:** This Act regulates the import, manufacture, distribution and sale of drugs in India. This Act was amended in 1962 to include cosmetics under its purview. It is now known as "Drugs and Cosmetics Act of 1940".

6. **The Drugs and Cosmetics Act, 1940:** This Act empowered the Central Government to form a Drugs Technical Advisory Board, and to establish a Central Drugs Laboratory, to help and advice the Governments for enforcing uniformity in the implementation of the different provisions of the Act, all over the Country. The Central Drug Laboratory analyses the purity and potency of imported and manufactured drugs. This Act was further amended to include Ayurvedic

and Unani drugs under its purview in 1964.

7. The Drugs and Cosmetics Rules, 1945:

The rules were framed under the provisions of the Drugs and Cosmetics Act of 1940 (former Drugs Act of 1940), which came into effect in 1945, known as Drugs and Cosmetics Rules of 1945, to regulate the import, manufacture, distribution and sale of drugs and cosmetics.

Under these rules, drugs are classified in certain schedules as follows:

Schedule C: Biological and special products;

Schedule E: List of poisons,

Schedule F: Vaccines and sera,

Schedule G: Hormone preparation,

Schedule H: Poisonous drugs which cannot be sold without a prescription,

Schedule J: List of drugs used to cure disease which should not be advertised, and

Schedule L: Antibiotics, antihistaminics and other chemotherapeutic agents.

[Schedule H and L drugs cannot be sold without the prescription.]

This rule also dictates the procedure of sale of medicine by the retailer. The retailer should maintain a register, which should contain the name and address of patient and prescribing doctor, name and ingredients of drug, the serial number and date of the sale should be recorded along with the name of manufacturer, batch number of the product and the expiry date of the drug enlisted in Schedule C, H and L.[5]

8. The Pharmacy Act, 1948:
It regulates the Pharmacy Councils and allows only the registered pharmacist to compound, prepare, mix or dispense any medicine on the prescription of doctor.

9. The Drugs Control Act, 1950:
It regulates the sale, supply, distribution and regulates the maximum price of a drug.

10. The Drugs and Magic Remedies Act, 1954:
It bans the advertisement of magic remedies in relation to: (i) abortion, (ii) prevention of conception, (iii) increase sexual potency/pleasure, (iv) treatment for menstrual disorders, (v) treatment and cure of venereal diseases, (vi) false or misleading information about a drug as to its nature and function.

11. Medicinal and Toilet Preparation Act, 1955:
This Act provides for payment of levy and excise duty for medicinal and toilet preparations containing alcohol, cannabis, opium and other similar drugs.[5]

12. Narcotic Drugs and Psychotropic Substances Act, 1985:
It repeals three Acts, namely The Opium Act, 1857 and 1878; and the Dangerous Drugs Act, 1930. This Act

i. Consolidates and amends the existing laws relating to narcotic.

ii. Strengthens existing control over drug of abuse.

iii. Makes stringent provision for the purpose of preventing, combating trafficking, and abuse of narcotic drugs and psychotropic substances.

To enforce the Act, Government of India had framed ND and PS Rules, 1985. Likewise, State Governments have also formed their own rules to enforce this Act within their jurisdiction.

A narcotic drug is one that produces narcosis or sleep. A **narcotic drug** includes cannabis, cocaine, opium, and their derivatives.

Psychotropic drugs are one that alters mental function by its action. "**Psychotropic substances**" means any substance or preparation of such substance that are included in the list of 77 psychotropic substances, e.g. hallucinogens—LSD, stimulants—amphetamines, hypnotic—barbiturate, tranquilizer—diazepam, meprobamate.

The Act prohibits the cultivation of poppy, cannabis and coca plants; however restricted cultivation is allowed for medicinal purpose. This Act also provides punishment of imprisonment for those dealing in these drugs and substance, for 10 years which may extend to 20 years with fine of ₹ 1 lakh extend to 2 lakhs.

Under Section 27, person who is found to be in possession of a small quantity of any drugs or substance for his personal use or who consume any material under this Act is punishable for a period of one year with fine or both.

IMPORTANT QUESTIONS

1. Classify poisons on the basis of their action. Describe general principles of treatment of poisoning.

2. Classify poison according to mode of poison. Enumerate the poisons which discolor/impart color to the skin and mucous membrane.

3. Write different actions of poison. Describe factors affecting absorption of poison.

4. Define antidote. Describe different types of antidote with their examples.

5. Write in brief about chelating agents with examples as an antidote.

6. Write indication and contraindication of emesis and stomach wash. Describe the procedure for stomach wash.

7. Describe the duties of doctor in case of poisoning.

8. Describe general guidelines or steps for diagnosis of poisoning in general.

9. How will you diagnose a case of poisoning during postmortem examination? What are the reasons for negative report from chemical analyser in a suspected case of poisoning?

10. A patient is brought in the hospital / casualty in an unconscious condition with history of poisoning. Discuss differential diagnosis and briefly outline the management in anyone of them.

SHORT NOTES/SAQs

1. Stomach tube
2. Laws related to poisons

3. Household emetics
4. Chelating agents
5. Universal antidote
6. Characteristic features of ideal suicidal and homicidal poisons
7. Physical antidotes with its examples, action and uses

SPECIFIC LEARNING OBJECTIVES

After reading this chapter, the reader should be able to:

- Define toxicology and related terms like poison and drugs
- Classify poisons with examples
- Enumerate the characteristics of ideal suicidal and homicidal poisons and their examples
- Understand different factors affecting the action of poisons
- Diagnose poisoning in living and in dead subject
- Understand the general principles of treatment of poisoning
- Recognize different antidotes and their examples
- Enumerate various indication and contraindication of emesis/ gastric lavage and to describe its procedure
- Enlist the examples of household emetics/ antidotes
- Enlist different chelating agents with their examples, dose and uses
- Enumerate different postmortem findings in suspected case of poisoning
- Understand the duties of doctor in poisoning cases

References

1. Toxicology. www.dictionary.com>browse>toxicology. Assessed on dated 5-11-17.
2. Origin and meaning of toxicology. https://www.etymonline.com>word>toxicology. Assessed on dated 5-11-17.
3. Biography of Mathieu Orfila (1787-1853). US National Library of Medicine. https:en.m.wikipedia.org>Toxicology. Assessed on 5-11-17.

4. Singhal SK. Singhal's Toxicology at a glance. 9th edn, National book depot, Mumbai. 2016: 1–24.

5. Nandy A. Principles of Forensic Medicine. New Central Book Agency (P) Ltd: Calcutta, 2nd edn Reprint, 2004: 438–53.

6. Pillay VV. Textbook of Forensic Medicine and Toxicology. Paras Medical Publisher: Hyderabad, 17th edn, 2016: 470–96.

7. Tripathi KD. Antiemetic, prokinetic and digestant drugs. In: Essential of Medical Pharmacology. 7th edn, Jaypee Brothers Medical Publishers (P) Ltd: New Delhi, 2014: 661–2.

8. Tripathi KD. Cholinergic system and drugs. In: Essential of Medical Pharmacology. Jaypee Brothers Medical Publishers (P) Ltd: New Delhi, 7th edn, 2014: 110–1.

9. Tripathi KD. Ethyl and methyl alcohols. In: Essential of Medical Pharmacology. Jaypee Brothers Medical Publishers (P) Ltd: New Delhi, 7th edn, 2014: 395.

10. Tripathi KD. Opioid analgesic and antagonists. In: Essential of Medical Pharmacology. Jaypee Brothers Medical Publishers (P) Ltd: New Delhi, 7th edn, 2014: 483.

11. Tripathi KD. CNS stimulants and cognition enhancers. In: Essential of Medical Pharmacology. Jaypee Brothers Medical Publishers (P) Ltd: New Delhi, 7th edn, 2014: 486.

12. Bardale R. Principles of Forensic Medicine and Toxicology. 1st edn, Jaypee Brothers Medical Publishers (P) Ltd: New Delhi. 2011: 413–31.

13. Dikshit PC. Textbook of Forensic Medicine and Toxicology. 2nd edn, PEEPEE Publishers and Distributors (P) Ltd. New Delhi. 2014:451–73.

14. Tripathi KD. Chelating Agents. In: Essential of Medical Pharmacology. Jaypee Brothers Medical Publishers (P) Ltd: New Delhi, 7th edn, 2014: 905–8.

Preservation of Viscera and Other Materials

In poisoning deaths, gastric content/viscera or blood is routinely preserved for toxicological analysis to know the type of poison. In some medicolegal case, the cause of death is not clear at autopsy and the viscera and blood is preserved for analysis to give a final opinion. Even in antemortem cases, the sample (like blood or stomach wash) is preserved to estimate the level of intoxicant. Apart from such routine poisoning cases, the viscera and other materials like skin, hair, tissue, bones, urine, blood, etc. are preserved in different cases for various reasons. So, the present chapter includes the preservation of samples/materials in different medicolegal cases like firearm, burns, drowning, hanging, disputed paternity, sexual offences, etc. apart from the poisoning cases. It also includes about preservation of tissue/material for biochemical, serological, microbiological, histopathological investigation and museum purpose.

The viscera and other material from the human body may be preserved for the following reasons/purposes:

a. Toxicological analysis (TA)—in poisoning, alcoholic intoxication, drug overdose.
- Detection of toxin—in food poisoning
b. Blood grouping—in homicidal cases, sexual offences.
c. Biological/immunological study—in snake-bites.
d. Detection of petroleum products—in burns.
e. Detection of residual and other material—in cases of firearm. Comparison of ligature fibres—in hanging/strangulation cases.
f. DNA fingerprinting—in disputed paternity and other cases.
g. Fingerprinting—in unknown persons for identification.
h. Diatoms detection—in drowning.
i. Biochemical estimation of certain elements and enzymes in poisoning (OP compounds), pathological condition and for time since death.
j. Microbiological examination: Culture and sensitivity in infections condition. Bacterial/protozoa detection in gastroenteritis and cholera.

k. Histopathological examination.
l. Histochemical examination.
m. Bone examination.
n. Wet specimen for museum purpose.

INDICATIONS OF VISCERA PRESERVATION FOR TOXICOLOGICAL ANALYSIS (TA)[1,2]

1. The doctor conducting the autopsy suspects poisoning.
2. The cause of death is not known at autopsy or where death occurred in suspicious circumstances all of a sudden.
3. The cause of death is established but there is also suspicion of poisoning.
4. The investigating officer requests for the same.
5. In traffic accidents especially of the driver when suspicion of alcohol consumption (blood for TA).
6. In homicidal deaths, to rule out any intoxication.

PRESERVATION OF ROUTINE VISCERA

In most of the poisoning cases, the poison is taken orally. It absorbs through stomach and intestines, metabolized in liver and excreted through kidneys in urine. Thus, the following viscera are routinely preserved at autopsy[3,4] (Table 2.1 and Fig. 2.1).

V1: Bottle No. 1: Stomach and intestinal loop and their contents.

V2: Bottle No. 2: Pieces of liver, ½ of spleen and ½ of both kidneys.

V3: Bottle No. 3: Blood 100 ml for TA.

Gallbladder should be preserved along with liver since majority of the drugs can be detected in it. Half of each kidney has to be preserved, as one kidney may be non-functional.

Sometimes gastric content, urine, vomitus and other materials are also preserved for toxicological analysis. These materials are sent to regional Forensic Science Laboratory (FSL) by the autopsy/treating doctor through the concerned police along with the related prescribed forms duly filled, signed and sealed.

Blood for grouping:[5] 2 ml blood from heart in 2 ml of 5% sodium citrate solution. However, it is preferred to prepare two blood stains of 5 cm diameter on sterile starch free cotton

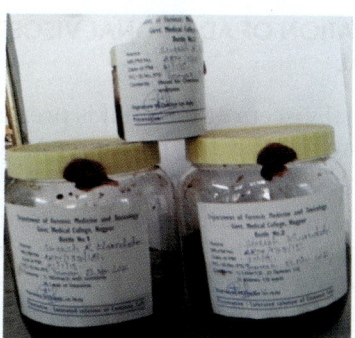

Fig. 2.1: Routine viscera for TA

cloth and send in an envelope after complete air drying. Starch from the cloth is removed by successive washing with plain water and then drying. **In routine practice, the stain for grouping is prepared over piece of cotton bandage.**

Dried blood stain over body for grouping: It is collected by taking stain scrapping if possible or transfer the dried stain onto the clean cotton cloth piece moistened with normal saline or distilled water, by gentle rubbing and send in an envelope after complete air drying.

Table 2.1: Guidelines for preservation of routine viscera in poisoning for TA[3,4]

Viscera	Quantity	Preservatives
1. V1: Stomach with its contents + intestinal loop with its contents	Whole stomach with 300 ml **or** whole, if less is available 1 meter (2 meters in children, whole in infants) 100 ml **or** whole if less is available	Saturated solution of **common salt (not used in acid poisoning)** or rectified spirit (but not used in alcohol, phosphorus, acetic acid, phenol, paraldehyde, formalin, chloroform, chloral hydrate, anesthetic agents, etc.)
2. V2: Liver + gallbladder, spleen, and kidney	500 gm or 1/3rd of liver (whole in infants) 1/2 of the spleen (whole in infants) 1/2 of each kidney (whole in infants)	Saturated solution of **common salt (not used in acid poisoning)** or rectified spirit (but not used in alcohol, phosphorus, acetic acid, phenol, paraldehyde, formalin, chloroform, chloral hydrate, anesthetic agents, etc.)
3. V3: Blood	100 ml (postmortem) 10 ml (antemortem)	30 mg of potassium oxalate + 10 mg of sodium fluoride/10 ml of blood
4. Urine	100 ml (postmortem) 30–50 ml (antemortem)	3 ml of concentration HCl or 2–3 ml chloroform/100 ml of urine or 100 mg of **sodium fluoride** per 10 ml of urine
5. Gastric aspirate vomitus	500 ml or whole, if less is available	No preservatives

In food poisoning cases, only the stomach content is preserved without any preservative for detection of toxins and sent to FSL, Mumbai

PRESERVATION OF ADDITIONAL VISCERA/MATERIAL

Additional viscera or material is preserved in a separate bottle for further analysis in following cases[3-9] (Table 2.2):

a. **In injection deaths:** The skin and muscles from injection site is preserved **for detection of suspected drugs.** A similar part from opposite side is preserved as control sample.

b. **In burn cases:** Skin, hair and clothes are preserved for the detection of **petroleum product** in cases where required. If clothes are present, then skin/hair is not required for CA as it does not add any advantage.

c. **In snakebite:** Skin from bite site along with blood is preserved for detection of venom. However, it is not detected on TA in almost all cases of poisonous snakebite due to neutralization of toxin.

d. **In electrocution cases:** A part of skin from the site of electrocution injury is preserved for the detection of **metallic residues**; and part of skin for histopathology.

e. **In hanging/strangulation cases:** Fibers of ligature material are collected by applying transparent cello tape over neck and then wrapped over the plain clean transparent glass slide for comparison.

f. **In spraying of insecticidal poison:** Nasal swabs, hand swabs, clothes, along with lungs and brain. The poison is not detected in routine viscera for TA.

g. **In cases of criminal abortion:** The uterus, cervix, bladder and rectum are preserved.

PRESERVATION OF MATERIALS IN SEXUAL OFFENCES

In case of victims, following samples/articles are preserved for Forensic Science Laboratory (FSL):

a. Blood for grouping

b. Blood for TA

c. Urine for TA

d. Seminal stain for grouping and identification

e. Nail scrapping for detection of epithelium of assailant

f. Pubic hair: Plucked/loose

g. Foreign material: Hair/cloth fibers/skin fragment

h. Vaginal swabs for detection of seminal fluid (acid phosphatase, etc.)

i. Anal/buccal swabs: For detection of semen.

j. Clothes—usually the undergarments for seminal stains.

In case of accused, following articles are preserved for FSL:

a. Blood for grouping

b. Blood for TA

c. Urine for TA

d. Nail scrapping for detection of epithelium of suspect

e. Pubic Hair: Plucked/loose

f. Foreign material: Hair/cloth fibers/skin fragment

g. Clothes

Apart from the above materials, the blood is preserved for culture; vaginal swab/smears for detection of spermatozoa; penis/urethral swab/smears for detection of vaginal epithelium. These materials should be sent to department of microbiology or examined by oneself, if facilities are available.

MATERIALS PRESERVED IN FIREARM CASE

In firearm case, the body is subjected to radiological examination prior to the autopsy for localization of projectiles (bullet/pellets) and for the track of firearm injuries.

Following materials are preserved in firearm cases and sent to FSL for further analysis[10] (Table 2.3):

1. Skin from the site of entry and exit.

2. Projectile or related material.

3. Wash sample: Swab moistened with distilled water.

4. Clothes

Table 2.2: Additional viscera/materials and body fluids to be preserved in other specific cases apart from routine viscera for different purposes[3–9]

Specimen	Indication/purpose	Quantity	Preservative
1. Blood[3–6]	Grouping[5,6]	2 ml (from cubital vein in AM cases) 2 ml (from heart in PM cases) **or** cotton bandage soaked in blood and dried* **or** two blood stains of 5 cm diameter on sterile cotton cloth* **or** plucked hair* **or** muscle (in saturated saline) **or** molar teeth* **or** bones*	2 ml of 5% sodium citrate solution prepared as (5 gm sodium citrate + 0.25 ml of 40% formalin + distilled water to make it 100 ml). *No Preservative, it is sent in an envelope after complete air drying.
	TA—for alcohol[9], poisoning cases[3,4]	10 ml (from cubital vein in AM cases) 100 ml (from heart in PM cases)	1 mg of sodium fluoride + 3 mg potassium oxalate/ml[7]
	Snakebite[5]	5–10 ml of blood	5% sodium citrate (i.e. 5 gm in distilled water)
	Volatile poisons or irrespirable gases (CO)	2–5 ml (from heart in PM cases)	A layer of liquid paraffin added to top of blood to avoid losses
2. CSF	Alcohol	As much as possible	10 ml of Na fluoride/ml CSF
3. Urine[3,7]	Alcohol	10 ml	30 mg phenyl mercuric nitrate or thymol per 10 ml of urine[7]
4. Brain[4]	a. Dog bite i. For HP ii. For Negri bodies	Piece of brain from hippocampus cerebral cortex, medulla and cerebellum	i. Formalin for HP ii. 50% glycerine in isotonic saline for Negri bodies
	b. Alcohol, CO, HCN, anesthetic drugs, opiates, strychnine, barbiturate	300 gm of brain tissue	Saturated solution of common salt
5. Spinal cord	Strychnine, gelsemium	Entire length	Rectified spirit
6. Lungs	Inhaled/volatile poison	One	Saturated solution of common salt
7. Skin with underlying tissue	a. Corrosive or injection death (insulin, cocaine, morphine, heroin)	5–10 gm of tissue around site **or** 2 × 2 × 4 cm area with muscle + control skin from opposite side	Common salt or rectified spirit
	b. Snakebite[5] (skin from bite site + control) + venous blood	5–10 gm of tissue around bite site + control skin 5–10 ml blood	Common salt 5% sodium citrate
	c. Electrocution[8]	From the site of electrocution injury for detection of metallic residues	Common salt
	d. Burns	Burnt site for detection of petroleum products	–
8. Heart	Cardiac poison	Complete	Saturated solution of common salt
9. Uterus with its appendages	Abortifacient agents in criminal abortion	Complete	Saturated solution of common salt

(Contd.)

Table 2.2: Additional viscera/materials and body fluids to be preserved in other specific cases apart from routine viscera *(Contd.)*

Specimen	Indication	Quantity	Preservative
10. Long bones[3]	Heavy metal poisoning	15 cm of length or 200–300 gm, **or** bone marrow from sternum/femur	–
11. Scalp hair[3]	Heavy metal	15–20 bands (20 gm) for detection of metals	–
	Burns	15–20 bands (20 gm) for detection of petroleum products	–
12. Pubic hair[5]	Suspected sex violence	Plucking or combing in sterile envelope after drying	Immediately dried in desiccators
13. Vaginal or anal swab/ fluid and foreign body[5]	Suspected sex violence	In test tube/slide immediately dried in desiccation and kept separated in TT	Sent in an envelope
14. Vomitus[3]	Poisoning cases	500 ml or whole, if less	–
15. Stomach wash (gastric aspirate)[3]	Poisoning cases	Wash with normal saline— 500 ml or whole if less	Nil—if wash with normal saline or otherwise with saturated sol of common salt
16. Nail scraping[5]	• Suspected sex assault • Homicidal/assault	Of all fingers, clipped without damaging underlying tissue to match with accused	–
17. Saliva[5]	Grouping	Few drops in sterile test tube, **or** two dried stains of 5 cm diameter on cloth	– Sent in envelope after drying
18. Soil	Exhumation articles	20 gm soil as much as possible	–
19. Clothes	Grouping—Homicidal Sexual offence Poisoning cases Burns	Blood stained cloth Undergarment or any stained cloth Soiled clothes For detection of petroleum products	Sent in envelope after complete air drying

MATERIALS TO BE PRESERVED FOR DNA FINGERPRINTING (Table 2.4)

In living person (Fig. 2.2)
1. Usually 1.5 ml of blood in 2 plastic tubes containing EDTA.
2. One drop of blood on FTA paper.

In dead person
1. Blood if available from heart.
2. Autopsy tissue usually spleen—2 gm.
3. Bone, usually femur/manubrium.
4. In fetus/neonate—blood/femur/sternum.

IN UNKNOWN PERSONS FOR IDENTIFICATION

Identification is the main concern of investigation in unknown bodies. It can be known from tattoo marks, scar, congenital or acquired peculiarities, clothes and belongings with ornaments. But fingerprints and dental charting is the ideal method for identification.

Materials Preserved but not Sent to FSL

1. **In dog bite cases[4]**—for detection of Negri bodies in brain, the samples should be sent to Director, Haffkine Institute for Training, Research and Testing, Acharya Donde Marg, Parel, Mumbai–400012. Phone: 022–24160947, 24160961–61, Fax: 022–24161787.

Table 2.3: Materials to be preserved in firearm cases[10]

Specimen	Quantity	Preservation technique
1. Skin	5–10 cm diameter around site or bearing shot holes	Keep in two plain white papers stapled to a thick cardboard and tied to another cardboard. Do not put in bottle or in any preservative
2. Pellets/fragments of bullet + other projectile like wad, etc.	As many as possible	Dried in air and put in bottle without any preservative
3. Bullet	Remove with finger or rubber tipped forceps	Dried and wrapped in cotton and put in a suitable container after putting identification mark on the base

4. Swabs
  a. Moist with distilled water
  b. Wet with 5% HNO_3
  c. Control samples of cotton, HNO_3 and distilled water
	From web and fingers of both hands separately in case of alleged firer	Dried in air and put in suitable container

5. Clothes	All or bearing shot holes	Dried in air and put in suitable container

Note: X-ray of the body is to be taken prior to the postmortem examination. Injury should be properly described, photograph with a scale attached or sketched and sent along with the articles to FSL for comparison purpose.

Table 2.4: Materials/tissue preserved for DNA profile[11, 12] (AM = Antemortem, PM = Postmortem)

Specimen	Quantity	Preservative	Container	Freezing
Blood liquid	1.5 ml in 2 tubes—AM 2–5 ml in tube—PM	EDTA	Plastic tube	Refrigeration
	1 drop on FTA paper—AM	Air-dried	Paper envelope	Dry freeze
Blood stain	5 cm radius on cloth—PM Cotton swabs moistened	Air-dried	Plastic container	Dry freeze
Buccal mucosa	3–4 swabs rubbed hard against cheek mucosa or mouth lining scraped with instrument and then smeared onto swab	Air-dried	Plastic container	Dry freeze
Swabs (oral/vaginal/rectal)	3–4 swabs	Air-dried	Plastic container	Dry freeze
Stain (blood, semen, saliva)	Cotton swab moistened with water or scrapped off if dried	–	Plastic container, paper envelope	Dry freeze
Seminal/vaginal fluid	1–20 ml or 1–2 drop	EDTA	Plastic tube	Refrigeration
Urine	60–100 ml	–	Plastic tube	Refrigeration
Saliva	A few drops	–	Plastic tube	Refrigeration
Hair	10–20 plucked hair	–	Paper envelope	Dry freeze
Autopsy tissue	2 gm (spleen, muscle, etc.)	–	Plastic container	Dry freeze
Bone/tooth	Femur, humerus, sternum	–	Paper	–
Bulk clothing	All	Air dried	Paper envelope	Refrigeration

Sometimes, the FSL person (along with kit) is accompanied for collection of blood for DNA profiling. So, if samples are collected and taken to the FSL on same day, then freezing is not required.

2. **Histopathological examination** of tissue, **biochemical** and hematological examination, and **microbiological examination are not done in FSL,** so such materials are not sent to FSL.

3. **For bone examination** in skeletonized or partially skeletonized body for ascertaining age, sex, etc. the bones should be sent to the Professor and Head, **Department of Anatomy**[4] (of authorized centers) Government Medical Colleges in Maharashtra.[13–15] However, in some states like MP, UP, Chhattisgarh, etc. the bones are examined in the Department of Forensic Medicine usually at medicolegal institute.

4. **For entomological examination to determine time since death**[16]: Live as well as dead eggs, larvae, maggots are collected in two vials. Half to be preserved in ethyl alcohol or formalin (if no other preservative is available) and other half should be kept alive to be reared out without any preservative. Container which contains preserved and living specimen should be properly labelled about date/time of collection, location of remains and the site of collection on the body.[17]

5. **Fingerprints for identification:** In Maharashtra, **Fingerprinting** is under the control of CID of the State (Home department) and **not done in FSL.** The fingerprints are taken by the police departments in unidentified persons.

MODE OF PRESERVATION, PACKING AND DISPATCH OF VISCERA/MATERIALS[3,18]

1. The collected viscera is preserved in a clean **wide mouth standard glass** or **preferably plastic** bottles **of ~1 liter capacity.** Blood is preserved in 30 ml bottle or plastic capped tubes of 5 ml. Sometimes bottles are supplied by the forensic science laboratory either in cleaned conditioned or it is to be cleaned with sulphuric acid—chromate solution, rinsed with distilled water and dried.

2. V1, V2, V3 should be preserved separately. The additional material should be preserved in separate bottles.

3. However, **bone, hair, nails, clothes, etc. are packed in polythene packet or plain paper.** But polythene bags or plastic containers are not used in volatile poison (which diffuse through it) and in corrosives poison (which corrode it). Lungs should be **preserved in nylon bags** for **volatile substance.**

4. The tissues are open/cut into small pieces before preservation.

5. The **preservative is added to each bottle, so as to completely dip the viscera to prevent decomposition**. A sample of preservative (100 ml rectified spirit or 25 gm common salt) is separately kept in a bottle and sent for analysis to exclude the possibility of contamination with poison.

6. However, container should not be filled completely and **one-third of the container should be kept empty,** so as to accommodate the gases liberated due to decomposition of viscera.

7. The bottle is made **air tight** by putting a lid on it. The lid is also **covered with** a piece of cloth, and tied with string or tape.

8. The bottle is then **properly labeled** and the ends of string/tape are **sealed.** The label contains the PM number; date and time of PM; name, age and sex of deceased; the viscera preserved; the preservative used and signature/seal of medical officer.

9. All sealed bottles containing viscera/materials are **handed over to** the concerned **police** immediately, **after taking due receipt.**

10. The forwarding **viscera form** requesting the chemical analyzer to examine the viscera/material, is to be **filled by the doctor** and **sent to FSL along with the viscera.** In the forwarding forms/letter to

the chemical analyser, the **specimen of seal** and copy of label on the material should be included along with the outward number, reference number and description of articles.

11. The **police then submit** the sealed viscera bottles and sealed viscera form to the concerned chemical analyzer and takes receipt. The copy of PM report is not required to submit the FSL.

At some places where **viscera box** is being provided by chemical analyzer's office, these sealed bottles are first kept in the viscera box. The box is then closed and locked. Cloth is tied on the lock and sealed. A label is put on the box mentioning the content of the box. The key of the box, viscera form, and a sample seal on a piece of paper corresponding to the seal used on bottles, lock and viscera form are kept in an envelope which is sealed and sent with viscera box.

Resealing/relabeling:[18] Sometimes the police bring back the viscera bottle stating that the seal of the bottle is detached or bursting of viscera bottle requesting to transfer the viscera to other bottle or resealing of viscera bottle. Sometimes the label is missing or soiled with the bottle contents, requesting to change the label.[18] In such case viscera bottles once sealed should not be resealed or transfer to other bottle, nor the new label be prepared. It is always better to **advice the police to prepare a panchnama of the damaged viscera bottle** and submit the viscera bottle after proper sealing/labeling to the chemical analyser's office with a copy a panchnama at the earliest. **To avoid soiling/** tampering of the label, it is to be coated with transparent adhesive tape or using plastic coated labels written by permanent marker pen.

DISPOSAL OF VISCERA[19, 20]

Viscera/any material or sample collected and preserved for FSL/other department should be **handed over to police** or investigating officer **immediately** after completing the autopsy. However, if the viscera is not collected by the police/investigating officer after autopsy even after due receipt without any information (unless advice to the contrary by the police), then it can be disposed off/ destroyed after 3 months[20] considering that it is no longer required.

It can also be disposed off

a. After taking written permission from magistrate or police.

b. When informed by the police/investigating officer in writing that the case is closed or viscera are not required for further investigation.

c. When informed by the police/investigating officer in writing about disposal of viscera.

Articles/materials which were sent to the FSL for analysis should be removed from the laboratory within 15 days from the date of issue of the report.[21] Similarly, the materials which were sent for the histopathological/ anatomical examination are also supposed to remove by the police within 15–30 days from the date of issue of report.

INTERPRETATION OF RESULT OF TOXICOLOGICAL ANALYSIS

a. Poison not found in bottles 1 and 2: Poison not detected or it was not a case of poisoning.

b. Poison found in bottle 1 and absent in bottle 2: Poison **not absorbed** or locally acting poison; death is not due to poisoning or locally acting poison or postmortem ingestion of poison.

c. Poison found in bottle 2 and absent in bottle 1: **Poison is absorbed** or **poisoning by other routes.**

d. Poison found in bottles 1 and 2: Poison is absorbed partially.
   +ve TA Report: When detected poison found in more than fatal level/dose.

   –ve TA Report: No poison detected or detected in less than fatal level.

REASONS FOR NON-DETECTION OF POISON IN VISCERA[22, 23]

Sometimes poison may not be detected on chemical analysis due to following reasons:

1. Delay in the examination of viscera and decomposition.
2. Improper preservation.
3. Tampering of preserved viscera.
4. Early disintegration or neutralization of the poison.
5. **Denaturation of protein**—example snake venom and bacterial toxins.
6. Use of wrong analytical technique.
7. Small amount of sample for analysis.
8. Lack of suitable chemical test for certain poison.
9. Complete metabolism of the poison in the body.
10. Removal/detoxification of poison during treatment.
11. Poison vomited or excreted out completely.
12. Delayed death after poisoning.
13. Some organic poisons such as alkaloids and glucosides, may, by oxidation during life or by putrefaction after death, be split up into other substances which have no characteristic reactions sufficient for their identification.
14. Lastly, due to the **unavailability of the standard** of specific poisons it will not be detected even if consumed. Example: **Vegetables and drug poison**. Also, there are various sub-types of insecticidal poison, if the person consumed some particular poison whose **standard is not available** with FSL, then that particular **poison will not be detected**/analyzed **in spite of the presence of poison** in stomach at autopsy. Moreover, if the level/concentration of poison is less than the fatal level, then also the chemical analyser's report is negative. The detection of poison/drugs in visceral material is also missed particularly when consumed in smaller quantities.[24]

Court question—about CA report and opinion in poisoning: In most of the admitted poisoning cases and other poisoning cases of vegetable/animal source, the poison is not detected on toxicological analysis (negative CA report).

In such cases the court will ask the autopsy doctor about the cause of death and the reason for non-detection of poison in the viscera.

In an **admitted case of poisoning**, it is advised **not to keep opinion reserved** for pending toxicological analysis, where the findings of poisoning were absent due to prolonged admission or gastric lavage or treatment. Rather, the **opinion** should be given at autopsy as "**PM findings are consistent with death due to poisoning**" in absence of any other findings suggestive of other cause of death. **Even in brought death or spot death of poisoning,** the opinion should be given at postmortem examination, if there are findings suggestive of poisoning in the stomach (like kerosene/insecticidal smell with hemorrhagic/eroded mucosa) or other specific findings to particular poisons (like fangs mark in snakebite).

In cases of poisoning, the opinion about cause of death is usually possible at autopsy either by way of positive findings of poisoning or by way of exclusion of findings suggestive of other cause of death. The toxicological analysis in such cases reveals only the type of poison, but in many cases it may not reveal any poisons on general and specific chemical testing. Similarly, in food poisoning cases, the toxin will not be detected on TA due to denaturation of toxin.

In snakebite cases, the **opinion (death due to snakebite)** should be given at postmortem examination. Toxicological analysis is almost always negative in such cases due to denaturation of venom. The **death** is usually due to **poisonous snakebite**, but **can also be possible in non-poisonous snakebite due to fear (neurogenic shock)**.

ALTERNATIVE TO ROUTINE VISCERA IN POISONING CASES

In **antemortem cases**, stomach wash, blood and urine are preserved in separate bottles for toxicological analysis in case of poisoning. But in **postmortem cases,** routine viscera from the dead body are preserved in two separate bottles and blood is preserved in third bottle for the detection of poison or intoxicants.

However, the purpose of detection of poison or intoxicant will be accomplished even if only the gastric content or washing (with normal saline) is sent in place of stomach and intestinal loop with content; blood in place of liver and spleen; and urine in place of kidneys. Moreover, there is no added advantage of sending routine viscera for TA. Thus, the alternative to routine viscera may be:

1st bottle	Gastric content or gastric washing with normal saline/plain water (100 ml or whole if less is available)
2nd bottle	Blood from heart—10 ml
3rd bottle	Urine—100 ml

FINGERPRINTING (DACTYLOGRAPHY)

In medicolegal deaths of unknown persons, the fingerprints are taken by the police departments; and analyzed by fingerprint expert. There are 4 types of fingerprints: Loops (65%), Whorls (25%), Arch (7%) and Composite (2–3%).

Method of fingerprinting: Fingerprints are taken with the help of printer's ink on non-glazed papers, after cleaning and drying the fingertips. It may be taken in two ways and are useful when the person is available.

1. **Plain method:** In this method, the inked finger is brought in contact with the paper and pressed gently. It is clearer and helps to check ridge pattern at a particular place, if the rolled impression is blurred at that place.

2. **Rolled method:** In this method, one side of the inked fingertip is gently pressed on the paper and rolled onto the other side without lifting finger. Maximum area of the impression is obtained and offer better study of the pattern of ridges, but sometimes may be blurred.

FINGERPRINTS FROM THE DEAD BODY

1. A few hours after death, tip of the fingers may get shrivelled in a dead body and may mask the picture. So to avoid this, **soak the fingers in alkaline solution**[25] **first and then take the print as mentioned above.**

2. Fingerprints can be taken from even the **highly decomposed bodies**, either from the **peeled off epidermis** of the fingers or **from the dermis** when epidermis is lost.[25]

3. Sometimes in dead bodies, the **skin and subcutaneous tissues of all the fingertips are dissected out** at the request of investigating officer and kept out in *weak alkaline solution* or normal saline **in ten different small clear bottles with markings** of initials of finger like RT, RI, RM (Right Thumb, Right Index, Right Middle), etc. respectively.

4. Sometimes in highly decomposed bodies, the skin of hand may be peeled off completely and come out as a **'gloves'** that may also be **preserved completely**. In this, fingerprints can be made by inserting the technician finger into the 'skin glove', inking the area to be printed and rolling.

Plastic fingerprinting are the fingertips impressions left on soft materials like dust, soap or wax. The fingerprints which are not visible as such but made visible are called **invisible fingerprinting or latent fingerprinting.**

Method of development and lifting of fingerprinting:[22, 25] The fingerprints which are not visible, are made visible by using various developing agents and the use of these agents depends on the type of surface needed to be searched for fingerprint.

a. **Physical/powder method:** For hard and non-absorbent surface (like glass, porcelain, painted or sun-mica covered surface, metallic articles) but light or dark surface, following powders are used:

   i. Light/white surface—black powder is used

   ii. Dark/black surface—grey powder/aluminum powder is used

   iii. Multicolored surface—fluorescent type of powder is used

   iv. Dragon's blood (a natural powder) may be used for both surfaces.

   v. Magnetic brush and powders are used to increase the efficiency in development of latent prints. The magnetic brush marks with magnetic powders are available in many colors like grey, black, red, yellow, etc.

Lifting of fingerprinting: Latent fingerprint on the paper or small articles can be preserved as such after development. But when they are on large immovable hard surface, the print can be lifted with transparent cello/adhesive tape of 1.5 or 2 inch width roll after being developed.

b. Chemical methods: For soft absorbent surface (like paper, cardboard, clothes, etc.), iodine vapor, silver nitrate and ninhydrin are used. While committing crimes or in nervous tension there is sweating from body including fingertips through the pores of the skin. When such person holds/touches any object, it produces invisible fingerprint due to moistness. This invisible fingerprint is made visible by different chemicals which react with NaCl, sulphates, phosphates, carbamates, lactic acid, fatty acid, glucose and urea present in the sweating.

The following methods (chemicals) are used

i. Iodine method: The iodine fumes reacts with the fatty acids of the print and appears yellowish brown or brownish.

ii. Silver nitrate method: It reacts with NaCl to form silver chloride, which is an unstable white substance that darkens, when exposed to light breaking into silver and chlorine that appear reddish brown.

iii. Ninhydrin method: It reacts with aminoacid and gives purple reddish brown stains. All the above methods are used for old prints.

iv. Osmium tetraoxide method: It is reduced to free osmium that is dark in color in presence of fatty substance.

Finder (fingerprint reader): It is a computerized automatic fingerprint reading system which can record each fingerprint data in half seconds. The light reflected from a fingerprint can be measured and converted to digital data which is classified, codified and stored in the computer.

Primary classification system of scoring: Scores are allotted for the presence of whorls in different finger of each hand.

Presence of whorls in finger	Scoring
Right thumb (RT)/right index (RI)	16
Right middle (RM)/right ring (RR)	08
Right little (RL)/left thumb (LT)	04
Left index (LI)/left middle (LM)	02
Left ring (LR)/left little (LL)	01

The scores are then arranged as follows and one is added for the purpose of calculation.

$$\text{Scores} = \frac{RT + RM + RL + LI + LR + 1}{RI + RR + LT + LM + LL + 1}$$

The score of numerator is multiplied with denominator. So, $32 \times 32 = 1024$ scores are possible, if whorls are present in all fingertips.

Federal Bureau of Investigation (FBI): USA maintains record of more than two crores fingerprints by systemic maintenance of separate files on the basis of presence of whorls in the finger. In 60% of the world population, there is no whorl in any finger, so according to primary classification, the score is one. On the basis of this scoring, 1024 divisions are made which are called **'pigeon holes'**. Depending on the scoring, final identification of any fingerprint is made by comparison.

DNA FINGERPRINTING

The technique of DNA fingerprint[26] was first developed by Sir Alex Jeffreys of Leicester University, UK in 1984 and developed in India in 1987. It was successfully used in sensational cases like Rajiv Gandhi assassination, famous Tandoori case and recently Madhumita murder case.[27]

Centers for DNA Fingerprinting

Initially it was done only in 'center for cellular and molecular biology' (CCMB), Hyderabad. Previously, all the samples were sent to Hyderabad from all regions of India. Now in Maharashtra, new center for DNA fingerprint is established in **Regional Forensic Science Laboratories at Mumbai and Nagpur.** These centers also provide the kit for collection (Fig. 2.2), preservation and dispatch of samples with prescribed forms.

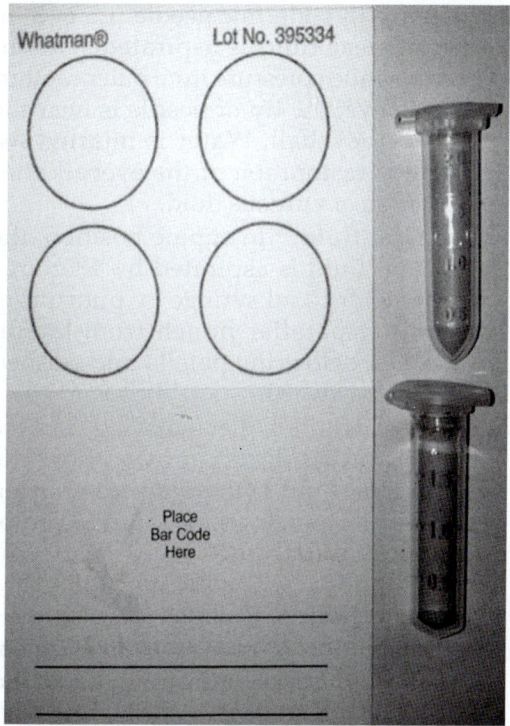

Fig. 2.2: Tubes and FTA paper for DNA profile

Materials used in DNA Profiling (Table 2.4)

DNA fingerprinting can be done from a wide range of biological specimens in both living and dead person. Biological specimens like blood, bone marrow, semen, hair root sheath, skin and any body tissue, fluid or secretion that contain nucleated cells are used. And cigarette butts, envelops, chewing gum and other articles which can contain saliva are amenable to PCR. Since DNA is very stable, the test can be done on very old stains (aged/dried stains) or specimens (mutilated/decomposed bodies).

Medicolegal Application

Here, the band of DNA is matched with the suspected source or individual.

1. Murder
2. Sexual offence
3. Paternity/maternity disputes: Blood from mother, baby and disputed father should be collected.
4. Mixed babies in hospitals
5. Identification of mutilated, dismembered or burnt bodies: The DNA fingerprinting obtained from such remains can be compared with those of close blood relatives of the deceased.
6. Missing person can be identified if his parents or children are available.

DIATOM TEST IN DROWNING

In 1904, Revenstorf was the first to attempt the use of diatoms in drowning. However, Hoffman discover them in lung fluid in 1896. The basic concept of diatom test is that when a person is drowned in water containing diatoms, the **diatoms which enter into the lungs may penetrate the alveolar walls and carried to distant target organs** such as brain, kidneys, liver and bone marrow.

If diatoms are demonstrated in the tissue of distant organs, then it goes strongly in support of death due to drowning, but there are certain fallacies. But still it is not conclusive in all cases, as it is present in the tissue even when the cause of death is other than drowning. At present the diatom test is used only as an indicative help and not as legal proof of drowning.[28]

Sample Used for Detection of Diatoms

1. Distant organ tissue like bone marrow (of femur), brain, kidneys: By acid digestion.
2. Test water where victim was drowned: Sedimentation, centrifuge and microscope examination.
3. Control water sample from place of testing: Sedimentation, centrifuge and microscopic examination.

Test: For tissue and bone **(sternum/femur)**[28, 29]

1. Bone marrow is exposed by cutting a small portion of bone or by crushing it.
2. Small portion (~10 ml) of marrow scooped out into a test tube/crushed tissue—TT.

3. Acid digestion: Add concentration 10 ml conc HNO_3 solution in TT × 24–48 hrs. Heat the solution till clear fluid is obtained.

4. Cool and centrifuge at 4000 rpm for 10 min.

5. Examine the sediment under microscope for diatoms.

Method to Detect Diatoms from Water (Not <30 Liters) Sent by Police

1. Immobilize the container/bucket containing water for 4–7 days.

2. Take out 30 ml of sediment with the help of pipette.

3. Centrifuge the fluid at 4000 rpm for 10 min.

4. Examine the sediment under microscope.

Result: Presence of diatoms

Tissue	Test water	Control water	Result
+	+	–	True positive
+	+	+	False positive
–	+	–	False negative

Fallacies of Presence of Diatoms

1. **False negative:** Diatoms may not be observed in the tissue even in antemortem drowning and the water in which drowned contained diatom.

2. **False positive:** Even if drowning was not antemortem, similar diatom may be present in both the test sample and the control sample, if the victim was habituated to drink water from the same source.

PRESERVATION OF MATERIAL FOR BIOCHEMICAL/HEMATOLOGICAL AND SEROLOGICAL ESTIMATION

1. **Blood:** 5–10 ml of blood is collected directly from heart during autopsy.

2. **Urine:** Obtained by catheter or suprapubic puncture with syringe and long needle before autopsy or by making incision on the anterior surface of bladder during autopsy. Preservative used is thymol 0.1 gm/100 ml urine.[30]

3. **CSF:** It can be obtained from three sites[31], namely lumbar puncture between L3 and L4 or cisternal puncture (posteriorly through atlanto-occipital membrane) or directly from lateral ventricles using long needle passed through the brain once the skull has been removed.

4. **Vitreous humor:**[32] It is obtained by using 20-gauge hypodermic needle. 1.5 to 2 ml crystal clear fluid is aspirated without exerting much pressure from outer canthus of each eye; the tip of needle is near the center of eyeball. Water is injected for cosmetic restoration of the eyeball after aspiration of vitreous fluid.

5. **Synovial fluid:**[33] In supine position, the synovial fluid is aspirated by 18-gauge needle with 10 ml syringe by puncturing the supra-patellar pouch from lateral sides just below the patella and pushed directly backward.

6. **Pericardial fluid:**[34] After removing sternum, the pericardial sac is cut by scissor. The pericardial fluid is then aspirated using sterile 10 cc syringe by taking care of contamination.

Above materials can be preserved in

1. Determination of time since death from the level of potassium in vitreous and synovial fluid[35], and from the level of enzymes in postmortem blood. In pericardial fluid, there is increase in enzyme activity of gamma-glutamyl transferase, creatinine phosphokinase, amylase and lactic dehydrogenase with increasing time interval.[34] However, these enzymes are also increased in cardiac, hepatic, pancreatic, muscular and malignant disorder.[36]

2. Different sudden/prolonged admitted cases like diabetes, uremia, hepatic failure, etc.

3. Poisoning deaths

a. Biochemical and Electrolyte Estimation (Table 2.5)

1. **In diabetes and hyperglycemia:** Serum glucose >600 mg/100 ml glucose is diagnostic of **diabetic**.[37] Level of >200 mg/100 ml in vitreous humor is significant for **hyperglycemia**[38]; whereas presence of ketone bodies >5000 µmol/L in vitreous is indicative of **diabetic acidosis.**[39]

2. **In renal failure:** Well demonstrated level of urea and creatinine in vitreous/ pericardial fluid is indicative of death due to renal failure/**uremia.**[40] **High serum or plasma potassium, uric acid, and phosphate** concentration usually indicate acute renal failure.

3. **Liver failure:** Raised serum bilirubin in postmortem sample is indicative of antemortem **jaundice.**

4. **Time since death: It can be estimated from potassium** level in vitreous and synovial fluid respectively as follows:[35]

Death interval (in hour) = 2.71 × potassium level – 20.19
Death interval (in hour) = 2.83 × potassium level – 15.41

There is linear rise of potassium level with increasing time interval after death.

5. **Toxic metabolic acidosis in severe poisoning:**[41] Measurement of serum/ plasma anion gap can be helpful in differentiating toxic metabolic acidosis (due to poisoning) from that of non-toxic metabolic acidosis. The anion gap is usually calculated as the difference between the sodium concentration and the sum of the chloride and bicarbonate concentrations. (Normally, it is ~10 mmol/L and corresponds to the sum of plasma potassium, calcium and magnesium concentration). This value is little changed in non-toxic acidosis. However, in toxic metabolic acidosis, the anion gap may exceed 15 mmol/L.

Table 2.5: Biochemical conditions in different poisoning[41]

Conditions	Poisoning
Hypoglycemia	Iron salts, ethanol, paracetamol
Hyperglycemia	Acetylsalicylic acid, salbutamol, theophylline
Hypokalemia	Acetylsalicylic acid, salbutamol, theophylline, barium
Hyperkalemia	Digoxin
Metabolic acidosis	Carbon monoxide, ethylene glycol, methanol, paraldehyde or acetylsalicylic. Poisoning with iron, ethanol, paracetamol and theophylline

b. Plasma Enzymes

1. **Time since death:** Peak levels of amylase and phosphatase are seen between 36 and 48 hrs after death. It is 48–60 hrs for transaminase and 4th day for lactic acid dehydrogenase.[42]

2. **Fall in serum cholinesterase** level is useful indicator in **organophosphate or carbamate** insecticide poisoning.[41]

3. **High plasma hepatic enzymes** are seen in poisoning due to **carbon tetrachloride, copper** salts, and paracetamol.[43]

4. **Increase gamma glutamyl transferase** activity is seen in **chronic alcoholism.**[44]

5. Presence of carboxyhemoglobin in blood can be used to assess the severity of CO poisoning and chronic dichloromethane poisoning.[41]

6. **Shock** coma and convulsions are often associated with nonspecific **increase in plasma** or serum activities of enzymes such as **LDH, aspartate aminotransferase, and alanine aminotransferase.**

c. Hemolytic

1. **Blood clotting:** Prolonged prothrombin time and clotting time is seen in snakebite poisoning (especially viper) and in acute poisoning with **hepatotoxic agents, rodenticides** containing anticoagulants.

2. **Anemia:** It is seen in chronic **lead, arsenic, copper, mercury and iron poisoning.** It is also seen in sickle cell disease with sickle shaped RBCs.

3. **Leucocyte count:** Leucocytosis is a feature of acute metabolic acidosis resulting from ingestion of **methanol and ethylene glycol.**[41, 43]

d. Serological Test

It is used in the following circumstances

1. **Infection:** For detection of antibodies like IgG for old infection and IgM for recent infection.

2. **Pregnancy test (hCG in urine):** For determination of suspected 1–2 months pregnancy in unmarried suicidal death.

3. Abortion cases up to 7–10 days of abortion for detection of hCG.

4. **Food poisoning/gastroenteritis:** For detection of toxin.

5. **Typhoid:** Widal test.

6. **Antigen test** for malaria.

7. **Dengue:** NS1 antigen.

8. **Viral and antibody test** for COVID-19

PRESERVATION OF MATERIAL FOR MICROBIOLOGICAL TEST

Microbiological Investigation

It is useful in

1. **Food poisoning/gastroenteritis:** Swab from small and large intestine for staining and culture/sensitivity of the bacteria.

2. **Cholera:** Stool sample for hanging drop preparation (for demonstration of motility).

3. **Malarial parasites:** Peripheral smear, spleen impression for malarial parasite.

4. **Sexual offences:** Vaginal swab/fluid for detection of sperms and sexually transmitted disease; blood for STD/HIV.

5. **Sudden death after trivial injury:** Skin tissue from the site of injury/injection should be cultured in Robertson cooked meat media for detection of Clostridium bacilli.[45] Blood is preserved for detection of toxins.

All samples for microbiological investigation must be collected using sterile instrument and placed in sterile containers.[31] The samples should be sent without delay to the microbiology or pathology department of Government Medical College or Virological Institute if needed. Different samples/swabs are required for bacteriological and virological study.

1. **Bacteriological examination: Blood for culture** must be obtained in septicemia before organs are disturbed either from heart through 3rd intercostals space or directly from vessels.[31, 46] It is also collected after opening **pericardial sac,** the anterior surface of right ventricle is seared with heated knife and 10 ml of blood aspirated using sterile needle and syringe.[46] The same technique may be used to remove material from other organs.

The most reliable method of collecting uncontaminated **cerebrospinal fluid (CSF)** is by spinal or cisternal tap.[46] It is collected even after opening **subarachnoid space** with sterile scalpel, a specimen is taken from a SA space by sterile syringe/dropper/swabs from which smears and cultures may be made.

Urine should be collected using a needle and syringe either through suprapubic puncture before autopsy or by direct puncture to bladder after abdomen is opened.[31]

For **culture of splenic tissue,** the surface of the organ is seared with a hot spatula, and the area is punctured with a sterile instrument and pulp is scrapped from which smears and cultures may be made.

Samples of gut contents should be taken as soon as possible preferably by tying off about 15 cm length of bowel and removing it, then emptying its contents into sterile container.[31]

Tissue representing smaller than 6 cm^3 is removed aseptically at autopsy and placed in a sealed plastic container and sent immediately or stored in a refrigerator at 4–6°C.[46]

2. **Virological examination:** A piece of **appropriate tissue** or swab is collected under sterile condition and the sample is **frozen or preserved in 80% glycerol**[47] in buffered saline.

3. **Feces:** 5–10 gm feces is preserved without any preservative for detection of **protozoa and helminthes**. In cholera cases, **hanging drop** preparation is prepared from the faecal matter to examine the darting motility of vibrio cholera.

4. **Smears of brain cortex and spleen:** Stained **for malarial parasite.**
Smears of bone marrow (ribs/sternum): stained **for blood dyscrasias.**
Smears from chancres and mucus patches: Stained or examined fresh by Darkfield **for STDs.**

PRESERVATION OF TISSUE FOR ENZYME HISTOCHEMISTRY

It is useful for

1. Determination of age of injury
2. To differentiate between antemortem and postmortem injury.

The injured tissue is stained for the presence of enzymes like:[48]

- Alkaline phosphatase (peak at 4–8 hours),
- Acid phosphatase (4 hours),
- Aminopeptidase (2 hours), and
- ATP-ases and esterase (1 hour).

Small pieces of tissues of size ½ × ½ inches from the site of injury with non-injured tissue are excised. The tissue is then cut into two pieces, one part is kept in formalin solution for histology examination and the other part is kept for enzyme histochemistry.

For enzyme histochemistry[49], the tissue is kept in two ice packs and preserved in a thermos flask containing liquid nitrogen.

The sections of 15–16 microns thick are taken in frozen section cryostat. The section is then placed over the slide and fixed with 10% neutral formalin at 4°C for 5 minutes.

Then the slide is washed with distilled water and is placed in the jar containing different chemical for specific enzyme in the incubator at 37°C for 1 hour.

After treating with various chemicals, the tissue is then examined under microscope for staining of the tissue.

PRESERVATION OF TISSUE FOR HISTOPATHOLOGICAL (HP) EXAMINATION

In some of the medicolegal cases, the tissue from the suspected pathology of the organ is preserved for histopathological examination. The microscopic examination of tissue not only helps to confirm the pathology on gross examination but also in a few other medicolegal cases while framing the cause of death.

The Tissue for HP Examination

It is preserved in

1. Pathological conditions

2. Injection deaths—part of the tissue at the site of injection is preserved to see local findings of anphylaxis
3. Electrocution/lightening cases
4. Dog bite cases[4]
5. Poisoning and drug abuse case for degenerative changes in the target organs.[50]

The tissues are best **preserved in 10% formalin or 70% ethanol.** For preservation of water soluble elements (such as mucus, glycogen, sodium urate crystals) **absolute alcohol** is the best preservatives.

Tissue size should not be more than 2 × 4 cm and 0.5–1.0 cm thick. Fixing fluid should be at least 25 times the volume of tissue. A typical portion of affected area seen on gross examination should be removed along with adjacent normal tissue. It should be cut into pieces of about 1–2 cm thickness and fixed in 10% formalin or 95% alcohol.

The tissue should be preserved in a jar, labeled and sealed as soon as possible. It should be **dispatched** to the department of pathology directly or **usually through police** along with histopathology form (Fig. 2.3).

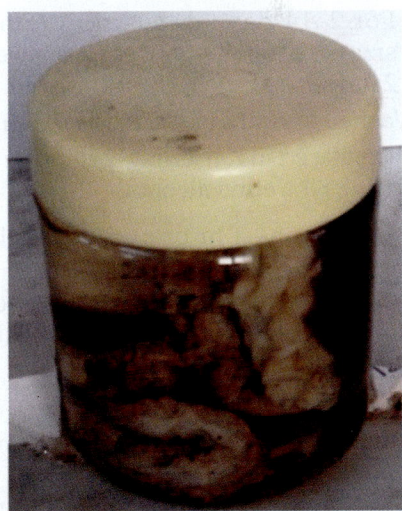

Fig. 2.3: Tissues preserved for histopathology

PRESERVATION FOR MUSEUM SPECIMEN

There is lot of disagreement whether it is legal to keep the organs removed during medicolegal autopsies for museum purpose. There are no valid guidelines in this regard as it is a medicolegal case and consent of the relatives is not taken for medicolegal postmortem. But, in surgical practice, if the ill organ with certain pathology or injury is removed, then it is either retained by the department for museum purpose or for histopathology or disposed of by incineration. In routine medicolegal practice, after completion of the autopsy, the particular organs having gross pathology or injury may be retained by forensic department for museum purpose, so that it will be useful for academic/teaching purpose for the students.

There are two methods[51] of preservation for museum specimen.

Method I: Kaiserling's Method (1897)

1. Firstly the tissue/organ is rinsed in cold water.

Then placed in Kaiserling-1 solution	
Potassium nitrate	10 gm
Potassium acetate	30 gm
Formalin	200 ml
Distilled water	1000 ml

- For 2–14 days depending upon the size of tissue (1 × 6 × 6 cm tissue kept for 2 days).
2. Washed in running water for 20 minutes.
3. Then placed in Kaiserling-2 solution (comprising 80% ethyl alcohol).

- For 10 mins–1 hr or until original color restored.
4. Again washed in running water and then placed in vacuum desiccators filled with Kaiserling-3 solution:

Potassium acetate	100 gm
Glycerine	200 ml
Formalin (40%)	50 cc
DW	1000 ml

and subject to a negative pressure of at least 50 mm Hg for 1 hr or more.
5. Mount the specimen in airtight museum jar filled with freshly filled Kaiserling-3 solution.

Method II: Dithionite method for restoration of natural colour

Tissue fixed for 3–4 days in Kaiserling solution or formalin can be recolorized.

1. Fixed or fresh tissue are again fixed in following solution for 3–4 days.

Formalin	1000 ml
Common salt	300 gm
Distilled water	5000 ml

2. They are thoroughly washed in tap-water for 1–3 hours.
3. Next treated with following solution for 2–3 days at least thrice.

Formalin	1000 ml
Distilled water	5000 ml
Sodium dithionite ($Na_2S_2O_4$)	100 gm
Potassium carbonate	30 gm
Pyridine	20 ml

4. Change the fluid or treat the tissue with above solution at least thrice.
5. They are finally mounted in glass or museum jar and filled with fresh solution.

IMPORTANT QUESTIONS

1. Describe mode of preservation, packing and dispatch of viscera for toxicological analysis. Add a note of negative chemical analyser report.

2. How will you preserve routine viscera for toxicological/chemical analysis in a case of poisoning? What are the indications of viscera preservation and their interpretation of the result?

3. Write about disposal of viscera not taken by the police after postmortem cases.

4. Describe the reason for non-detection of poison in viscera. How will you frame opinion as to the cause of death in such cases?

5. Describe the method for collection, preservation and dispatch of samples for DNA fingerprinting.

6. Discuss about removal of material after autopsy but are not required to be forwarded to FSL for further examination.

7. Write about preservation of tissue for histopathological examination.

8. Describe the utility for preservation of material/postmortem sample for biochemical and microbiological investigation at autopsy.

9. Describe methods of preservation of organ for museum purpose.

SPECIFIC LEARNING OBJECTIVES

After reading this chapter, the reader should be able to:

- Delineate the guidelines for preservation of routine/additional viscera for toxicological analysis
- Enumerate the different indications of preservation of viscera in poisoning cases
- Recognize the different materials preserved in sexual offences, firearms, DNA profiling, identification, etc
- Understand the procedure of packing and dispatch of viscera/materials
- Explain the method of disposal of viscera
- Recognize the alternative to routine viscera in poisoning cases
- Enlist reasons for non-detection of poison in the viscera/material
- Enumerate different materials for preservation in biochemical and serological estimation for various medicolegal cases
- Enumerate different materials for preservation in microbiological and histopathological examination in various medicolegal cases
- Summarize the steps involved in preservation of viscera for museum specimen

References

1. S.G's Circular Memo No. PML46/4868/11850/B dated 9th May 1968. In: Maharashtra Civil Medical Code. Chapter 13: Forensic Science Laboratories, Para 13.5 (A)(i) . Vol 1, 1977: 106–22.

2. Home Department Circular No. PRO 2360/57359/IX dated 12th JAN 1962. In: Maharashtra Civil Medical Code. Chapter 13: Forensic Science Laboratories, Para 13.5 (A)(i). Vol 1, 1977: 106–22.

3. SG's Memorandum No. PLM-4863/6224 Dated 22nd March 1963; and SG's Circular Memo No PML/18/467/14809/B dated 7th July 1969. In: Maharashtra Civil Medical Code. Chapter 13- Forensic Science Laboratories, Para 13.5 (A)(ii). Vol 1, 1977: 106–22.

4. Forensic Science Laboratories. In: Maharashtra Civil Medical Code. Chapter 13, Para 13.5 (A)(iii). Vol 1, 1977: 106–22.

5. Forensic Science Laboratories. In: Maharashtra Civil Medical Code. Chapter 13, Para 13.5 (B). Vol 1, 1977: 106–22.

6. Govt Letter UDPH and HD No HD/FSL 3064/29239/4263G Dated 9 Dec 1965. In: Maharashtra Civil Medical Code. Forensic Science Laboratories. Chapter 13, Para 13.5 (B). Vol 1, 1977: 106–22.

7. Bardale R. Inebriant poison. In: Principles of Forensic Medicine and Toxicology. 1st edn, Jaypee Brothers Medical Publishers (P) Ltd: New Delhi. 2011: 511–27.

8. Forensic Science Laboratories. In: Maharashtra Civil Medical Code. Chapter 13, Para 13.5 (A)(iv). Vol 1, 1977: 106–22.

9. Forensic Science Laboratories. In: Maharashtra Civil Medical Code. Chapter 13, Para 13.5 (D). Vol 1, 1977: 106–22.

10. Forensic Science Laboratories. In: Maharashtra Civil Medical Code. Chapter 13, Para 13.5 (C). Vol 1, 1977: 106–22.

11. Kagne RN, Ambade VN, Pathak AG. DNA fingerprinting: Collection, preservation and dispatch of biological sample. Souvenir of Formedicon 2004, XIIth Annual Conference of Medicolegal Association of Maharashtra, 2004, 39–42.

12. Knight B. DNA profiling. In: Forensic Pathology. 2nd edn, Arnold: London. 1996: 597–8.

13. Government Resolution No FSL 1966/6724–XXII, dated 12th May 1967, Government of Maharashtra, regarding examination of medicolegal cases by Anatomy.

14. Government Resolution No. CRA-697 dated 6 Feb 1998, Home Department, Government of Maharashtra, regarding authorization of centers for bone examination.

15. Ambade HV, Kasote AP, Fulpatil MP, Meshram MM. Medicolegal Cases for Bone Examination: 11-Year Retrospective Study. Journal of Indian Academy of Forensic Medicine. 2018; 40(1):102–6. DOI: 10.5958/0974-0848.2018.00017.9

16. Rosilawati R, Baharudin O, Syamsa RA, Lee HL, Nazni WA. Effects of preservatives and killing

methods on morphological features of a forensic fly, Chrysomya megacephala (Fabricius, 1794) larva. Tropical Biomedicine. 2014; 31(4): 785–91.

17. Lord WD, Rodriguez WC. Forensic Entomology: The use of Insects in the investigation of Homicide and Untimely death. Winter 1989: 41–8.

18. SG Circular Memo PML/18/467/14809/H dated 7th July, 1969. In: Maharashtra Civil Medical Code. Chapter 13: Forensic Science Laboratories, Para 13.5 (A) (iii), 1977: 106–22.

19. Para No 123 and 145 (2) of Police Manual, Home Department, Maharashtra. In: Maharashtra Civil Medical Code. Chapter 13: Forensic Science Laboratories, Para 13.5 (A) (iii), 1977: 106–22.

20. SG Endorsement No 1662/1072/D, dated 17 Sept 1962 on IGP's Letter to the SG. In: Maharashtra Civil Medical Code. Chapter 13: Forensic Science Laboratories, Para 13.A(iv), 1977: 106–22.

21. Forensic Science Laboratories. In: Maharashtra Civil Medical Code. Chapter 13, Para 13.6, Vol 1, 1977: 106–22.

22. Mathiharan K, Patnaik AK. Chapter 1 Section II. Toxicology. In: Modi's textbook of medical jurisprudence and toxicology, 23rd edition, Lexis Nexis: New Delhi. 2006: 26.

23. Bardale R. Toxicology Medicolegal consideration. In: Principles of Forensic Medicine and Toxicology. 1st edn, Jaypee Brothers Medical Publishers (P) Ltd: New Delhi. 2011: 432–6. Non-detection of poison on CA

24. SG's Circular No PML 4863/6224/B dated 2nd June 1967. In: Maharashtra Civil Medical Code. Chapter 13: Forensic Science Laboratories, Para 13.5 (A) (iv), 1977: 106–22.

25. Nandy A. Identification of an individual. In: Principles of Forensic Medicine. 2nd edn, Reprint. New Central Book Agency (P) Ltd: Calcutta. 2004: 93–7: Fingerprints.

26. Jeffreys AJ, Brookfield JFY, Semenoff R. Positive identification of an immigration test case using human DNA fingerprints. Nature. 1985; 317: 818–9.

27. DNA profiling in Justice delivery system. Central Forensic Science Laboratory, Kolkata. Ministry of Home Affairs, Government of India. 2007. Assessed on: *wbja.nic.in › wbja_adm › files › dna profiling cfl*

28. Knight B. Diatoms and diagnosis of drowning. In: Forensic Pathology. 2nd edn, Arnold: London. 1996: 404–6.

29. Nandy A. Violent asphyxial deaths. In: Principles of Forensic Medicine. 2nd edn, Reprint. New Central Book Agency (P) Ltd: Calcutta. 2004: 331–3; Diatoms

30. Karmakar RN. Forensic Medicine and Toxicology: Theory, oral and practical. Academic Publishers: Kolkata. 5th edn, 2015: 68–72. For urine preservatives.

31. Sheaff MT, Hopster DJ. Post Mortem Technique Handbook. 2nd edn. Springer-Verlag London Ltd: USA. 2005: 326–31.

32. Tumram NK, Ambade VN, Dongre AP. Thanotochemistry: study of vitreous humour potassium. Alexandria J of Medicine, 2014, 50:365–8.

33. Tumram NK, Ambade VN, Dongre AP. Thanotochemistry: study of synovial fluid potassium. Alexandria J of Medicine, 2014, 50:369–72.

34. Dalbir Singh and Rajendra Prasad. Relationship between the postmortem intervals and the pericardial enzyme activities in subjects of Chandigarh zone of India—A preliminary study. J Indian Acad Forensic Med. 2009; 31(1): 30–6.

35. Tumram NK, Bardale RV, Dongre AP. Postmortem analysis of synovial fluid and vitreous humor for determination of death interval. Forensic Sci Int. 2011; 204: 186–90.

36. Sagar Vidya, Berry V, Chaudhary RJ. Diagnostic value of serum enzymes—A review on laboratory investigations. Internat. J Life Sci and Pharma Res. 2015; 5(4): 8–12.

37. Arieff AI, Carroll HJ. Hyperosmolar nonketotic coma with hyperglycemia: abnormalities of lipid and carbohydrate metabolism. Metabolism 1971;20:529–38.

38. Coe JI. Postmortem chemistry update: Emphasis on forensic application. Am J Forensic Med Pathol. 1993; 14(2):91–117.

39. Pounder DJ, Stevenson RJ, Taylor KK. Alcoholic ketoacidosis at autopsy. J Forensic Sci. 1998 Jul; 43(4):812–6.

40. Palmiere C, Mangin P. Urea nitrogen, creatinine, and uric acid levels in postmortem serum, vitreous humor, and pericardial fluid. Int J Leg Med. 2015 Mar;129(2):301–5.

41. Flanagan RJ, Braithwaite RA, Brown SS, Widdop B, de Wolff FA. General Laboratory findings in clinical toxicology. In: Basic Analytical Toxicology. WHO in collaboration with UNEP and International Labour Organisation: Geneva. 1995: 13–7.

42. Nandy A. Death and postmortem changes. In: Principles of Forensic Medicine. 2nd edn, Reprint. New Central Book Agency (P) Ltd: Calcutta. 2004: 168–71.

43. Pillay VV. Modern Medical Toxicology. 4th edn, Jaypee Brothers Medical Publishers (P) Ltd: New Delhi. 2013: 581–2.

44. Teschke R. Gamma-glutamyltransferase and other markers of alcoholism. In: Seitz HK, Kommerell B (eds). Alcohol related diseases in gastroenterology. Springer, Berlin Heidelberg, New York. 1985: 48–64.

45. Ananthanarayan R, Paniker CKJ. Textbook of Microbiology. 6th edn. (reprint). Hyderabad: Orient Longman Private Ltd. 2002: 229.

46. Ludwig Jurgen. Special Methods. In: Current methods of autopsy practices. 1st edn. WB Saunders Company: Canada. 1979: 207–16.

47. Johnson FB. Transport of viral specimens. Clinical Microbio Reviews. 1990. P. 120–31.

48. Knight B. The pathology of wounds: Histochemical changes in injured tissues. In: Forensic Pathology. 2nd edn, Arnold: London. 1996: 165–6.

49. Drury RAB, Wallington EA. Enzyme Histochemistry. In: Carleton's Histological Technique. 5th edn, Oxford University Press: Oxford, New York. 1980:298–322.

50. Patel F. Ancillary Autopsy–Forensic histopathology and toxicology. Med. Sci and law, 1995; 35: 25–30.

51. Drury RAB, Wallington EA. Museum and injection techniques. In: Carleton's Histological Technique. 5th edn, Oxford University Press: Oxford, New York. 1980:474–88.

Forensic Science Laboratory and Analytical Methods Including Psychoanalysis

Forensic science laboratories (FSLs) are the laboratories working under Union Government or State Government for the examination of physical evidences sent either by doctors after clinical examination/postmortem examination or recovered from the scene of crime in different criminal and civil cases. Thus, it helps to link the victim/accused to the crime or incident. As the person (chemical analyser) working in FSL are using different analytical methods for the analysis of different physical evidences to link the suspect to the scene, they should be rightly called "Forensic Scientist" instead of "Forensic Expert".

Almost all the states have their FSL to carry out analysis of physical evidences. In Maharashtra[1], there are four FSLs at Mumbai (1958), Pune (1979), Aurangabad (1981) and Nagpur (1968). Two more laboratories have been started at Nashik (2004) and Amravati (2009).

FSL is having following sections for different purposes:[2]

1. **Toxicology section:** For toxicological analysis of viscera and other body fluids/materials or suspicious articles in different poisoning cases.

2. **Biology/serology section:** For blood group estimation and identification of body fluids, hair and plant material in murder, assault, rape and disputed paternity case. It also helps in food poisoning and skull superimposition cases.

3. **Physics (including photography) section:** For examination of trace materials in murder, theft, vehicle accident, etc. by spectrographic, X-ray, thermoanalytical, photomicrographic method.

4. **Ballistic and explosive section:** For microscopic examination and chemical analysis of firearms and explosive material.

5. **General analytical and instrumentation (GAI):** It deals with chemical analysis of petroleum products, explosive material, dyes, chemicals, drugs of abuse in murder, arson, theft, cheating, etc. with the help of chromatography and spectrophotometer.

6. **Prohibition and excise section:** It helps to detect blood alcohol concentration in consumption/possession cases under Bombay Prohibition Act. It also examines ganja, charas, bhang, opium, etc.

7. **Document analysis:** For examination of handwriting, typewriting, forged documents and currencies.

8. **Photography section:** Evidences from various exhibits and materials.

It also has following sections with the advancement of crime:

1. **Tape authentication and speaker identification (TASI):** It helps to determine whether any audio/video tape is edited, tampered or altered. Every human being has a unique voice like fingerprint; thus helps to identify the speaker and record certain characteristics in his/her voice by using advanced computerised method.

2. **DNA fingerprinting section:** For identification of individual. It is a costly method but has a broad application in forensic

investigation like paternity dispute, murder, rape, etc.

3. **Cyber forensic:** It helps to extract important data from computer, mobiles, SIM cards, debit/credit cards. So it helps not only to crack cyber crimes but also in murder, accidents, etc. from location of the mobiles.

4. **Polygraphy section:** For lie detection.

5. **Narcoanalysis and brain mapping:** For extracting truth.

6. **Mobile evidence collection unit:** For collecting different evidences from the crime spot directly under the supervision of police.

PHYSICAL EVIDENCE

It includes weapons, knives, blunt instruments, firearms, bullets, cartridge cases, wads, blood, seminal stains, saliva, epithelium, hair, poisons, fingerprints and foot/shoe prints, broken pieces of glass, vehicles paint, oil, grease, soil, clothes, documents, and cigarette butts, etc. It is useful to prove the crime and also connects with the suspect.

Examples

1. In Poisoning

In poisoning, stomach wash, blood, urine, feces and vomitus apart from routine viscera at autopsy are sent for chemical analysis. In food poison, only the stomach contents are preserved without any preservative and should be sent to chemical analyzer for detection of toxin.

a. Toxicological analysis of viscera/body fluids to know nature of poison.

b. Analysis of food/utensils, bottle/clothes, etc.—provides corroborative evidence in food poisoning.

2. In Assault and Murder

In homicide, examination of certain object/material from the body or scene helps to detect crime and for identification of accused/victim.

a. Blood grouping from blood stains on victim, hair in victim's hand, saliva on cigarette butts for identity of assailant.

b. Clothes examination for identification.

c. Examination of weapon/object to detect crime.

3. In Burn Deaths

In this, the clothes and hair are sent to chemical analysis for detection of petroleum product (like petrol, kerosene).

However, examination of metallic objects, teeth and bones also helps in identification of the charred body.

4. In Sexual Offences

In this, the examination of different samples is collected for chemical analysis. It helps to know whether the offence has been committed and to identify the accused.

a. Examination of vaginal fluid, blood/seminal stains—to check whether crime has been committed.

b. Examination of hair, epithelium, blood grouping for identity of accused.

c. Examination of clothes—site of offence, identity of accused.

5. In Vehicular Accident

a. Blood for CA for alcohol detection (especially driver)

b. Blood grouping for identification/matching

c. Tyre marks to compare with the type of offending vehicle.

d. Grease, mud, blood, tissues, glass pieces, hair, paint, etc. on vehicle to indicate offending vehicle.

e. Examination of clothes/site to identify accused.

6. In Firearm Injuries

a. Examination of projectile (bullet/pellet) to know the nature and type of firearm.

b. Examination of markings on bullet—to know which gun was used in firing by comparison method.

7. In Explosion and Blast

Examination of the material/soil from the core of blast for detection of explosives material.

8. In Hanging/Strangulation

For matching of ligature material used in hanging and strangulation.

a. The fibers of ligature on the neck are taken by applying transparent cellotape over the mark and then stuck onto a clean glass slide. It is then compared with the fibers of ligature material used.

b. Also the epithelial tissue adherent over the ligature should be compared with the tissue of the victim.

9. Identification

Identification is the main concern in unknown, decomposed and skeletonized bodies. It can be known from fingerprints, footprints, clothes, tattoo marks, scar, or any acquired or congenital malformation. This can also be possible by DNA fingerprinting, fingerprints, superimposition technique and reconstruction of face.

10. Disputed Paternity/Identity

The cases can be settled by blood grouping and DNA fingerprinting. DNA matching can be done by collecting amniotic fluid/chorionic membrane or by collecting blood from the umbilical cord and matching with suspected biological father. Recently, it can also be done by just collecting maternal blood for fetal cells.

11. Drug Addiction/Drug Trafficking/Drug Reaction

This can be known from detection of drugs in tissues and vials/specimen along with blood for CA.

ANALYTICAL METHODS USED IN TOXICOLOGY

In any particular case of poison, it is important either to know the nature/type of poison (**qualitative analysis**) or to know both type and concentration of poison in the body (**quantitative analysis**). The preservation of proper sample is the most important step in any toxicological analysis. The result of any analytical method depends on the amount and purity of the extract obtained from different biological materials (like viscera, stomach wash/vomit, urine, blood and tissue sample). The method for isolation/extraction of the poison not only depends on type of poison (pesticide, volatile, drugs, alkaloids, metallic, etc.) but also on the type of biological material[3]. After the isolation/extraction of the poison from biological material kept for toxicological analysis, screening/color test for different poisons can be done before any analytical method for quantitative estimation.

1. QUALITATIVE ANALYSIS

I. Screening/Color Tests (Table 3.1)

Table 3.1: Screening/chemical test used for detection of different poisons

Names of test	Procedure	Result	Indicates
1. **Chemical test: Acid**[4–6]	$BaCl_2 + H_2SO_4 \rightarrow BaSO_4$ $H_2SO_4 + FeSO_4 + HNO_3$ $AgNO_3 + HCl \rightarrow AgCl$ $BaCl_2 + TM*$	White precipitates Junction: Brown ring White curdy ppt White barium oxalate crystals	H_2SO_4 HNO_3 **HCl** **Oxalic acid**[5]
Ferric chloride test[7]	1 ml of 10% ferric chloride + 2 ml TM (urine)	Blue color substance/persistent purple color	**Phenol,** phenothiazines, phenylbutazone, or salicylates
Ferric chloride test[6]	2 ml of TM + few drops of $FeCl_2$	Red color → disappear on HCl	**Acetic acid**
2. **Chemical test: Alkalies**[8]	Hydroxides + $AgNO_3$ Carbonates + HCl	Yellow precipitates White precipitates	**Alkalies**

*TM: Test material

(Contd...)

Table 3.1: Screening/chemical test used for detection of different poisons *(Contd...)*

Names of test	Procedure	Result	Indicates
3. **Metallic poison:** Marsh's test[9]	**TM is placed in a hydrogen generator** → Arsine is formed which comes out through the narrow mouth of a generator and burns with a blue or greenish flame and gives garlicky smell.	If the porcelain plate is plate at the top of the flame, then greyish metallic arsenic is deposited, which is soluble in hypochlorite solution	**Arsenic**
Reinsch test[6,9]	20 ml TM (stomach content) in conical flask + 10 ml HCl + strip of copper—heated × 1 hr in a boiling water bath inside a fume cupboard. Copper is removed and examined.	• Silvery deposit • Black deposit • Bluish black	**Mercury** **Arsenic (dull black) or bismuth (shiny black)** **Antimony**
Gutzeit test[10]	TM in large TT + Pure Zn+ 3 drops of dil HCl + Pot iodide. A plug of absorbent cotton wool is inserted in the upper part of TT and mouth of TT is covered with a filter paper moistened with concentrated solution of silver nitrate.	Filter turns yellow Filter turns brown or black	**Arsenic** **Antimony**
Ammonia test	TM in TT + few drop of NH_4OH	Deep blue precipitate	**Copper**
HCl acid test[6]	1 ml TM in TT + 1 ml dil HCl	White ppt, dissolves on boiling and reappears on cooling	**Lead**
Ammonium sulphide test[11]	Ammonium suphide + TM containing ferric/ferrous salt →	Black precipitate, soluble in dil. HCl	**Iron**
Ferro-cyanide test[12]	50 ml of filtered stomach content + 100 ml HCl + 50 ml potassium ferrocyanide solution.	Deep blue precipitates	**Ferrous or ferric iron**
4. **Agricultural poisons:** OP: KOH test[6]	A fraction of extracted residue in 1 ml ethanol in micro crucible + 1 ml KOH (10%) and heated	Yellow color	p-nitrophenol derivative like parathion, chlorthion
OC: Sulfuric acid test[6]	Test extracted residue + Toluene + 2 drops of fuming sulfuric acid reagent	Red color	OC
Carbamate: HCl test[6]	Mixture of extracted residue + 5 drops ethanol applied over Whatman paper No 1 and dried, exposed to vapor of HCl	Steel blue color spot on paper	Carbamate
Silver nitrate test[13]	Patient is asked to breath in and out through a piece of filter paper impregnated with 0.1N $AgNO_3$ sol × 5–10 min	Filter paper turns black due to presence of phosphine in breath	• Aluminium/zinc phosphide • Hydrogen sulphide

TT: Test tube

(Contd...)

Table 3.1: Screening/chemical test used for detection of different poisons *(Contd...)*

Names of test	Procedure	Result	Indicates
Dithionate test:[12]	1 ml of test sample + 0.5 ml of aqueous ammonium hydroxide (2 mol/L). Mix for 5 sec + 20 mg of solid sodium dithionate.	Blue to **blue black color** Yellow-green color	**Paraquat** Diquat
5. **Veg Irritant:** Marquis test[6]	Dried residue of extract in TT + 1 drop of Marquis reagent	Brown color Pink color	Ergot Abrus
NaOH test[6]	2 ml of extract in alcohol + 2 ml NaOH	Brownish red ring	*Croton tiglium*
Sulfuric acid test[6]	2 ml of residue of extract + 1 ml H_2SO_4	Pink/purple color	*Calotropis gigantea*
6. **Somniferous poison:** Marquis test[6]	One drop of mixture (3 ml conc H_2SO_4 + 3 drops formalin) on a blotting paper soaked with TM (gastric fluid)	Purple color that gradually turns blue	**Opium/morphine**
7. **Inebriant poison:** Dichromate test[12]	Filter paper soaked with potassium dichromate is placed at the mouth of test tube containing test material (urine). Heat × 1 min.	Color of filter paper changes from orange to green.	**Alcohol**
Phosphoric acid-sodium bisulfite— chromotropic acid test[6]	0.5 ml distillate in TT + 0.2 ml phosphoric acid + 0.2 ml $KMnO_4$. Add sol of sod bisulfite till brownish color persist. 1 drop phosphoric acid + 1 drop sod bisulfite + 5 ml chromotropic acid	Violet color	**Methyl alcohol**
Chromotropic acid test[6]	0.5 ml distillate in TT + 5 ml chromotropin acid. Heated on hot water bath at 60°C × 30 min and cooled	Violet color	**Formaldehyde**
8. **Deleriant:** Gerrard's test[6]	2 ml of 2% mercuric chloride in 50% alcohol added to extract.	Red color Yellow color	**Atropine** **Hyoscyamine**
Fast blue B test[6]	Residue of extract in TT + small amount of FBB reagent + 1 ml chloroform → shake	Purple red color	**Cannabis**
9. **C. Depressant:** Silver nitrate test[14]	Br + $AgNO_3^-$	**Whitish**/yellowish ppt, soluble in potassium cyanide	**Bromides**
Fujiwara test (1 ml each in all three test tubes)[12]	**TT-A:** Sample + NaOH + Pyridine **TT-B:** Putrified water + NaOH + Pyridine **TT–C:** Trichloroacetic acid +NaOH + Pyridine → Heat in boiling water bath × 2 m	A. Red/purple color B. No color C. Red/purple color	**Chloral hydrate, chloroform, TC Ethylene**
10. **Spinal:** Manganese dioxide test[6]	2 drops extract in acetic acid in porcelain dish + pinch of Mn dioxide. Lines drawn with rod dipped in MnO_2 and H_2SO_4	Play of color from blue-violet-purple-red and finally yellow	**Strychnine**

(Contd...)

Table 3.1: Screening/chemical test used for detection of different poisons *(Contd...)*

Names of test	Procedure	Result	Indicates
11. Cardiac poison: Lee-Jones test:[15]	5 ml gastric fluid + few crystals of $FeSO_4$ + 5 drops of 20% NaOH—boil and cool. Then add 8–10 drops of 10% HCl	Greenish blue color Purple color	**Cyanide** **Salicylates**
Test for digitalis[6]	TM + conc H_2SO_4	Green color Yellow to brick red Red color	**Digitoxin** **Digitalin** **Digitonin**
Keller test[6]	Ether extracts in viscera + 1 ml GAA. Put over mixture (100 part of conc H_2SO_4 + 1 part $FeSO_4$)	Blue color on GAA Violet color on H_2SO_4 layer	*Cerbera thevetia*
Mayer's reagent test[6]	Dried residue acidified with AA + 2 drops of reagent	White/yellowish ppt	**Nicotine**
Palet's reaction test[6]	1 ml extract in acetic acid in dish. Heated and dried. Drops of Phosphoric acid + sod molybdate is added. Heated	Violet color vapor appears	**Aconitine**
Test for CO poisoning[16]	1 ml of test blood + 10 ml water	If >20% sat of CO turns pink	**CO**
12. Food poisoning: Nitric acid test[6]	5 ml adulterated mustard oil + 5 ml Nitric acid → shake the test tube	Orange yellow color	**Argemone**
Melzer's test[17]	Spores of mushroom are stained with 1 drop of Melzer's reagent and viewed under microscope.	Spores turn to bluish black color	**Amanita phalloides** of toxic mushrooms
Tensilon test[18]	In sudden paralysis, 10 mg edrophonium is given IV.	• If dramatic recovery • If no recovery	Myasthenia gravis Botulism
Melxner test[19]	Squeeze a drop of juice from the fresh tissue onto a piece of pulp paper or mash it on a paper and encircle it with a pencil and dry it. Put few drops of conc HCl.	Blue color within a few minutes	**Amatoxin present in mushrooms**
Drugs: Dille-Koppanyl test[6]	TM extract on spot plate + 4 drops cobaltous acetate + 4 drops iso-propylamine sol (5%)	Reddish-purple	**Barbiturates**
Marquis reagent test[6]	1 ml of TM extract in TT + few drops of marquis reagent	Yellow or orange color	**Benzodiazepines**
Trinder's test[12]	2 ml urine + 100 ml Trinder's reagent × mix for 5 sec	Violet/purple color If turns darkens	**Salicylates** **Negative test**

Trinder's reagent: 40 g mercuric chloride in 850 ml water + 120 ml of aqueous HCl mixed with 40 g hydrated ferric nitrate diluted to 1 L with warm water. If the test sample is other than urine like stomach contents, etc. then it should first be hydrolyse by heating with 0.5 mol/L HCl in a boiling water bath × 2 min, and neutralise with 0.5 mol/L sodium hydroxide

| FPN test:[12] | 1 ml of test sample (urine/stomach content) + 1 ml FPN reagent | Color from pink, red violet to blue Green/blue color | Phenothiazines. Tricyclics |

(Contd...)

Table 3.1: Screening/chemical test used for detection of different poisons *(Contd...)*

Names of test	Procedure	Result	Indicates
FPN Reagent: 5 ml Ferric chloride + 45 ml perchloric acid + 50 ml HNO_3			
O-Cresol test:[12]	0.5 ml test sample + 0.5 ml conc HCl → heat in boiling water bath × 10 min and cool. Then add 1 ml aqueous o-cresol solution (1 gm/L) + 0.2 ml test mixture + 2 ml ammonium hydroxide (4 mol/L)—mix × 5 seconds	Blue or blackish color	**Paracetamol or Phenacetin**
Forrest test:[12]	0.5 ml test sample + 1 ml forrest reagent × 5 seconds	Yellow green color deepening to blue	**Imipramine and related compound**

Forrest reagent: 25 ml pot. Dichromate + 25 ml H_2SO_4 + 25 ml perchloric acid + 25 ml HNO_3

II. Thin Layer Chromatography (TLC)

TLC is a simple, and widely used, inexpensive qualitative technique, which involves movement by capillary action of a liquid phase through a thin, uniform layer of stationary phase (usually silica gel) held on a rigid support.

2. QUANTITATIVE ANALYSIS

If the positive result of any suspected poison is obtained from the qualitative analysis (chemical/bed side test), then its estimation is carried out by quantitative analysis (Table 3.2). This can be done with the help of the following methods:

1. Ultraviolet spectrophotometry (UVS)
2. Gas chromatography (GC)
3. High performance liquid chromatography (HPLC) and high performance thin layer chromatography (HPTLC)
4. Mass spectrometry (MS)
5. Radioimmunoassay (RIA)
6. Enzyme-mediated immunoassay technique (EMIT)
7. Atomic absorption spectrophotometry
8. Neutron activation analysis (NAA)

Table 3.2: Comparison between GC, HPLC and HPTLC

Comparison points	GC	HPLC	HPTLC
1. Stationary phase	Solid	Liquid	Solid
2. Mobile phase	Gaseous	Liquid	Liquid
3. Conditioning phase	–	–	Gas
4. Samples should be	Volatile	Non-volatile	Non-volatile
5. Sample	Invisible	Invisible	Visible
6. System	Closed	Closed	Open
7. Separating medium	Tubular column	Tubular	Planar (plate)
8. Analyzed at a time	1 sample	1 sample	up to 20 × 5
9. Automation	Full	Full	stepwise
10. Operation required	High temperature	High pressure	Room T and P
11. Sample clean up	Essential	Essential	Not essential
12. Maintenance	Medium	High	Low
13. Running cost	Medium	Very high	Low
14. Samples/shift	5–25	5–25	up to 100

ANALYTICAL TECHNIQUES

1. Chromatography

It is a technique to separate mixture of substances, based on differences in the relative affinities of the substances for **two different media—one, a moving fluid (the mobile phase) and other, a porous solid/gel/liquid, coated on a solid support (the stationary phase or sorbent).** The speed at which each substance is carried along by the mobile phase depends upon its solubility and on its affinity for the sorbent. It is used to **detect poisons and chemicals.**

a. Thin Layer Chromatography (TLC)

In TLC, the stationary phase is a thin layer of absorbent, e.g. silica gel coated on a rectangular plate and the mobile phase is a solvent mixture. The sample is applied to a spot on the plate which is made to stand in solvent. As the solvent rises through the absorbent, the components of the sample are carried along at different rates and can be visualized as a row of spots, after the plate is dried and stained or viewed under UV light.

b. Paper Chromatography

It is similar to TLC. But the stationary phase is a sheet of special grade filter paper.

c. Column Chromatography

It is a type of chromatography using a sorbent packed in a column. The sample dissolved in a solvent, is poured on the top. Some components are retained in the column bound to the sorbent. They are then washed out in suitable solvents.

d. Gas Chromatography (GC)

It is a more sophisticated system of quantitative analysis. It offers a way of simultaneously separating, identifying, and measuring drugs and other organic poisons.

It is a type of chromatography in which the sample dissolved in a solvent is vaporized and carried by an inert gas through a column packed with a sorbent to any of the several types of detectors. Each component of sample, separated from others by passage through the column, produces a separate peak in the detector output, which is graphed by a chart recorder. The sorbent may be an inert porous solid (gas-solid chromatography) or a nonvolatile liquid coated on a solid support (gas-liquid chromatography).

e. High Performance Liquid Chromatography (HPLC)

This is similar to GC, except that it is not restricted only to volatile compounds. It can be used to separate and analyze complex mixtures as well.

f. High Performance Thin Layer Chromatography (HPTLC)

This is the fastest of all chromatography methods. It can analyze about 100 samples of 5–10 different types per shift. It is a visual technique where the chromatogram (separated sample after chromatography) is visible. In this, the stationary phase is solid, whereas in HPLC, the stationary phase is liquid. TLC is the method of choice for **impurity analysis of pharmacopeias.** It is not useful for the detection of unknown poison. Rather it is helpful to find out the impurities in known pharmacological samples.

2. Electrophoresis (Electrochromatography)

It is a technique used to separate mixture of ionic solutes in an applied electric field. The speed at which the solutes are separated depends on the difference in their rate of migration. The original method in which the movement of the solvent is unrestricted is termed **moving boundary electrophoresis,** because all the particles of a single species move at the same rate, maintaining a sharp boundary. This method involve a support medium such as paper, cellulose acetate, agarose gel, starch gel or polyacrylamide gel, which prevents convective motion of the solvent; this is called **zone electrophoresis.** The electrically charged protein components move on the phase plate. The plate is then treated with coloring agent which causes appearance of **visible characteristic bands specific for a particular protein.**

3. Spectroscopy

Every substance absorbs light of specific wavelength thus producing dark bands in specific zones. With the help of spectroscope, the light of specific wavelength is propagated through the medium/solution and then analyzed. Thus, it helps in the **identification of various forms of hemoglobin.**

4. Spectrophotometer

It estimates the quantity of coloring matter in the solution by the quantity of light absorbed after passing through the solution by means of spectrophotometer.

a. Colorimeter

Using filters, the light of specific wavelength is allowed to pass through the test substance, and the rays absorbed are detected.

b. UV/IR Spectrophotometry

This technique is based on the principle that many drugs when in solution will absorb ultraviolet (UV)/infrared (IR) radiation. The degree of absorption depends on the chemical structure of the drug, its concentration in the solution, and the wavelength of the rays. The amount of UV/IR radiation that passes through the solution is measured by the photocell.

This technique is ideal to quantitative blood levels of paracetamol and salicylates, as well as urine levels of phenothiazines. A major disadvantage of UV spectrophotometry is the possibility of interference in multiple drug overdoses.

c. Mass Spectrometry (MS)

The testing material in minute amount is placed in high vacuum chamber, and is bombarded with electrons. The molecules of the material, lose electrons, get positively charged, and break into fragments, which get separated according to their mass in an electromagnetic field. The same is recorded as lines in a graph.

This is usually **combined with gas chromatography (GS-MS)**, and is considered to be the best technique for quantitative analysis of

wide variety of chemicals, but its expense greatly restricts its use.

d. Emission Spectrophotometry

Every element on being excited emits light spectrum which can be separated and recorded by photography.

e. Atomic Absorption Spectrophotometry (AAS)

The element is vaporized and through this radiations from a light source are passed. This displaces the electrons of the atoms resulting in emission of energy which is recorded graphically.

This is the **best method for detecting inorganic elements (arsenic, lead, mercury, thallium, etc.).** However, it requires a large sample of blood for accurate analysis. The organic matrix is combusted and the metal forms a cloud of atoms, which absorbs a fraction of the radiation in proportion to the concentration of metal in the sample.

5. Neutron Activation Analysis (NAA)

It is based on the principle that many substances become radioactive when exposed to bombardment by neutrons. It can be used for the **estimation of any** of the 90 naturally occurring **elements** from antimony to zinc.

This is highly sophisticated and **expensive method of detection of a variety of inorganic elements** to analyze very small quantity of matter. **It is carried out in firearm cases to detect firearm residue.**

ACRO-Reaction Test

It is done in **electric current** death for **detection of metallic residue (pearls)** at the site of entry.

6. Radioimmunoassay (RIA)

It is slow and expensive method of detecting drugs in the blood, but is highly accurate. It involves mixing known quantities of drug-specific antibody with known amount of radioactively labeled drug that allows analysis of the precipitate with a gamma counter. It is excellent for the **detection of drugs in extremely low blood concentration** (cannabis, LSD, paraquat, digoxin, etc.).

7. Enzyme-mediated Immunoassay Technique (EMIT)

It is a fast, expensive method with good accuracy. It works on the principle that the amount of drug present is proportional to the inhibition of an enzyme-substrate reaction.

A known quantity of a drug is labeled by chemical attachment to an enzyme. Drug-specific antibodies added to the specimen bind the drug–enzyme complex, thereby reducing enzyme activity. Free drug in the specimen competes with enzyme labeled drug and limits the antibody-induced enzyme inactivation. Enzyme activity correlates with the drug concentration in the specimen as measured by absorbance change resulting from the enzyme catalytic action on a substrate.

EMIT is preferred over other RIA methods because of its simplicity and speed in providing information on toxic drug concentrations.

There are two main disadvantages

1. Negative result does not exclude the ingestion of a drug that may be present in undetectable quantities.
2. Antibodies cross-reactions can produce false positive results.

8 Microscope

a. Comparison Microscope (Color Contrast Microscope)

It is an instrument which permits simultaneously viewing of parts of images of two separate specimens involving **two microscopes bridged together with a comparison eyepiece** or one microscope, with two body tubes and lens systems.

b. Darkfield Microscope (Ultra Microscope)

It is a microscope with a central stop in the condenser, permitting diversion of light rays and illumination of the object, from the sides, so that details appear light against a dark background.

c. Electron Microscope

It is the microscope in which an electron beam, instead of light, forms an image for viewing, allowing much greater magnification and resolution. The image may be viewed on fluorescent screen or may be photographed.

d. Fluorescence Microscope

It is the microscope, used for the examination of specimens stained with fluorochromes, e.g. fluorescein labeled antibody which fluoresces in UV light.

e. Polarizing Microscope

It is a microscope, equipped with polarizer, analyzer and means for measurement of the alteration of the polarized light by the specimen.

f. Scanning Microscope/Electron Microscope

It is a microscope, in which a beam of electrons scans over a specimen, point by point and builds up an image on the fluorescent screen of a cathode ray tube.

g. X-ray Microscope

It is a microscope in which a beam of X-ray is used instead of light, the image usually being produced on film.

9. Psychoanalytical Test (DDT Test)

With the increase in crime incidence, the police interrogation techniques play a vital role in extracting the truth from the suspect. The scientific methods have been developed for extracting confession. Following scientific tests also known as **deception detection tests**[20] (DDT) are used as police interrogation tools:

a. Lie detector or the polygraph test

b. P300 or the brain mapping test

c. Narcoanalysis or the truth serum test

d. The brain electrical oscillation signature (BEOS)

The polygraph test was among the first scientific tests to be used by the interrogators. These psychoanalytical tests are also used to interpret the behavior of the criminal (or the suspect) and corroborate the investigating officers' observations.

a. Polygraph or Lie Detector Test

It records various physiological responses represented by mechanical or electrical impulses, such as **respiratory movements, pulse wave, blood pressure and skin sensitivity**[21] **(psychogalvanic reflex).** Such phenomenon reflects emotional reactions which are of use in detecting deception.

Polygraph test is conducted in three phases:[21] **A pretest interview, actual test (chart recording) and post-test interrogation/diagnosis.** The pre-test interrogation consists of a medical/personnel history, and educational background of the examinee. After that the examiner (a clinical or criminal psychologist) prepares a **set of test questions** (not more than 12 questions to avoid any discomfort to the examinee)[21] depending upon the relevant information about the case provided by the investigating officer, and reviews them with the examinee in the same sequence as they will be put during the test. After explaining about the instrument and attaching the different components of the instrument to the body, the actual test is started by asking from the set of test questions. All questions must be asked in moderate tone without any inflexion of the voice. The procedure is repeated after allowing time for the subject to relax. Post-test interrogation is done for the purpose of obtaining further information.[21]

Polygraph is based on the theory that when a person tells a lie, there is a fear that his lie would be detected. It results in stimulation of symphathetic nervous system resulting in physiological and behavioral changes. These changes can be recorded in the polygraph. However, these changes may also be triggered by anxiety, fear, confusion, hypoglycemia, psychosis, depression, etc.[20] Hence, the reliability has been repeatedly questioned.

b. P300 or the Brain Mapping Test or Brain Fingerprinting

This test was developed and patented in 1995 by neurologist Dr. Lawrence A. Farwell, Director and Chief Scientist "Brain-wave Science", IOWA.[22] Dr. Farwell has published

that a Memory and Encoding Related Multifaceted Electroencephalographic Response (MERMER) is initiated in the accused when his brain recognizes noteworthy information pertaining to the crime.[22] These stimuli are called the **target stimuli**.

In this method, called the "brain-wave fingerprinting" the **accused is first interviewed** and interrogated to find out whether he is concealing any information.

Then **sensors are attached** to the subject's head and the person is seated before a computer monitor. He is **then shown certain images or made to hear certain sounds.**

The **sensors monitor electrical activity** in the brain and register P300 waves, which are generated **only, if the subject has connection with the stimulus,** i.e. picture or sound. It measures the changes in the electrical field potentials produced by the sum of neuronal activity in the brain by means of sensors.[20] The changes directly related to specific perceptual or cognitive events.[23] Thus, brain generates a unique brain-wave pattern when a person encounters a familiar stimulus.[24]

The subject is **not asked any questions.** In a nutshell, brain fingerprinting test matches information stored in the brain with information from the crime scene. Studies have shown that an innocent suspect's brain would not have stored or recorded certain information, which an actual perpetrator's brain would have stored.

The Forensic Science Laboratory in Bangalore is the first center in India, which conducts the brain-mapping or brain-fingerprinting test.

In the USA, the FBI has been making use of "Brain-mapping technique" to convict criminals.

c. Narcoanalysis or Truth Serum Test

It is one of the scientific tools of interrogation for extracting confessions/truth after giving certain anesthetic and sedative drugs by putting a subject into a hypnotic state. This lowers a subject's inhibition in the hope that the subject will more freely share information and feelings.

Historical background

The term *narcoanalysis* was coined by Horseley. Narcoanalysis first reached the mainstream in 1922, when Robert House, a Texas obstetrician used the drug scopolamine on two prisoners.[22]

Narcoanalysis was rather unheard in India till recent past. It was first used in 2002 in the Godhra carnage probe. It was again in news in the Telgi stamp paper case in December 2003 at a government hospital in Bangalore. Later on, it was done in number of criminal cases like Nithari serial killing case, Talwar murder case, etc.

Principle and theory

This is based on the principle that **at a point close to unconsciousness the person cannot resist questions and also not be able to speak lie,** which he had been to conceal his crime.

The **underlying theory** is that a person is able to lie by using his imagination. In the narcoanalysis test, the subject's imagination is neutralized by making him semiconscious. The subject is not in a position to speak up on his own but can answer specific and simple questions. In this state, it becomes difficult for him to lie and his answers would be restricted to facts, he is already aware of. His answers are spontaneous as a semiconscious person is unable to manipulate his answers.

Drugs[25] and dose

1. **Scopolamine hydrobromide**
2. Sodium amytal or **sodium pentothal**
3. **Sodium seconal**

The narcoanalysis test is conducted by mixing 3 g of sodium pentothal or sodium amytal dissolved in 3000 ml of distilled water.[22] Depending on the person's sex, age, health and physical condition, this mixture is administered intravenously along with 10% of dextrose over a period of 3 hours with the help of an anesthetist.[22] The rate of administration is controlled to drive the accused slowly into a hypnotic trance, resulting in a lack of inhibition.

The team

In India, the narcoanalysis test is done by a **team**[26] comprising of an **anesthesiologist, a psychiatrist, a clinical/forensic psychologist, an audio-videographer, and supporting nursing staff.** The forensic psychologist will prepare the report about the revelations, which will be accompanied by a compact disc of audio-video recordings.

Procedure

It is completed in four stages[25]

i. **Pre-test interview:** Giving all the information to the subject about the test and consent is taken.

ii. **Pre-narcotic state:** Drug is being given to maintain pre-narcotic state throughout the interview.

iii. **Semi-narcotic state:** When the subject appears to be flushed with slurred speech and nystagmus, the forensic expert/psychiatrist facilitates the interview, the subject is allowed to sleep off and allow to wake up.

iv. **Post-test interview:** In this, the subject got relax after the interview.

The complete procedure of interrogation is recorded in audio-visual format and the report is prepared by the experts, which helps in the process of collecting evidence.

This procedure is conducted in government hospitals after a court order is issued instructing the doctors or hospital authorities to conduct the test. Personal consent of the subject is also required.

Reliability

Although inhibitions are generally reduced, people under the influence of truth serums are **still able to lie** and even tend to fantasize.

Different aspects of narcoanalysis test

1. It helps a lot in crime prevention and detection.
2. It also helps in getting clinching evidence and is an effective and non-hazardous method of inducing hypnosis.

3. If a criminal was put under narcoanalysis then he would reveal about the crime committed, where he had hidden the weapons used in committing the crime and why did he do it?

4. This would help in getting the motive for the crime and collect other evidence needed for prosecution.

5. Narcoanalysis is also considered by many to be definitely better than third degree treatment to extract truth from an accused.

But on the other hand, it has following drawbacks:

1. It required highly qualified physician for administration of drug and its analysis.

2. Dose depends on individual physique and mental attitude and will power, so difficult to determine correct dose.

3. Wrong overdose may lead the individual into coma or even death.

4. If the subject is an abuser of other intoxicants/narcotics, the test could be false due to cross tolerance.

d. Brain Electrical Oscillation Signature (BEOS)

An Indian Scientist, Champadi Raman Mukundan as developed a technology called Brain Electrical Oscillation Signature test.[27] The concept behind this electroencephalography (EEG) technology is that, it is able to show like as functional MRI, activated areas of the cortex which are then localized and the implications are determined. It deals with the experiential knowledge of the person. The Visual and Auditory Stimulus Programming (VASP) system allows recording and compilation of the probe like in different scenarios, marking events, etc. as well as creating video presentation for priming the subject. The probes are presented in a predefined manner by the VASP computer. They are sequentially interlinked and are designed after extensive interviews with the investigation officers and the suspects. Noncontroversial information is used as 'control probes'. The 'neutral probes' are used for

baseline correction. When the experiential knowledge is consistently present for relevant sequence of event, the test findings are said to be forensically significant.

Legal Aspect on DDTs

The interrogation of the accused by the police plays an important role in collecting evidence. But, if the culprit remains silent and does not answer any questions of the investigating agencies, then to what extent the investigating agencies can force the accused to extract truth. Moreover, any confession made to the police is not considered valid in the court of law; and police torture is not acceptable to extract truth as per human rights and ethics. So, in such circumstances can investigation agencies use DDT to extract information about crime.[20]

There are many who support that such tests often help the investigation agencies to extract truth. But others reject it as a clear violation to constitutional provisions.

These psychoanalytical methods as a tool of police interrogation also raises serious concerns related to the professional ethics of medical personnel involved in the administration of these techniques and violation of human rights of an individual.[28] In this regards, National Human Rights Commission had published Guidelines in 2000 for the Administration of Polygraph test.[20]

In a landmark judgment[29], the Madras High Court ordered that investigating agency is required to complete investigation within a reasonable time. If not completed, the benefit is given to the accused. If the accused fails to cooperate with the investigation process during custodial interrogation, then scientific investigation methods may have to be carried out to find the truth.[29]

On May 5, 2010 the Supreme Court in India[28] in Smt. Selvi and other vs. State of Karnataka declared brain mapping, lie detector tests and narcoanalysis to be unconstitutional, violating Article 20 (3) of Fundamental Rights. These techniques cannot be conducted forcefully on any individual and requires consent for the same. When they are conducted with consent, the material so obtained is regarded as evidence during trial of cases according to Section 27 of the Evidence Act.[20]

IMPORTANT QUESTIONS

1. Describe different divisions of forensic science laboratories of the state and its function.

2. Describe different screening test for metallic poison or agricultural poison. Add a note on 'non-detection of poison' in the viscera sent after postmortem examination.

3. Describe different scientific methods of interrogation for extracting confession from the criminals by police.

4. Describe different psychoanalytical method (Deception Detection Test) of investigation for extracting truth from the culprits. Discuss legal point of view in such investigation.

SPECIFIC LEARNING OBJECTIVES

After reading this chapter, the reader should be able to:

- Understand the purpose of different sections of FSL
- Enlist various chemical tests for the detection of different poisons
- Enumerated different analytical techniques
- Describe different psychoanalytical tests (Deception Detection Tests) like polygraph, narcoanalysis, brain mapping.
- Understand legal aspects of DDTs.

References

1. Forensic Science Laboratories. In: Maharashtra Civil Medical Code. Chapter 13, Para 13.1, Vol 1, 1977: 106–22.

2. Forensic Science Laboratories. In: Maharashtra Civil Medical Code. Chapter 13, Para 13.4,. Vol 1, 1977: 106–22.

3. Jaiswal AK, Millo T. Extraction/isolation and Clean-up methods. In: Handbook of Forensic Analytical Toxicology. 1st edn, Jaypee Brothers Medical Publishers (P) Ltd: New Delhi. 2014: 45–79.

4. Qualitative analysis test for identifying organic functional groups of homologous series of molecules identification—for anions identifying negative ions hydroxide (alkalis) identification. http://www.docbrown.info/page13/ChemicalTests/ChemicalTestsa.htm#Sulphate.

5. Reddy KSN, Murthy OP. The Essential of Forensic Medicine and Toxicology. 32nd edn, Om Sai Graphics: Hyderabad. 2013: 503–9.

6. Jaiswal AK, Millo T. Screening/spot/color test for different poisons. In: Handbook of Forensic Analytical Toxicology. 1st edn, Jaypee Brothers Medical Publishers (P) Ltd: New Delhi. 2014: 81–174.

7. Pillay VV. Textbook of Forensic Medicine and Toxicology. Paras Medical Publisher: Hyderabad, 17th edn, 2016: 497–520.

8. Nandy A. Corrosive Agents. In: Principles of Forensic Medicine. 2nd edn, Reprint. New Central Book Agency (P) Ltd: Calcutta. 2004: 455–66. (For alkalies)

9. Nandy A. Metallic chemical irritant. In: Principles of Forensic Medicine. 2nd edn, Reprint. New Central Book Agency (P) Ltd: Calcutta. 2004: 475–90. (For metallic poison)

10. Sanger CR, Black OF. The quantitative determination of arsenic by the Gutzeit method. Proceedings of the American Academy of Arts and Sciences. 1907; 43(8): 297–324.

11. Dikshit PC. Textbook of Forensic Medicine and Toxicology. 2nd edn, PEEPEE Publisher and Distributors (P) Ltd., New Delhi. 2014: 482–500. (For iron).

12. Analytical Toxicology: Flanagan RJ, Braithwaite RA, Brown SS, Widdop B, de Wolff FA. Qualitative tests for poison. In: Basic analytical toxicology. WHO in collaboration with UNEP and International Labour Organisation: Geneva. 1995: 34–49.

13. Bardale R. Principles of Forensic Medicine and Toxicology. 1st edn, Jaypee Brothers Medical Publishers (P) Ltd: New Delhi. 2011: 490–9.

14. Reddy KSN, Murthy OP. The Essential of Forensic Medicine and Toxicology. 32nd edn, Om Sai Graphics: Hyderabad. 2013: 557–9.

15. Lee-Jones M, Bennett MA, Sherwell JM. Cyanide self poisoning. Brit Med J. 1970; 4; 780–1.

16. Pillay VV. Textbook of Forensic Medicine and Toxicology. Paras Medical Publisher: Hyderabad, 17th edn, 2016: 640–54.

17. Leonard LM. Melzer's Lugol's or Iodine for identification of white-spored Agaricales. Mcllvainea, Spring 2006. 16(1): 42–51.

18. Pascuzzi, Robert M. The edrophonium test. *Seminars in Neurology*.2003; 23 (1): 83–8.

19. Melxner. The Melxner test for Amatoxins in Mushrooms. Mycena News. 1979; 29(9): 74. In: Clinical toxicology. 1980;16(3):401–2.

20. Math SB. Supreme Court judgement on polygraph, narcoanalysis and brain mapping: boon or bane. Indian J Med Res. 2011; 134(1): 4–7.

21. Camps FE. The Polygraph (Lie Detector). Gradwohl's Legal Medicine. 2nd edn, John Wright and Sons Ltd: Bristol. 1968: 545–7.

22. Nagaraja MR. 3rd degree torture by doctor and police: SOS e Voice for justice _ e- news weekly. 24/10/2015. Vol 11 (43). https://sites.google. com/site/sosevoiceforjustice/3rd-degree-torture-by-doctors-police. Assessed on 08/10/2019.

23. Lefebvre CD, Marchand Y, Smith SM, Connolly JF. Use of event-related brain potentials (ERPs) to assess eyewitness accuracy and deception. Int J Psychophysiol. 2009;73:218–25.

24. Dickson K, McMahon M. Will the law come running? The potential role of "brain fingerprinting" in crime investigation and adjudication in Australia. J Law Med. 2005;13:204–22.

25. Sharma BR. Scientific Criminal Investigations. 1st Edn. 2006, University Law Publication: New Delhi. pp. 60–1.

26. Barnwal AK, Sole AN Development of narco Analysis Test as Investigation Technique In The Criminal Justice System: An Indian Perspective *IOSR Journal Of Humanities And Social Science (IOSR-JHSS). 2016; 21(7): 97–102.*

27. Rose NS. Reading the Human Brain: How the Mind Became Legible. Body and Society. 2016; 22(2), 1–36.

28. Selvi, Ors vs State of Karnataka. Judgment on 5 May 2010. (Criminal Appeal No. 1267 of 2004). Assessed on 10/10/2019. http://supremecourtofindia.nic.in/

29. Dinesh Dalmia vs. State of Tamil Nadu, Crl. R.C. No. 259 of 2006. Madras High Court.

Corrosives

Corrosives refer to any chemical (strong acids or alkalies) that dissolves or destroys the structure of an object. However, caustic (sometimes used as a synonym) refers only to the strong bases, particularly alkalies and not to the acids. Thus, corrosives are the substance which corrode and damage the tissue on contact causing *chemical burns.* In dilute form, they act as an irritant. Strong acids react violently with water and generate heat and fire.[1] So, never pour water in it and when diluting, always add it slowly to the water. Sulfuric acid, nitric acid and hydrochloric acid are the examples of inorganic strong acid; and oxalic, carbolic and acetic acids are examples of organic strong acid. Hydroxide and carbonates of sodium, potassium, calcium and ammonium are the examples of strong alkalies.

Actions

1. Destruction and corrosion by burning of tissues on contact with acids.
2. Coagulation of tissue protein
3. Fixation of tissues
4. Extraction of water from the tissues (hygroscopic) and liberate heat[2,3]
5. Convert hemoglobin into acid hematin[4]
6. Carbonization of organic matter

SULPHURIC ACID	NITRIC ACID	HYDROCHLORIC ACID
Synonyms	**Synonyms**	**Synonyms**
Oil of vitriol, battery acid.	Red spirit of nitre, aqua fortis	Muriatic acid, spirit of salts
Chemically: H_2SO_4	**Chemically:** HNO_3	**Chemically:** HCl
Source Industries, commercial, laboratories	**Source** Industries, commercial, laboratories	**Source** Industries, commercial, laboratories, household
Uses <ul><li>Wet batteries</li><li>Diatom test</li><li>Fertilizer manufacturing</li><li>Ore processing</li><li>Oil refining, drain cleaner</li></ul>	**Uses** <ul><li>Used by goldsmith,</li><li>In explosives: Picric acid, nitrocellulose</li><li>In fertilizer</li></ul>	**Uses** <ul><li>Cleaning of ceramic surface</li><li>Preparation of chlorine</li><li>Treatment of achlorhydria</li><li>In hemoglobin estimation</li><li>In leather processing</li></ul>
Properties[1,2] 1. Colorless 2. Odorless	**Properties**[6,7] 1. Colorless/yellowish tinge 2. Pungent[7]/choking odor[8]	**Properties**[9,10] 1. Colorless 2. Pungent odor

(Contd...)

3. Non-fuming	3. Fuming	3. Non-fuming
4. Burning sour taste	4. Burning sour taste	4. Burning sour taste
5. Carbonises organic matter[5] It chars tissue and blackened organic matter	5. Xanthoproteic reaction[8]: Nitric acid reacts with organic proteins to cause nitration of phenyl group and forms picric acid to cause yellow discoloration	
6. Oily, heavy and hygroscopic	6. Powerful oxidizing agent dissolves all metals except gold and platinum	

Clothes: Burns instantly, black	**Clothes:** Yellow staining[4]	**Clothes:** Whitish or grey stain
Action: Locally corrosives	**Action:** Locally corrosives	**Action:** Locally corrosives
Fatal dose: 5–10 ml	**Fatal dose:** 10–15 ml	**Fatal dose:** 15–20 ml
Fatal period: 12–24 hours	**Fatal period:** 12–24 hours	**Fatal period:** 12–24 hours

Clinical features

1. Intense burning pain, difficulty in speech and deglutition, dyspnea (edema of larynx), vomiting, thirst, excessive salivation with blood and mucous, hoarseness of voice (inflammation of epiglottis and larynx), abdominal pain, **constipation,**[5, 11] suppression of urine and dehydration followed by shock
   - The vomitus is strongly acidic mixed with altered blood (brown or black due to hematin), mucous and mucous membranes
2. There is erosion of mucosa from lips to stomach. There is also erosion of skin along line of trickling of acid from the mouth due to constant drooling of saliva or acid spillage while swallowing.[12]

Erosion: Blackish color	Yellowish color	Grey color[12, 13]
3. **Teeth:**[4] Chalky white	Yellowish	Not significant
4. **Perforation:** Common	Less common	Uncommon

5. **On inhalation:** Irritation of the eyes, lacrimation, photophobia, burning sensation in the throat, cough and dyspnea.[1,7] Immediate death can result due to suffocation.

Causes of death: Shock, laryngeal spasm, perforation peritonitis, septicemia, malnutrition

Treatment

1. Emetics and gastric lavage are contraindicated (perforation of stomach).
2. Drinking of plenty of plain water or wall scrapping or toothpaste or non-flatulent antacids[11].
3. Weak solution of non-carbonated alkalies like CaO, MgO (4TSF in a pint of water or milk) and lime water, aluminum hydroxide
4. Demulcent drinks like milk, egg albumin, vegetable oil, ghee, butter, starch, etc.
5. Supportive treatment for pain, dehydration and shock.
6. Tracheostomy and artificial respiration is required for laryngeal edema; laparotomy and surgical repair for perforation.
7. Wash the affected part with water and soap or sodium/potassium carbonate; followed by application of thick paste of magnesium oxide or sodium carbonate.[5]

Postmortem findings: It depends upon the concentration of corrosive and the period of survival.

A. In early deaths

Gross corrosion of skin and mucous membrane of mouth, tongue and lips with discoloration

Stomach: Wall—soft, swollen,

Mucous membrane (MM)—desquamated, ulcerated, hemorrhagic with discoloration

Contents—acidic, altered blood, mucous, epithelium shreds

(Contd...)

Corrosion color:[3] Blackish	Yellowish	Brownish
Gastric perforation and peritonitis:		
Very common	Common	Uncommon

B. In late deaths: Signs of repair or infection may be present

Medicolegal aspect:

1. **Suicide:** Mostly used for suicide
2. **Homicide:** Rarely used for homicide, especially on children. It is also used for acid bath murder (hydrochloric acid/sulphuric acid).[13, 14]
3. **Accidental poisoning:** May occur in laboratory or goldsmith shop, mistaken with liquid paraffin or castor oil. It also occurs due to inhalation of acid fumes/vapor in factories.
4. **Abortifacient:** Sometimes used to procure criminal abortion.
5. **Vitriolage:** They are commonly used for throwing on other person.
6. **Punishment for adultery/infidelity** by putting acids in the vagina of a woman.[4, 11]
7. **For forgery purpose:** Hydrochloric acid is used to erase writings.[15]

Material preserved:	**Material preserved:**	**Material preserved:**
Routine viscera in rectified spirit	Routine viscera in rectified spirit	Routine viscera in rectified spirit
Stained scrapping—no preservative	Stained scrapping—no preservative	Stained scrapping—no preservatives
Clothes: No preservatives	**Clothes:** No preservatives	**Clothes:** No preservatives

Diagnosis

1. Chemical test:[4, 5, 16]

$BaCl_2 + H_2SO_4 \rightarrow BaSO_4$ (white ppt.)

$H_2SO_4 + FeSO_4 + \underline{HNO_3}$ brown ring at the junction of two fluids

$AgNO_3 + HCl \rightarrow AgCl$ (white curdy ppt.)

2. Blue litmus paper test:[3,16] Acid turns blue litmus paper red

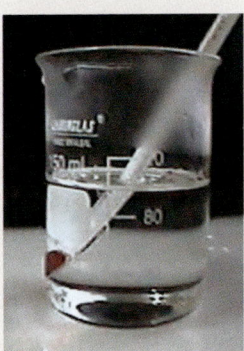

Fig. 4.1: H_2SO_4

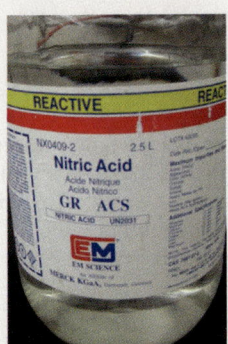

Fig. 4.2: HNO_3

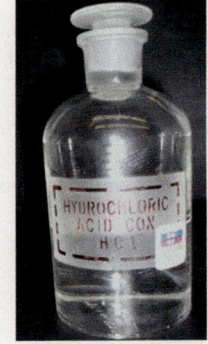

Fig. 4.3: HCl

VITRIOLAGE

Definition: It is throwing of any corrosive substance (usually acids) on other person out of jealousy or to take revenge with the intension to cause injury, disfigurement or death. Since sulphuric acid (oil of vitriol) is commonly used, hence the name Vitriolage. Acid filled in old electric bulbs are usually used for vitriolage.

Substances used: Sulphuric acid, nitric acid, hydrochloric acid, sodium/potassium hydroxide, and marking nut juice.

Features of vitriolage

1. Chemical burns: In the form of disfigurement of face or body with burn injury. It is characterized by:

  a. Discoloration and staining of clothes and body

  b. Absence of vesicles/blisters

  c. Trickling marks of an acid

  d. No red line of demarcation

2. Eye: Blindness, corneal destruction or conjunctival edema

Cause of death: Neurogenic shock or septicemia

Treatment

1. Wash the affected part with plenty of water and soap or sodium/potassium carbonate.

2. Apply thick paste of magnesium oxide or sodium bicarbonate.[5]

3. Eyes are irrigated with water or dilute solution of sodium bicarbonate.[5]

4. Treat like a case of burns, using antibiotic and steroid ointments and eyedrops.

Medicolegal aspect

Grievous injury due to disfigurement of any part of the body by throwing of an acid.[17] It is also due to permanent privation of hearing and vision of either side as per Section 320 IPC.[18]

OXALIC ACID	CARBOLIC ACID	ACETIC ACID
Synonyms: Acid of sugars	Phenol, phenic acid, phenyl alcohol	Glacial acetic acid (100% conc.), vinegar (4–5%)[19]
Chemically: $C_2H_2O_4$	**Chemically:** C_6H_5OH	**Chemically:** CH_3COOH
Source Industries, commercial, laboratories, household (metal cleaning, stain remover)[11], vegetables—onion, spinach, cabbage, radish, carrot, beet	**Source** Industries, commercial, laboratories, household (disinfectants), it is a coal tar derivative	**Source** Industries, commercial, laboratories, household (vinegar)
Uses • To erase writing and signature for forgery purpose[5] • For ink/rust stain removal • For calicoprinting[4] • For metal/glass cleaning • In bleaches (esp. pulp wood)	**Uses** • Used as disinfectant/antiseptic • Accepted as snake repellant • In cosmetics/sunscreen, hair dyes, skin lightening preparations	**Uses** • Used in food • Medicinal use in superficial ear infection, jelly fish sting and bladder irrigation
Properties[20] 1. Colorless, transparent, shining crystals (resemble $MgSO_4$ and $ZnSO_4$) 2. Odorless/irritating smell 3. Burning sour taste 4. Hygroscopic 5. Vaporizes on heating and sublimates on cooling[11]	**Properties**[21] 1. White small needle like crystals, on exposure to air, it becomes light pink liquid 2. Sweetish acrid odor 3. Burning sweet taste 4. Hygroscopic 5. Crude carbolic is **phenyl**, which is dark brown in color	**Properties**[22] 1. Colorless liquid, when freezes becomes crystalline solid 2. Vinegar, pungent smell 3. Burning sour taste 4. Volatile liquid
Action 1. **Locally:** Corrosives	**Action** 1. **Locally:** Corrosion, necrosis and	**Action** 1. **Locally:** Corrosives

2. **Systemic:** It causes hypocalcemia by utilization of serum calcium to form oxalate.
3. Nephrotoxicity—oxaluria

Gangrene of the local area.
2. **Systemic:** CNS—first stimulate and then depresses
3. Nephrotoxicity—carboluria

2. Respiratory distress

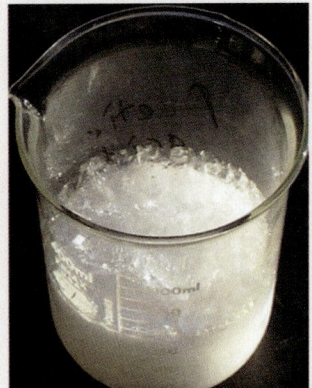

Fig. 4.4: Oxalic acid

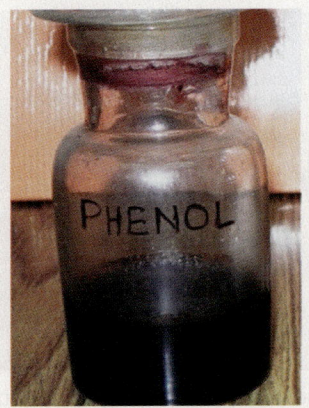

Fig. 4.5: Phenol

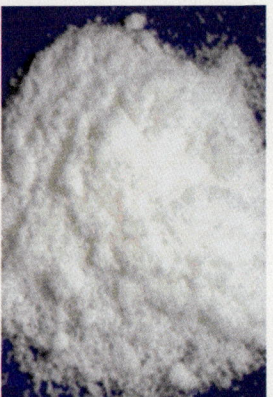

Fig. 4.6: Acetic acid

Fatal dose: 10–15 gm **Fatal period:** 2–12 hrs	**Fatal dose:** 10–20 gm **Fatal period:** 2–12 hrs	**Fatal dose:** Uncertain **Fatal period:** Uncertain
Clinical features **Locally:** There is corrosion of mucosa of mouth, tongue and lips—whitish or yellowish. Skin—Whitish or yellowish discoloration[12,20]	**Clinical features:** (Carbolism) **Locally:** There is corrosion of mucosa of mouth, tongue and lips—grayish white. Skin—reddened, necrosis and gangrene.	**Clinical features** **Locally:** There is corrosion of mucosa of mouth, tongue and lips. Skin—no corrosion, redness, blisters[22]

1. **GIT:** Intense burning pain, difficulty in speech and deglutition, dyspnea (edema of larynx), vomiting, abdominal pain, thirst, excessive salivation with blood and mucous, hoarseness of voice (inflammation of epiglottis and larynx), **diarrhea** and pain at anus, suppression of urine and dehydration followed by shock. The vomitus is strongly acidic mixed with altered blood (brown, black or coffee color due to acid hematin), mucous and mucous membranes

2. **CNS:** Due to hypocalcemia, there is tetany characterized by twitching of face and extremities with tonic muscle spasm, cramps and convulsions, with positive *Chvostek's sign and Trousseau sign*[12] 3. **Kidney:** Oxaluria characterised by hematuria and oliguria with calcium oxalate crystals in urine which is octahedral in shape.	2. **CNS:** Dyspnea, dizziness, delirium, convulsion, collapse, coma 3. **Kidney: Carboluria** characterized by hematuria and oliguria, with casts in urine, which on exposed to air for 20–30 sec turns greenish due to the oxidation of its metabolic product like hydroquinone and pyrocatechol 4. These metabolites may get deposited in cartilages and ligaments or cornea[3]/sclera[12] producing dark pigmentation—called **ochronosis** 5. Pupils constricted	2. **CNS:** Not specific 3. **Kidney:** Oliguria and hematuria 4. **RS:** Respiratory distress due to trickling of vomitus or leakage of acid

Chvostek's sign:[23] When the facial nerve is tapped in front of tragus the facial muscles on the same side of the face will contract momentarily (typically a twitch of the nose or lips) because of hypocalcemia

Trousseau sign:[23,24] There is spasm of the muscles of the hand and forearm. The wrist and metacarpophalangeal joints flex, the DIP and PIP joints extend, and the fingers adduct (Fig. 4.7).

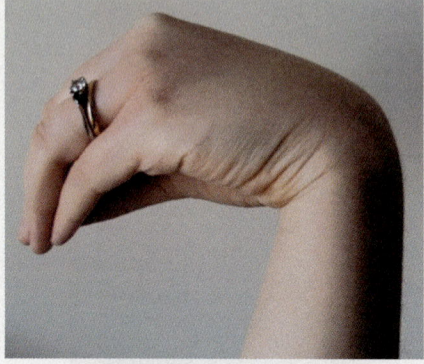

Fig. 4.7: Hand being held similar to Trousseau signs in latent tetany due to hypocalcemia

Treatment	Treatment	Treatment
1. Emetics	1. Emetics	1. Emetics
2. Gastric lavage with calcium lactate (2 TSF), chalk, CaO. Warm water should not be used since it will dissolve oxalic acid	2. Gastric lavage with sodium/magnesium sulfate solution[25]	2. Gastric lavage
3. Purgatives and demulcents	3. Demulcents	3. Demulcents
4. **Antidotes:** Chalk powder, lime or wall scrapping (all contain calcium carbonate) can be given orally or 10 ml of 10% calcium gluconate is given IV[5]	4. **Antidotes:**[25] Sodium/magnesium sulfate	4. **Antidotes:** Not specific
5. **Supportive:** IV fluids—25% glucose; acidosis—NaHCO$_3$	5. **Supportive:** IV fluids—25% glucose acidosis—NaHCO$_3$ Digitalis for circulatory shock Artificial respiration + oxygen inhalation	5. **Supportive:** IV fluids—25% glucose acidosis—NaHCO$_3$ Artificial respiration + oxygen inhalation
6. Restrict Na/K salts[11]	6. **For methemoglobinemia:** If >30%—methylene blue (1–2 mg/kg) If >70%—exchange transfusion.[25]	

PM findings	PM findings	PM findings
1. **Local:** Skin irritation with whitish or yellowish discoloration[12, 20]	1. **Local:** Skin necrosis, gangrene	1. **Local:** Nil
2. MM of mouth/tongue—corroded, swollen/sodden, bleached appear whitish/yellowish[12]	2. MM of mouth/tongue—corroded, first appear greyish white	2. MM of mouth/tongue, lips-corroded
3. **Stomach:** **Wall:** Soft, swollen **MM:** Congested, desquamated, hemorrhagic, Scalded yellowish[12] but becomes brownish due to acid hematin **Contains:** Brownish, blood mixed with mucus	3. **Stomach:** **Wall:** Tough, thick, leathery brown,—"**Leather bottle appearance**". (Fig. 4.9) **MM:** Congested, desquamated, hemorrhagic **Contains:** Brownish, blood mixed with mucus + Phenolic Smell	3. Stomach: **Wall:** Soft, swollen **MM:** Congested, desquamated, hemorrhagic **Contains:** Brownish, altered blood + mucus shreds + vinegar smell
		4. All visceral organs are congested
		5. Kidneys are congested
		6. Respiratory tract—congested, inflamed due to leakage of acid in RT. Lungs edematous

4. All visceral organs are congested	4. All visceral organs are congested	
5. Kidneys are congested with presence of calcium oxalate crystals	5. Kidneys are congested, enlarged and cortical hemorrhagic	
6. Visceral organs show cloudy areas due to deposition of calcium oxalate	6. Surrounding structure/organs appeared necrosed and hardening with greyish white staining of the viscera	
Preservation of viscera: V1 + V2 **Preserved in:** Rectified spirit	**V1 + V2 preserved in** saturated salt solution and **not in rectified spirit**	**V1 + V2 preserved in** saturated salt solution and **not in rectified spirit**
Medicolegal (ML) aspects 1. **Suicide:** Sometimes used for suicide 2. **Homicide:** Rarely used 3. **Accidental poisoning:** Mistaken with magnesium or zinc sulfate (Table 4.1) in children. 4. **For forgery purpose:** It is used to erase writing and signature[5]	**ML aspects** 1. **Suicide:** Commonly used for suicide (household poison) 2. **Homicide:** Rarely used where it is mixed with rum 3. **Accidental poisoning:** Mistaken with drakshasava (Ayurvedic drug), usually in children, chronic exposure due to its use or industrial exposure 4. **Abortifacient:** Used to procure criminal abortion	**ML aspects** 1. **Suicide:** May be used for suicide (household poison) 2. **Homicide:** Rarely used— detectable smell 3. **Accidental poisoning:** Mostly in children when taken by mistake, chronic industrial exposure
Diagnosis 1. **Chemical test:**[5,11] $BaCl_2$ + Oxalic = white Barium Oxalate crystals 2. **Blood:** Low serum calcium level	1. **Chemical test:**[12,21] 1 ml of 10% Ferric Chloride + 10 ml urine containing Phenol → blue color substance 2. Urine test-carboluria 3. Typical odor	1. **Chemical test:** Acid + drop of phenophthalein → pink color + drop of 0.1 N NaOH → pink color disappears 2. Typical odor

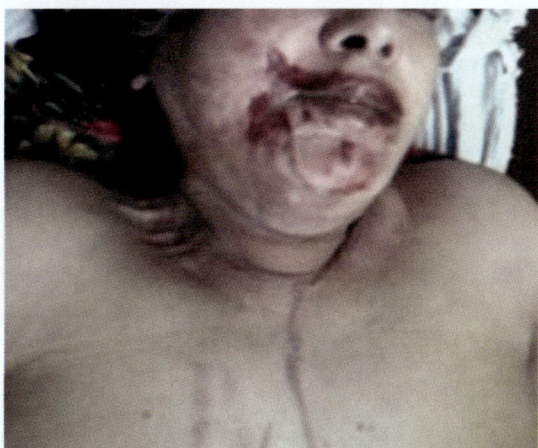

Fig. 4.8: Corrosion around mouth in carbolic acid

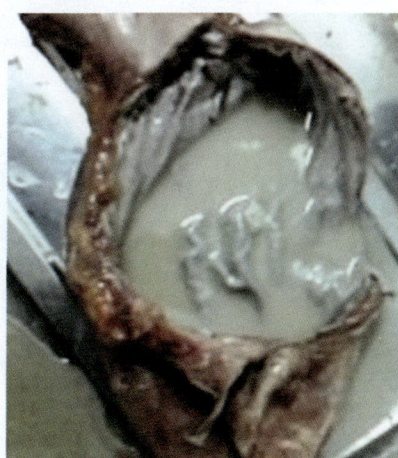

Fig. 4.9: Stomach in carbolic acid: Tough, thick and leathery bottle appearance

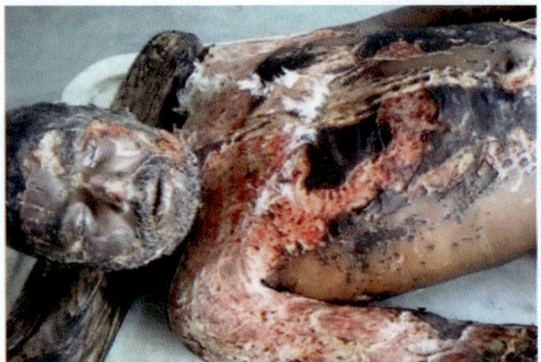

Fig. 4.10: Burns due to fall of sulfuric acid

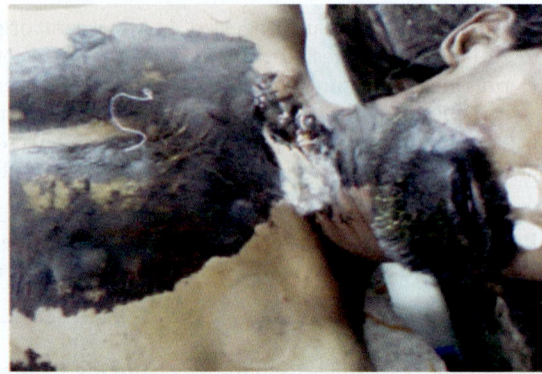

Fig. 4.11: Blackish corrosion of skin due to consumption of sulfuric acid

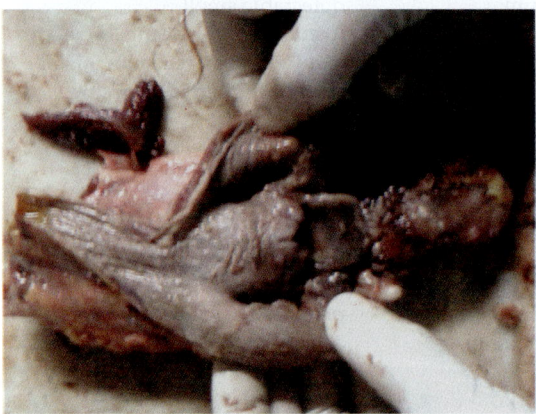

Fig. 4.12: Corrosion of tongue, epiglottis and esophagus due to consumption of hydrochloric acid

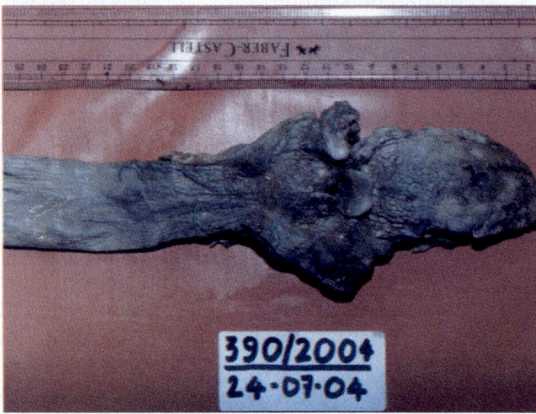

Fig. 4.13: Black corrosion of tongue, epiglottis and esophagus due to consumption of sulfuric acid

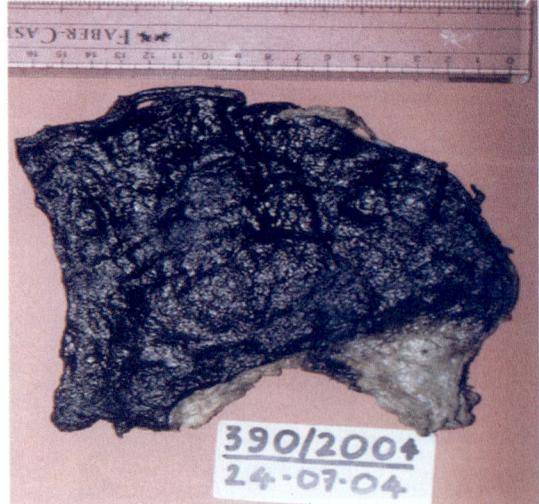

Fig. 4.14: Blackish corrosion of stomach in sulfuric acid poisoning

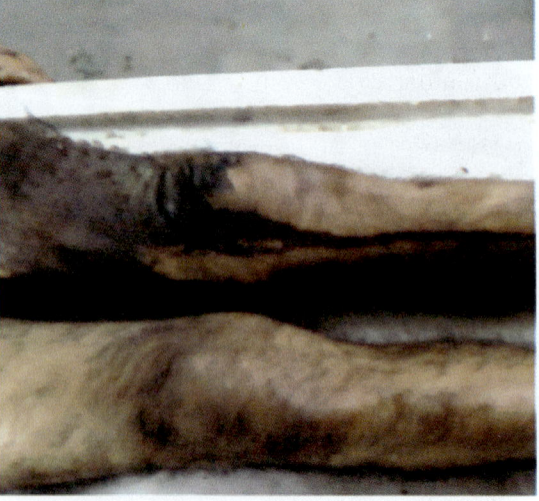

Fig. 4.15: Trickling mark of acid over legs

Table 4.1: Difference between oxalic acid and magnesium sulfate and zinc sulfate

Differences	Oxalic acid	Magnesium sulfate (epson salt)	Zinc sulfate
1. Taste	Sour	Bitter	Bitter
2. Reaction	Acidic	Neutral	Acidic
3. On heating	Vaporizes	–	–
4. With $NaCO_3$	Effervescences, no ppt.	White ppt.	White ppt.
5. Stain	Removed	–	–
6. Figure			

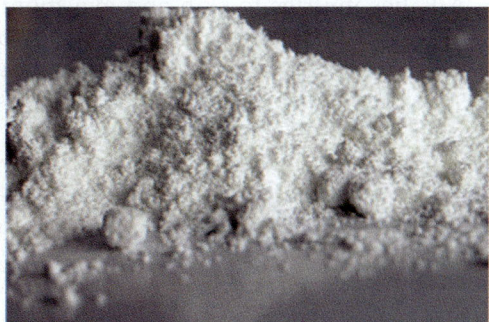

ALKALIES

Examples

1. **Hydroxide:** Ammonium, potassium, sodium, calcium.
2. **Carbonate:** Ammonium, potassium, sodium.

Source: Industries, laboratories.

Uses, fatal dose and period (Table 4.2)

Properties

- Most of these occur as white powder.
- Odorless
- Burning irritating taste
- Ammonium hydroxide is a liquid, having ammoniacal smell.
- Hygroscopic in nature[11]

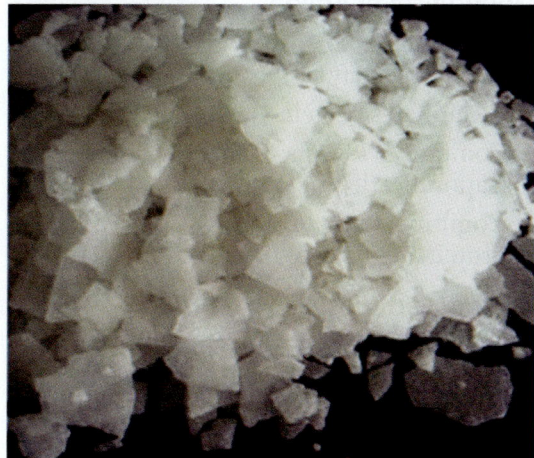

Fig. 4.17: Sodium hydroxide (caustic soda)

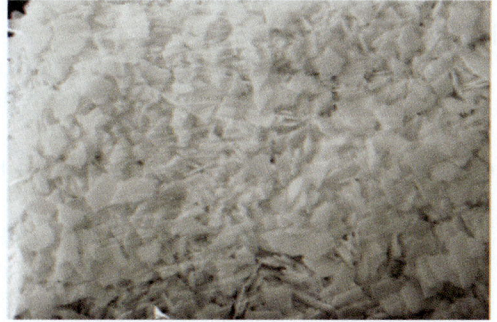

Fig. 4.16: Sodium carbonate (washing soda)

Fig. 4.18: Potassium hydroxide (caustic potash)

Table 4.2: Different alkalies and their uses

Alkalis	Chemical formula	Common name	Uses[12]	Fatal dose	Fatal period
Ammonium hydroxide	NH_4OH	Aqua ammonia	Cleaning agents, plastic/rubber manufacture	30 gm	24 hours
Sodium hydroxide	$NaOH$	Caustic soda	Drain cleaner, oven cleaner	5 gm	24 hours
Potassium hydroxide	KOH	Caustic potash	Drain cleaner, hearing aid batteries	5 gm	24 hours
Calcium hydroxide	$Ca(OH)_2$	Slaked lime	White washing	–	–
Ammonium carbonate	$(NH_4)_2CO_3$	Baker's ammonia	Baking powder, fire extinguisher	30 gm	24 hours
Sodium carbonate	Na_2CO_3	Washing soda	Household cleaning agent, detergent	30 gm	24 hours
Potassium carbonate	K_2CO_3	Pearl ash	To make soap, in fire extinguishers	15 gm	24 hours

Lye: It is a mixture of caustic soda and washing soda, used for washing purpose[4]

Mechanism of Action

Locally: Act as corrosives. They dissolve the protein and saponify fats, hence cause deeper burns.

- Precipitates protein
- Combine with fats to form alkaline soaps (saponification of fats)
- Combine with protein to form alkaline proteinates (causes **liquefaction** necrosis).[5]

Clinical Features

a. Intense burning pain in mouth and throat and abdomen with **acrid, caustic and soapy taste,** difficulty in speech and deglutition, dyspnea, vomiting, thirst, excessive salivation with blood and mucous, hoarseness of voice, diarrhea, suppression of urine and dehydration followed by shock.

b. The vomitus is **strongly alkaline** mixed with altered blood (brown or black due to hematin), mucous and mucous shreds. Stool is mixed with blood and mucus.

c. There is erosion of mucosa from lips to stomach, reddish brown color.

  There is also erosion of skin **(greyish, soapy)** necrotic area[5,12] along line of trickling of alkalies from angle of the mouth.

d. Perforation may occur

e. With ammonia vapors—congestion and watering of eyes, sneezing, coughing and choking. There may be edema glottis, pneumonia and death.

Treatment

1. Emetics and gastric lavage are contraindicated (perforation of stomach).
2. Drinking of plenty of plain water.
3. Weak vegetable acids like 3–5% acetic acid (vinegar), citric acid (lime/orange juice), 0.5% HCl
4. Demulcent drinks like milk, egg albumin, vegetable oil, ghee, butter, soap solution, etc.
5. Supportive treatment similar to acid burns.
6. Keep airway patent in ammonia inhalation
7. Antibiotic to prevent infection.
8. Alkalies injuries to skin and eye should be washed with water or saline for 20–30 minutes. Topical antibiotics and steroids may be helpful.[12]

Cause of Death

Shock, perforation, peritonitis and laryngeal spasm, infection, stomach, esophageal stricture.

PM Findings

1. Gross corrosion of skin with soapy, greyish discoloration.

2. Corrosion of mucous membrane of mouth, tongue and lips with brownish discoloration present.
3. Stomach
   Wall: Soft, swollen
   MM: Desquamated, ulcerated, hemorrhagic, brownish (alkali hematin)
   Contents: Alkaline, altered blood, mucous, epithelium shreds
4. Gastric perforation may lead to peritonitis
5. Signs of repair with scarring present in late deaths.

Medicolegal Aspects

Poisoning by alkali is rare.

1. **Suicide:** Rare.
2. **Homicide:** Rare.
3. **Accidental poisoning:** Sometimes may occur due to mistaken for medicine, by children, or due to ingestion while pipetting the fluid usually in laboratory.
4. **Vitriolage:** They are commonly used for throwing on body, usually caustic soda.

Chemical Test[11]

Hydroxides + $AgNO_3 \rightarrow$ yellow precipitates
Carbonates + $HCl \rightarrow$ white precipitates

IMPORTANT QUESTIONS

1. **Classify corrosives with examples. Describe clinical manifestation, treatment and medicolegal significance of poisoning with anyone inorganic strong acid. Add a note on carboluria.**

2. **Describe vitriolage with its medicolegal importance. Describe clinical features, treatment, postmortem findings and medicolegal aspect in death due to carbolic acid poisoning.**

3. **Enumerate examples of organic corrosives. Describe clinical features, treatment, postmortem findings and medicolegal aspect in death due to oxalic acid corrosion.**

4. **Enumerate different alkalies. Describe clinical features, treatment, autopsy findings, medicolegal significance in alkalies corrosion. Add a note on its chemical test.**

SPECIFIC LEARNING OBJECTIVES

After reading this chapter, the reader should be able to:

- **Classify corrosives with examples and their actions**
- **Enlist various uses of different acids/ alkalies**
- **Describe clinical features, treatment, postmortem findings and medicolegal aspects in HCl/H_2SO_4/HNO_3 poisoning**
- **Explain clinical features, treatment, post-mortem findings and medicolegal aspects in carbolic/oxalic/acetic acid poisoning**
- **Define vitriolage and explain its features, treatment and medicolegal aspect**
- **Enumerate different chemical tests for strong acids/alkalies**
- **Explain clinical features, treatment, post-mortem findings and medicolegal aspects in alkalies poisoning**
- **Delineate the difference between acid and alkali poisoning with respect to clinical features and treatment**

References

1. Sulfuric acid, concentrated (>51% and < 100%). Source: ILO-ICSC.
   http://www.ilo.org/dyn/icsc/showcard. display? p_version=2&p_card_id=0362
   Description: International Chemical Safety Cards (ICSC) are data sheets intended to provide essential safety and health information on chemicals in a clear and concise way. © ILO and WHO 2017
2. Sulfuric acids in: PubChem CID: 1118. https:// pubchem.ncbi.nlm.nih.gov/compound/sulfuric_ acid#section=Top. Assessed on 18-11-2018.
3. Bardale R. Principles of Forensic Medicine and Toxicology. 1st edn, Jaypee Brothers Medical Publishers (P) Ltd: New Delhi. 2011: 437–44.
4. Dikshit PC. Textbook of Forensic Medicine and Toxicology. 2nd edn, PEEPEE Publisher and Distributors (P) Ltd. New Delhi. 2014: 474–81.
5. Reddy KSN, Murthy OP. The Essential of Forensic Medicine and Toxicology. 32nd edn, Om Sai Graphics: Hyderabad. 2013: 503–9.

6. Nitric acid in PubChem CID: 944 https://pubchem.ncbi.nlm.nih.gov/compound/nitric_acid#section=Top

7. Nitric acid (>70% in water). Source: ILO-ICSC http://www.ilo.org/dyn/icsc/showcard.display?p_version=2&p_card_id=0183 Description: International Chemical Safety Cards (ICSC) are data sheets intended to provide essential safety and health information on chemicals in a clear and concise way. © ILO and WHO 2017.

8. O'Neil, MJ (ed.). The Merck Index—An Encyclopedia of Chemicals, Drugs, and Biologicals. Whitehouse Station, NJ: Merck and Co., Inc., 2006., p. 1138.

9. Hydrochloric Acid In: PubChem CID: 313. https://pubchem.ncbi.nlm.nih.gov/compound/hydrochloric_acid#section=Physical-Description

10. Hydrogen chloride. Source: ILO-ICSC. http://www.ilo.org/dyn/icsc/showcard.display?p_version=2&p_card_id=0163.

    Description: International Chemical Safety Cards (ICSC) are data sheets intended to provide essential safety and health information on chemicals in a clear and concise way. © ILO and WHO 2017.

11. Nandy A. Principles of Forensic Medicine. New Central Book Agency (P) Ltd: Calcutta, 2nd edn Reprint, 2004: 455–66.

12. Pillay VV. Textbook of Forensic Medicine and Toxicology. Paras Medical Publisher: Hyderabad, 17th edn, 2016: 497–520.

13. Claydon SM. An Acid Bath Murder. Acta Medicinæ Legalis Vol. XLIV 1994 pp 231–3.

14. Modi NJ. Examination of mutilated bodies or fragments. In: Modi's Textbook of Medical Jurisprudence and Toxicology. NM Tripathi Private Ltd: Bombay. 20th edn, 1977: 78–9.

15. Singhal SK. Singhal's Toxicology at a glance. 9th edn, National book depot: Mumbai. 41–9.

16. Qualitative analysis test for identifying organic functional groups of homologous series of molecules identification—for anions identifying negative ions hydroxide (alkalis) identification. http://www.docbrown.info/page13/ChemicalTests/ChemicalTestsa.htm#Sulphate.

17. Criminal Law Amendment Act, 2013.

18. Reddi PR. Section 320 IPC. In: Criminal major Acts. 28th edn, Hyderabad: Asia Law House. 2018: 156.

19. Rentoul Edgar, Smith Hamilton. Toxic Hazards. In: Glaister's Medical Jurisprudence and Toxicology. 13th edn, 1973. Churchill Livingstone: Edinburgh. 517–709.

20. Oxalic Acid In: PubChem CID: 971. https://pubchem.ncbi.nlm.nih.gov/compound/oxalic_acid#section=Color

21. Phenol in: PubChem CID: 996. https://pubchem.ncbi.nlm.nih.gov/compound/phenol#section=Physical-Description

22. Acetic Acid In PubChem CID: 176. https://pubchem.ncbi.nlm.nih.gov/compound/acetic_acid#section=Boiling-Point

23. Jesus JE, Landry A. Images in clinical medicine. Chvostek's and Trousseau's signs. The New England Journal of Medicine. 2012; 367 (11): e15. doi:10.1056/NEJMicm1110569. PMID 22970971.

24. Kumar, Abbas, Fausto. *Pathologic Basis of Disease, 7th edition.* Philadelphia: Elsevier-Saunders, 2005. 1188.

25. Barclay PJ. Phenols. In: Viccellio P (ed). Handbook of Medical Toxicology. 1st edn, 1993. Little, Brown and Company: Boston. 264–70.

Mechanical Irritants

Mechanical irritants are the substances which causes irritation of the GIT at the site of contact. As such they are not poisons and do not cause any toxic effect. Glass powder, hair and fiber, diamond powder and metallic chips/pins are the examples of mechanical irritants (Figs 5.1 to 5.6).

MECHANICAL IRRITANTS

1. *Glass powder/broken glass pieces*

    Bigger pieces can cause injury and hemorrhage in GIT. But smaller pieces fortunately do not get adhered to the wall of GIT and rather pass out the whole length of the tract by peristaltic movement[1]

    Medicolegal aspects

    a. **Accidental:** Usually with jam, jelly, etc. contaminated with broken piece of their container. It also occurs to showmen while performing their show and may face problem

    b. **Homicidal:** May be used, where it is mixed with food/drink

    c. **Cattle poisoning:** Occasionally used.[2]

2. *Hair and fibers*

    They may stick on the wall of stomach and intestine and remains undigested in the stomach. The hair ball may cause irritation (inflammation and pain) and lead to ulceration, GIT bleeding, perforation and obstruction.[3] This collection of mass of hair in the stomach is called Trichobezoar. (Phytobezoar is due to collection of vegetable fibers in the stomach, particularly in patients who have gastric stasis.)[4]

    Medicolegal aspects:

    a. It is almost exclusively found in female psychiatric patients, often young due to ingestion of hair.[4]

    b. **Homicidal:** Very rare, where it is mixed with food

3. *Diamond dust or powder*

    It is really harmful due to the presence of minute spike on the surface of the diamond powder. These spikes get stuck and impregnated the wall of intestine and cause perforation, hemorrhage, inflammation and peritonitis.

    Medicolegal aspects

    a. **Accidental:** Poisoning may occur due to chronic exposure to diamond cutters

    b. **Homicidal:** Used in ancient period by slow poisoning the king

    c. **Suicidal:** Rarely used

4. *Metallic chips/nails and pins*

    Minute piece do not pose any problem but bigger piece may cause injury, hemorrhage and perforation of GIT. But the sharpness of the corner of metal piece is reduced due to the action of digestive enzymes.[1]

    Medicolegal aspect

    Accidental: Mostly to children and also to magician (showmen) while performing their show

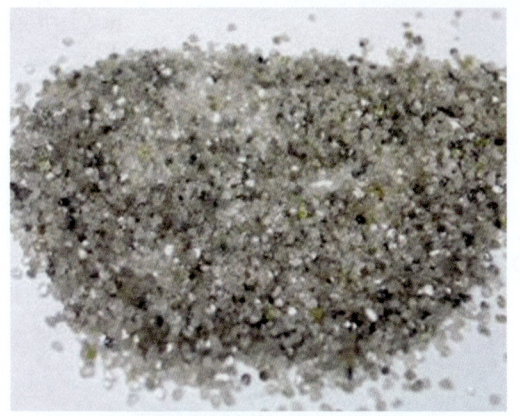

Fig. 5.1: Diamond powder

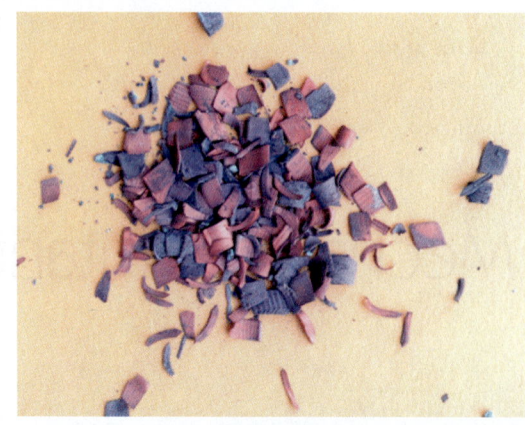

Fig. 5.2: Metallic chips

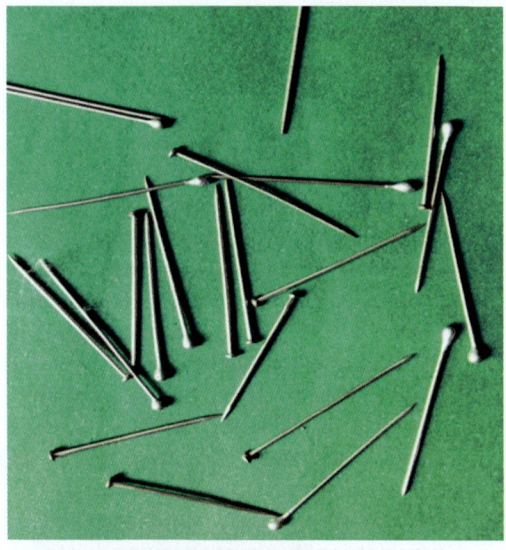

Fig. 5.3: Nails/pins

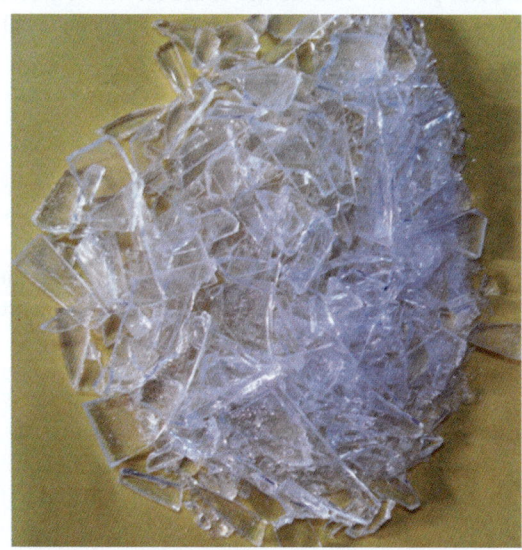

Fig. 5.4: Glass pieces

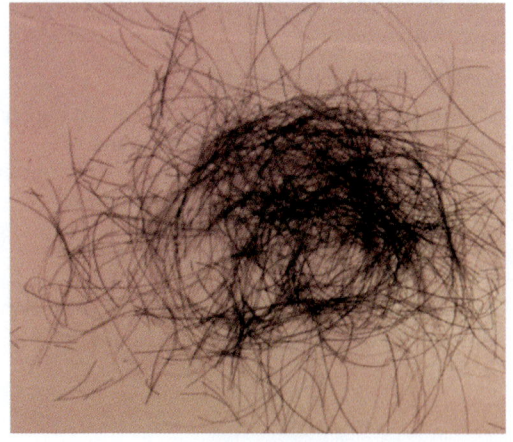

Fig. 5.5: Hair

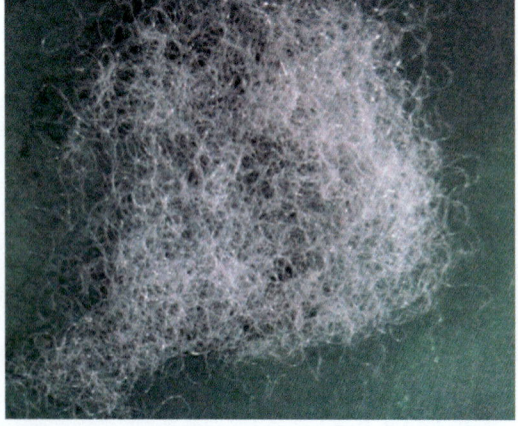

Fig. 5.6: Fibers

Treatment of mechanical irritant poisoning

1. Bulky foods like banana, mashed potato, boiled rice, etc.

2. Demulcents: Starch, milk, barley water, oil, ghee, butter, egg albumin, etc.

3. High fiber diet, Metamucil or lactulose.[5]

4. Removal of swallowed foreign body through upper gastrointestinal endoscopy is also safe.[5]

5. Surgical intervention if required.

IMPORTANT QUESTIONS

1. **What are mechanical irritants? Describe clinical manifestation, treatment in case of ingestion of anyone of mechanical irritant. Write its medicolegal aspect.**
2. **Enumerate mechanical irritants. Describe hair and fiber as mechanical irritant with its medicolegal significance. Write treatment in mechanical irritant.**
3. **Describe Trichobezoar and Phytobezoar with its medicolegal aspect.**

SPECIFIC LEARNING OBJECTIVES

After reading this chapter, the reader should be able to:

- **Enumerate different mechanical irritants with their examples and medicolegal aspects**
- **Recognize the treatment of mechanical irritant poisoning**

References

1. Nandy A. Principles of Forensic Medicine. New Central Book Agency (P) Ltd: Calcutta, 2nd edn Reprint, 2004:467–74.

2. Reddy KSN, Murthy OP. The Essential of Forensic Medicine and Toxicology. 32nd edn, Om Sai Graphics: Hyderabad. 2013: 521–3.

3. Levy NEJM, Levy Ronald M, Komanduri, Srinadh M. Trichobezoar. New England Journal of Medicine. 2007; 357 (21): e23. doi:10.1056/NEJMicm067796. PMID 18032760.

4. Williams NS, Bulstrode CJA, O'connel PR (editors). Bailey and Love's Short Practice of Surgery. 25th edn, Edward Arnold (publishers) Ltd: United Kingdom. 2008: 1077.

5. Al Shehri GY, Al Malki TA, Al Shehri MY, Ajao OG, Jastaniah SA, Haroon KS, Mahfouz MM, Al Shraim MM. Swallowed foreign body: Is interventional management always required? Saudi J Gastroenterol. 2000; 6:84–6.

Non-Metallic Inorganic Chemical Irritants

These are the inorganic chemicals which not only exert their toxic effect on contact but also cause systemic poisoning. Phosphorus and halogens like iodine, chlorine, bromine, and fluorine are the examples of non-metallic inorganic chemical irritant.

PHOSPHORUS

Properties and uses:[1, 2] It exists in 2 forms— white or yellow and brown or red (Figs 6.1 and 6.2). White phosphorus is highly toxic and poisonous, causes burns when contact with skin. Red or brown phosphorus is non-toxic, inert and is prepared when white phosphorus is heated at a temperature of 280°C, in the atmosphere of nitrogen (Table 6.1).

Table 6.1: Difference between white and red phosphorus

Differences[1]	Yellow phosphorus	Red phosphorus
Color	White, which on exposure to air becomes yellow	Red or brown
Appearance	Crystalline, translucent, soft, waxy, cylindrical	Amorphous, solid
Smell	Garlicky	Odorless
Taste	Garlicky	Tasteless
Luminosity	Luminous in dark	Non-luminous
Exposed to air	Ignites at 30°C and emits white fumes	Inert, non-fuming
Storage under water	Required	Not required
Toxicity	Highly toxic	Non-toxic
Uses	• It is used in chemicals, fertilizers, manufacture of phosphates and organophosphorus, rodenticide, insecticide. • It is also used in fireworks and gunpowder (smoke bombs and incendiary bullets), i.e. firearm ammunition.	• It is used on the sides of matchbox, where it is mixed with glass. • It is also used in matchstick head, where it is mixed with potassium chlorate [$KClO_3$] and antimony sulphide [AnS].

Initially, white phosphorus was being used for the manufacture of Lucifer Matches, but due to its toxicity, it was banned in European countries[2] after 1872 and present day safety match came into being after 1910.

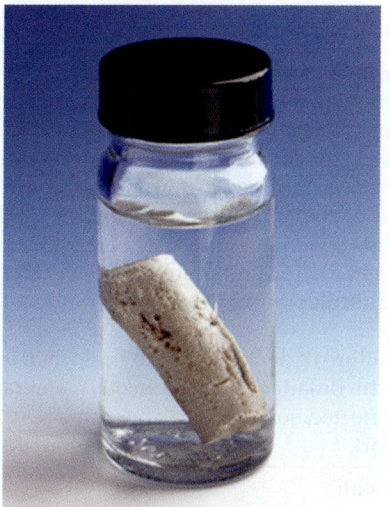

Fig. 6.1: White phosphorus

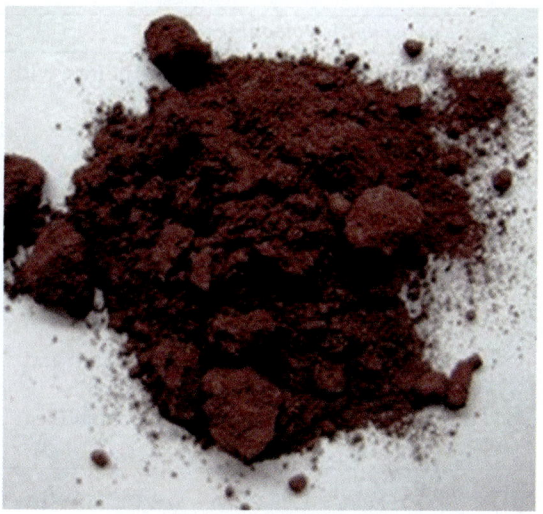

Fig. 6.2: Brown phosphorus

Mechanism of action

Locally, it destroys or burns the tissue (skin/ mucosa) on contact.

It is a **protoplasmic poison**[3], hampers tissue oxidation and causes fatty infiltration and **necrosis**[4, 5]

1. In acute poisoning: It causes hepatic dysfunction resembling ischemia known as **necrobiosis**, which results in disturbance in carbohydrate and fat metabolism

2. In chronic poisoning: There is excessive bone formation at the epiphyseal end (sequestration) with necrosis

3. Phosphine (PH_3) causes respiratory distress

| **Fatal dose:** 60–120 mg | **Fatal period:** Variable, 12 hours to 1 week |

Absorption, metabolism, excretion

Absorbed through mucous membrane, quickly when stomach is empty or contains fatty foods. After absorption, it is distributed in all the organs and metabolized to hypophosphate and excreted through urine. Small part is excreted as such through feces and respiration

Clinical manifestation depends upon

1. Dose
2. Period of exposure
3. Nature/type of poison
4. Routes: Contact/ingested/inhaled

I. Acute phosphorus poisoning	*II. Chronic phosphorus poisoning*
1. Local: Necrosis of epidermis of skin after 1–2 days of its contact. Burned when ignited and becomes ulcerated (very painful and heals slowly) **2. GIT:** Burning pain, vomiting, diarrhea, garlicky smell, intense thirst, salivation, and abdominal pain, followed by dehydration Vomitus and stool is dark, garlic smell, luminescence **3. CNS:** Headache, insomnia, vision impaired, deafness, restlessness, delirium, tremor, convulsion, coma	**It occurs due to** i. Exposure/inhalation of fumes in industries where phosphorous is used ii. Consumption of sea fish containing high quantity of phosphorus There is a **triad** of manifestation **1. GIT/general disturbances:** Nausea, vomiting, loss of weight/appetite, pain in abdomen, alternate constipation and diarrhea, irritability, fatigability, lack of interest/concentration, weakness

Acute phosphorus poisoning	Chronic phosphorus poisoning
4. **Liver:** Jaundice, pruritis, bleeding points, with hepatosplenomegaly 5. **Kidney:** Oliguria, albuminuria, hematuria, with sugar and bile salt present 6. Bleeding from gums, nose, in skin, and under surface of visceral organs 7. **Priapism**[6] (painful persistent erection of penis) 8. The patient usually presents with acute hepatic failure, coagulopathy, deranged liver function and acute renal failure.[7] 9. There is also decrease granulocyte count and bone marrow biopsy shows considerable decrease in cellular mass with degenerative changes.[8]	2. **Cirrhosis of liver** 3. **Phossy jaw:**[9] It is the necrosis of mandible[10] and sequestration (due to increased bone formation) and discharge of foul smelling pus by sinus formation. It is seen in 3% of industrial workers exposed to phosphorus. It is characterized by: • Pain/swelling/loosening of teeth with osteomyletis and necrosis of lower jaw with multiple sinuses discharging foul smelling pus. • Failure of dental socket to heal when teeth fall with inflammation of mucous membrane • Affected bone glowed greenish white color in dark[11]

Treatment:
1. Emesis
2. Stomach wash with **antidote:**
   0.1% $CuSO_4$ (forms copper phosphide)
   0.5% $KMnO_4$ (oxidizes phosphorus to phosphates)
3. **Demulcents are contraindicated** as they dissolve phosphorus
4. Non-fatty purgatives—$MgSO_4$
5. Restriction of fats, demulcents, morphine due to liver damage
6. **Dehydration or shock:** IV fluids and glucose
7. Vit K, B-complex and vit C—hypoprothrombinemia
8. For external lesion: Washing with warm water or 1% $CuSO_4$ solution, followed by application of bland and antibiotic ointment[12]
	Treatment:
	1. Prevent further exposure
	2. **Regular dental care:** Mouthwash with $NaHCO_3$
	3. Plenty of oral calcium
	4. Protect liver
	5. Prevent intercurrent infection
	6. Use of exhaust fans in working area
	7. Working area sprayed with turpentine oil vapor

PM findings: 1. Locally, skin-necrosis, ulcerated 2. Mucous membrane of mouth eroded 3. Gum swollen with bleeding points 4. GIT stomach wall—soft, swollen; MM—eroded, desquamated, hemorrhagic; Contents—dark, garlic smell, luminous 5. **Liver:** In early stage, it is **enlarged**, soft, friable, greasy due to **fatty degeneration (necrobiosis).** In late stage it is **shrunken**, leathery, gritty, dirty yellow due to **necrosis (acute yellow atrophy)** (Table 6.2) 6. Yellowish discoloration of skin and petechial hemorrhage 7. **Kidneys:** Tubular degeneration 8. Fatty degenerative changes in heart and kidney	**PM findings:** 1. Phossy jaw 2. Liver cirrhosis 3. Poor oral hygiene

Table 6.2: Liver findings in phosphorus poisoning and acute yellow atrophy

Phosphorus poisoning	Acute yellow atrophy
Usually enlarged, may be contracted later	Smaller, irregular
Marbled color	Bright yellow color
Soft, friable, greasy	Very soft and friable
Fatty degeneration	Necrosis of cell

Medicolegal aspects

1. **Suicide:** Not preferred (due to painful death)
2. **Homicidal:** Not used (due to its smell and taste)
3. **Accidental poisoning:** Children are attracted by luminosity, or when they chew the matchstick heads or side. It also occurs:
   - Due to industrial exposure.
   - Through consumption of rodenticidal agents containing phosphorus
4. **Abortifacient:** Used both locally or general administration
5. **Arson:**[4,13] It is used for causing outbreak of fire without being suspected. For this, phosphorus is wrapped in moist cow dung or moist rag and is kept/thrown on the roof of a house. When dung/rag becomes dry, the phosphorus gets ignited, producing fire on the thatched roof
6. To destroy undesired letters that has been posted
7. It is also used to create smoke screen in war field[14] so as to infiltrate in the enemy side.
8. **Greek fire/Fenian fire[15]:** In this, phosphorus dissolved in carbon disulfide may be thrown on other person or property *with malicious intention.* The phosphorus burst into flames when carbon disulfide evaporates.

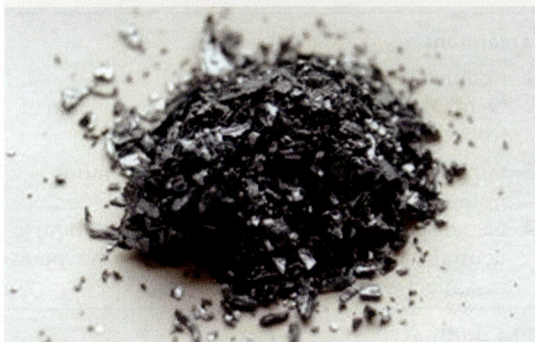

Fig. 6.3: Iodine crystals

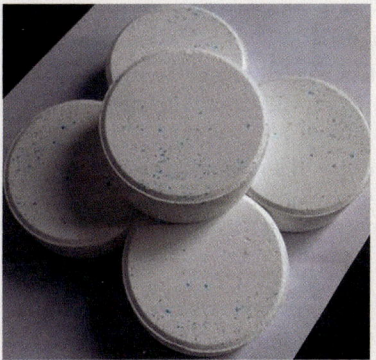

Fig. 6.4: Chlorine tablets

HALOGENS

IODINE POISONING	CHLORINE POISONING
Physical characteristics: Solid, bluish-black scaly shining crystals emitting violet vapors (Fig. 6.3).	Greenish yellow gas, pungent smell
Uses: 1. In radio-opaque dyes. 2. For dressing, e.g. tincture of iodine, Lugol's iodine or povidone iodine.	**Uses:** 1. Chlorine tablets (Fig. 6.4) for water purification in well and swimming pool 2. Bleaching agent 3. Sewage treatment[12]
Fatal dose: ~ 2 gm	**Fatal dose[12]:** >50–100 ppm
Fatal period: 12–24 hours	**Fatal period[14]:** 5 min to 12 hours
Actions: • It precipitates the protein • Irritation of GIT and RT	**Actions:** • It is extremely active oxidizing agent causing destruction of organic tissue.[12] • **Irritation to GIT and RT:** Combine with water to form HCl and hypochlorus acid.

Clinical features

There may be sudden death due to anaphylaxis in sensitive people or it may cause chronic poisoning (Iodism) due to exposure of its vapor over long period.

- Inhalation of vapor causes increased nasal and bronchial secretions, salivations, conjunctivitis, parotitis with cough and dyspnea.
- Burning pain in upper GIT with nausea, vomiting, abdominal pain, diarrhea.
- Vomitus/stool is bluish or violet with smell of iodine.
- Urine is scanty and reddish brown with albuminuria and painful micturation.[14]
- Cold calmy skin, fall of BP/respiration, weak pulse.
- Headache, giddiness, muscle cramp, delirium, collapse, shock.

Clinical features

- Inhalation of gas causes increased nasal and bronchial secretions, salivations, lacrimation with cough and dyspnea.
- It may also result in laryngeal edema, pulmonary edema.
- Nausea, vomiting, abdominal pain, diarrhea with increased BP and respiration rate.
- Vertigo, headache, ventricular ectopic beats and metabolic acidosis.[12]
- Chronic exposure may cause corrosion of teeth[12] anemia, loss of weight and appetite, bronchitis and emphysema[14]

Treatment

1. **Emetics:** Gastric lavage[14] with 5% sodium thiosulfate or with starch or egg albumin
2. **Demulcents**
3. **Antidote:**[14] 5% sodium thiosulphate 100–150 ml orally to reduce free iodine to nontoxic iodides.
4. **Supportive:** For shock, dehydration, low BP, glottic edema.

Treatment

1. Removal of patient to fresh air
2. O_2 inhalation + artificial respiration + suction of frothy fluid form air passage.[14]
3. Supportive treatment for shock, dehydration, pulmonary edema, acidosis.
4. Nebulised sodium bicarbonate (3.75% solution) to neutralized the acid formed when chlorine comes in contact with water in air passage.[12]

PM findings

i. **Mucosa of upper GIT:** Inflamed.
ii. Stomach contents are blue and emit smell of iodine.
iii. Degeneration of heart, liver and kidney.

PM findings

RT: Massive pulmonary edema with denudation of epithelium. Peculiar odor of chlorine from brain ventricle

All organs are congested

Medicolegal aspects

1. **Suicide:** Rare.
2. **Homicide:** Rare.
3. **Accidental poisoning:** When mistaken with $KMnO_4$, tincture iodine.
4. **Vitriolage:** It is used for vitriolage.

Medicolegal aspects

1. **Suicide:** Not possible
2. **Homicide:** Rare
3. **Accidental:** Commonly due to domestic or industrial exposure.
4. It is used in World War I as chemical warfare agent.

IMPORTANT QUESTIONS

1. Write difference between yellow and red phosphorus. Add a note on phossy jaw.
2. Describe mechanism of action, clinical features, treatment, postmortem findings and medicolegal aspect in acute phosphorus poisoning.
3. Enumerate non-metallic chemical irritant. Write in brief about clinical findings in chronic phosphorus poisoning.
4. Describe clinical manifestations, treatment and medicolegal aspect in iodine or chlorine poisoning. Add a note on different uses of iodine and chlorine.

SPECIFIC LEARNING OBJECTIVES

After reading this chapter, the reader should be able to:

- **Enumerate difference between white and red phosphorus**
- **Understand the mechanism of action of phosphorus**
- **Explain clinical manifestations, treatment and postmortem findings in acute phosphorus poisoning**
- **Explain clinical manifestations, treatment and postmortem findings in chronic phosphorus poisoning**
- **Understand the basis of phossy jaw with medicolegal aspect of phosphorus poisoning**
- **Enlist the uses of iodine and chlorine**
- **Describe clinical manifestation, treatment, postmortem findings and medicolegal aspect in iodine/chlorine poisoning**

References

1. Pubchem: Phosphorus. In:PubChem CID: 5462309. https://pubchem.ncbi.nlm.nih.gov/compound/5462309#section=Chemical-and-Physical-Properties

2. Crass MF, Jr.. "A history of the match industry. Part 9" (PDF). Journal of Chemical Education. 1941; 18 (9): 428–31.

3. Tenenbein M. Position statement: Whole bowel irrigation. American Academy of Clinical Toxicology; European Association of Poisons Centres and Clinical Toxicologists. J Toxicol Clin Toxicol.1997;35:753–62. [PubMed]

4. Nandy A. Principles of Forensic Medicine. New Central Book Agency (P) Ltd: Calcutta, 2nd edn Reprint, 2004: 467–74.

5. Bardale R. Principles of Forensic Medicine and Toxicology. 1st edn, Jaypee Brothers Medical Publishers (P) Ltd: New Delhi. 2011: 445–8.

6. Singhal SK. Singhal's Toxicology at a glance. 9th edn, National book depot: Mumbai.2016: 50–1.

7. Mauskar A, Mehta K, Nagotkar L, Shanbag P. Acute hepatic failure due to yellow phosphorus ingestion. Indian J Pharmacol. 2011 May-Jun; 43(3): 355–6. doi: [10.4103/0253-7613.81500]

8. Tafur A J, Zapatier J A, Idrovo L A, Oliveros J W, Garces JC. Bone marrow toxicity after yellow phosphorus ingestion. Emerg Med J. 2004; 21: 259–60. doi: 10/1136/emj.2003.007880

9. Hughes J P, Baron R, Buckland D H, Cooke M A, Craig J D, Duffield D P, Grosart A W, Parkes PW, Porter A. Phosphorus Necrosis of the Jaw: A Present-Day Study: With Clinical and Biochemical Studies. British Journal of Industrial Medicine. 1962; 19 (2): 83–99.

10. Marx Robert E. "Uncovering the Cause of "Phossy Jaw" Circa 1858 to 1906: Oral and Maxillofacial Surgery Closed Case Files—case Closed". Journal of Oral and Maxillofacial Surgery. 2008 66 (11): 2356–63. doi:10.1016/j.joms. 2007.11.006. PMID 18940506.

11. Workshops of Horror. New Zealand Department of Labour. Archived from the original on 20 June 2007. https://web.archive.org/web/20070620223046/http://www.osh.govt.nz/kidz/gore/jphossy.shtml

12. Pillay VV. Textbook of Forensic Medicine and Toxicology. Paras Medical Publisher: Hyderabad, 17th edn, 2016: 511–27.

13. Reddy KSN, Murthy OP. The Essential of Forensic Medicine and Toxicology. 32nd edn, Om Sai Graphics: Hyderabad. 2013: 521–3.

14. Dikshit PC. Textbook of Forensic Medicine and Toxicology. 2nd edn, PEEPEE Publisher and Distributors (P) Ltd. New Delhi. 2014: 522–7.

15. Naill W, Whelehan Niall (9 August 2012). The Dynamiters: Irish Nationalism and Political Violence in the Wider World, 1867–1900. Cambridge University Press. p. 58. ISBN 9781139560979. Retrieved 3 March 2018.

Irritants: Inorganic Metallic Poison

These are the inorganic metallic compounds causing local irritation to the GIT. It includes toxic compounds of the metals. From the forensic point of view, important inorganic metallic poisons include compounds of arsenic, lead, copper and mercury. Pure metallic form (Figs 7.1 to 7.4) of arsenic, mercury and copper is not poisonous and not absorbed through GIT, but their compounds (Tables 7.1 and 7.2) are toxic.

Table 7.1: Toxic compounds of arsenic and lead

Arsenic	*Lead*
1. **Arsenic trioxide** (*sankhya, somalkhar*): White amorphous powder, colorless, odorless, tasteless, sparingly soluble in water	1. **Lead acetate, lead sub-acetate**—white crystalline salt, sweet astringent taste (Fig. 7.2)
2. **Arsenic hydride** (*Arsine*) (AsH$_3$): Highly toxic gas, burns with blue flame, garlic smell	2. **Lead carbonate**—white fine dusty powder used in paints
3. **Copper arsenite** (*Scheele's green*) and **copper acetoarsenite** (*Paris green*): Greenish color powder	3. **Lead tetraoxide** (*vermillion, sindoor, shondoor*)—scarlet/safron color crystalline powder (used on Hanuman idol)
4. **Arsenic trisulfide** (*orpiment, multani mitti, harital*)—bright yellow solid	4. **Lead sulfide** (*surma, kajal*)—black powder
5. **Arsenic bisulfide** (*Realgur*)—brick red powder	5. **Lead monoxide**—brick red
6. **Arsenic trichloride:** Highly toxic liquid having pungent smell and irritant to eyes	6. **Tetraethyl lead** (added to petrol)
	7. **Other:** Lead chloride, lead nitrate, lead chromate, lead bromide, lead iodide

Table 7.2: Toxic compounds of mercury and copper

Mercury	*Copper*
1. **Mercuric chloride** (corrosive action)—colorless crystalline powder, odorless, burning metallic taste, highly toxic. Used in medicines, laboratories, industries, and as preservatives. *Mercurous chloride (ras kapoor) is non-toxic, used as purgatives.*	1. **Copper sulfate** (CuSO$_4$—blue vitriol, blue stone)—greenish blue crystals/powder, odorless, metallic taste, soluble in gastric juice, absorbed in water
2. Mercuric **cyanide**—used in medicine	2. Copper **subacetate** (verdegris)
3. Mercuric **sulfide**—[vermillion, sindoor, kumkum, kunku]—scarlet red crystalline powder	3. Copper **chloride**—white crystals
4. Mercuric **sulphate**—white crystalline powder	4. Copper **carbonate**—white dusty powder
5. **Phenyl mercuric acetate**—used as fungicidal agent and preservation of seeds	

Other: Mercuric nitrate, mercurous nitrate, mercuric cyanide, mercury fulminate, mercury thiocyanate and mercurochrome

Mercury exists in three forms:[1,2]
1. Elemental mercury/vapor
2. Inorganic mercury (mercuric and mercurous salts)
3. Organic mercury (ethyl/methyl mercury, mercurochrome).

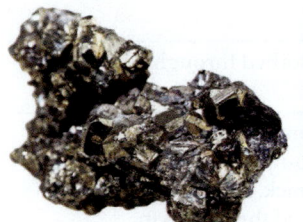

Fig. 7.1: Arsenic

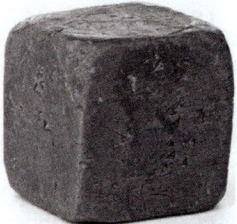

Fig. 7.2: Lead

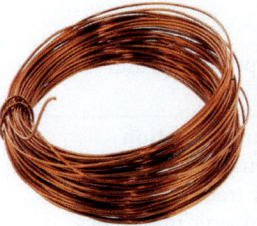

Fig. 7.3: Copper

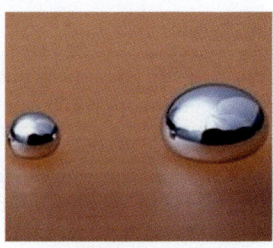

Fig 7.4: Mercury

Table 7.3: Fatal dose and fatal period of metallic poison

Metals	Fatal dose	Fatal period
Arsenic	White arsenic = 200 mg	24 hrs to 7 days
Lead	Lead acetate = 20 gm, Lead carbonate = 30 gm	24 hrs to 7 days
Mercury	Mercuric chloride = 400–500 mg	Few hrs to 3–7 days
Copper	Copper subacetate = 15 gm, Copper sulphate = 30 gm	Few hrs to 3–7 days

Table 7.4: Source and uses of metallic irritant poison

Arsenic	Lead	Mercury	Copper
Source: Industrial, domestic, commercial, agricultural	**Source:** Industrial, commercial, domestic	**Source:** Industrial, commercial, domestic	**Source:** Industrial, commercial, domestic, agricultural
Arsenic is also found in *soil and air,*[3] *drinking water,*[4] *sea fish and crustaceans*[5]			
Uses: • Depilatory/cosmetic agents • Paints, calico printing, Fruit spray • Colouring agents—toys • Insecticidal, weed killer, rodenticide • In fly paper/powder • In medicine—as Fowler's solution[6] in intermittent fever, general tonic, syphilis.	**Uses:** • Water pipes • Batteries • Paints, hair dye • Vermillion • Petrol • Glass blowing on the surface of ceremic articles • Pencil lead contains a mixture of graphite and clay, and not lead • Projectiles—bullet • Shielding from radiation	**Uses:** • As preservatives Vermillion • BP apparatus • Thermometer • Medicine, antiseptic and disinfectant • **Snake tablet** (Mercury Thiocyanate) in Diwali • **Amalgam (dental filling)** • *Embalming* • *Fingerprint powder*	**Uses:** Copper sulphate • Emetic agent • Antidote for phosphorous • Paints • Laboratory—test for fragility of RBC • Coloring agents—used to impart colour to peas, vegetable, stone • It is used as fungicide, and pesticide • Household appliances—copper utensils • *Copper IU devices*

Mechanism of action of metallic irritant[7]

1. Inhibits sulphydryl group of enzymes, thereby interfering with cell metabolism and oxidation.
2. Interfere with mitochondrial oxidative phosphorylation.

ARSENIC	LEAD
Pure metallic arsenic is not poisonous and not absorbed through GIT.	Pure metallic lead is absorbed through GIT.

Absorption, distribution, and excretion	**Absorption, distribution, and excretion**
• Absorbed through mucous membrane of GIT, intact skin, or respiratory tract • The absorbed inorganic arsenic undergoes methylation mainly in liver to monomethylarsonic acid and dimethylarsinic acid, which are excreted in urine. [6] • Deposited in liver, kidneys, bones, hair, nails. • Excreted through urine, hair and nail. Small amount is also eliminated through feces, saliva, bronchial secretions, and milk	• Usually absorbed through GIT. Lead dust/fumes through respiratory track. Lead tetraoxide/ tetraethyl lead aboerbed through skin. • After absorption, it is stored in bones as phosphate and carbonate.[8] • Lead is a cumulative poison and deposited in bones, liver and kidneys. • It is excreted through urine, bile and nails

ACUTE ARSENIC POISONING	ACUTE LEAD POISONING

Clinical features
• Burning sensation, metallic taste, difficulty in speech and swallowing, excessive salivation, thirst with abdominal pain, vomiting, diarrhea with painful defecation and micturition. This is followed by dehydration, muscle cramps, convulsion, collapse, and coma
  – Vomiting initially contains stomach contents mixed with blood and finally mucoid, watery with streaks of blood
  – Diarrhea initially contains foul smelling fecal matter mixed with blood[5] and finally colorless, odorless mucoid and watery **like rice-water stool of cholera** (due to rupture of vesicles formed under the mucosa)[9]
• Scanty urine containing blood and albumin
• There is jaundice, anemia, hepatomegaly.
• **Hematological abnormalities:**[5] Hemoglobinuria, intravascular coagulation, bone marrow depression, severe pancytopenia, and normocytic normochromic anemia and basophilic stippling.
	Clinical features
	• Burning sensation, metallic taste, difficulty in speech and swallowing, excessive salivation, thirst with abdominal pain, vomiting, diarrhea with painful defecation and micturition. This is followed by dehydration, muscle cramps, convulsion, collapse, and coma
	  – Vomiting—curdy white (lead chloride)
	  – Diarrhea—black (lead sulfide)
	• Scanty urine containing lead, albumin, copro-porphyrin 3 (**red colored urine**).[9]
	• **CNS manifestations:** Headache, insomnia, drowsiness, dizziness, muscular cramps, tremor, convulsions, collapse, coma, rarely paralysis

Treatment	**Treatment**
1. **Emesis** 2. **Stomach wash:**[6] With freshly prepared ferric oxide (45 ml $FeCl_2$ + 15 gm MgO)—filtering the ppt 3. **Demulcent** 4. **Purgatives:** Magnesium sulfate 5. **Antidotes:** BAL[10]/ferric oxide[6] 6. **Supportive:** For shock/dehydration Liver protection—vitamin/amino acids Renal failure—dialysis Blood transfusion, if required	1. **Emesis** 2. **Stomach wash:**[6] With magnesium/sodium sulfate (forms insoluble lead sulfate) 3. **Demulcent** 4. **Purgative:** Mg/Na sulfate 5. **Antidotes:** Calcium edetate/BAL or penicillamine or Mg/Na sulphate 6. **Supportive** Shock/dehydration—IV fluids Liver protection—vitamins D, and C/Thiamine Renal failure—dialysis Pain in abdomen—morphine Abdominal colic—calcium gluconate and atropine

Antidote

1. **Chemical:**[6, 8] Freshly prepared **ferric oxide** precipitate (prepared by adding 45 ml ferric chloride and 15 gm magnesium oxide then filtering the precipitate). Dose is 15 gm ppt in glass of water. It forms ferric arsenite—which is a harmless salt
2. **Pharmacological:**[10] BAL, dimercaptosuccinic acid (It forms BAL—arsenic complex that is excreted out by the kidney). Dimercaprol is considerably more toxic than Succimer or Penicillamine

Antidote

1. **Chemical:** Sodium sulfate and magnesium sulfate
2. **Pharmacological**[10]**: Calcium edetate** CaNa$_2$ EDTA (Calcium disodium ethylene diamine tetra acetic acid), it excretes lead from circulation and bones. *For dose: Refer to Chapter 1: Chelating agents* BAL or penicillamine are also used.

PM findings

- MM of mouth/esophagus—inflamed.
- **Stomach: Red-velvety appearance**[11]
  Wall—soft, swollen
  MM—inflamed, hemorrhagic, and reddened
  Contents—blood with mucous shreds present arsenic powder or watery fluid mucoid and blood streaks
- Surrounding viscera—soft, inflamed, congested.
- Visceral organs congested
- **Large intestine:** Contains mucoid, watery material
- Heart—subendocardial hemorrhage
- Hemorrhages on larynx, trachea, lungs and abdominal organs
- Usually, it retards decomposition.

PM findings

- MM of mouth—inflamed
- **Stomach**
  Wall—soft, swollen
  MM—congested, greyish, sometimes eroded
  Contents—curdy white material
- Visceral organs congested
- **Large intestine:** Stools are black

In decomposed body, yellowish discoloration occurs in stomach and surrounding tissue due to the formation of arsenic sulphide in arsenic poisoning. [arsenic +H$_2$S = arsenic sulphide].

CHRONIC ARSENIC POISONING

It occurs due to:
1. Industrial or agricultural exposures.
2. Contaminated food or drinks.
3. Arsenical medicines
4. Consumption of repeated small doses.
5. Consumption of contaminated drinking water, particularly arsenic laced tube well water in early 1980s in West Bengal.[12]

CHRONIC LEAD POISONING (PLUMBISM, ALSO KNOWN AS SATURNISM):

It occurs due to:
1. Inhalation of dust/vapors in people working in factories/industries (e.g. paint industry, plumbing, glass—blowers, electric wire industries, batteries, toys, hair-dye and gasolene industries)[9]
2. Contaminated food and drinks with lead (stored/cooked in tins or lead vessels)[6]
3. Prolonged use of vermillion, dye and cosmetic containing lead
4. One who handled petrol

Clinical features:

Stage I: General loss of health and gastrointestinal disturbances

Irritability, fatigability, lack of interest and concentration, loss of weight and appetite, abdominal pain, alternate constipation and diarrhea, gums inflamed and tooth loosened

Clinical features [C-LEAD-P]:

C → Constipation, colicky pain
The colic is intermittent, spasmodic and relieved by pressure and is associated with constipation
L → Lead line (**Burtonian line**[6]—bluish discoloration over gingival surface of gums)

Stage II: Nasolacrimal and bronchial catarrhal changes

Inflammation of conjunctiva, with watering from eyes and nose, photophobia, hoarseness of voice, cough with expectoration. (Features as of common cold)

Ulceration of nasal mucosa

Stage III: Cutaneous/keratin involvement
  i. **Pigmentation of skin:** Rain-drop appearance—pin-point brownish pigmentation of the skin.
     Milk rose complexion—generalized brownish pigmentation due to vasodilatation
     Dark pigmentation with thickening of palm and soles
 ii. **Nails**—brittle, 'Mee's lines' present (transverse, white streak at growing part of nail)
iii. **Hair**—dry, alopecia, pigmented (yellow or brown)

Stage IV: Neurological involvement
Headache, irritability, fatigability, lack of interest and concentration

Tingling and numbness, tremor, cramps, muscle weakness and paralysis

Other manifestations
Liver damage—jaundice, pruritis
Kidney damage—albuminuria, hematuria, renal failure
Bone marrow aplasia and **basophilic stippling of RBC**

E → Encephalopathy: It leads to irritability, fatigability, lack of interest/concentration, delirium, convulsion, collapse, coma.

A → Alopecia, anemia with punctate basophilia. Anemia is due to:
  i. Impaired hemesynthesis.
 ii. Increase fragility of RBC due to loss of potassium due to increase cell permeability[8]
iii. Antithrombin effect of lead leads to defective clotting

There is also **basophilic stippling of RBC** due to condensation of iron containing RNA near mitochondria.[8] The RBC shows dark blue spots due to metabolic products of porphyrin.

Other features seen on peripheral smear examination are:
  a. Reticulocytosis
  b. Decreased platelets
  c. Increased monocytes
  d. Anisocytosis
  e. Poikilocytosis

D → Degenerative effect, lead deposited. Degenerative effect on:
  Reproductive system—leads to sterility.
  CVS in arteries—hypertension.
  Kidneys—chronic interstitial nephritis.
  Peripheral nerves—peripheral neuritis.
  Eye changes—retinal stippling and optic atrophy leading to blindness.

  Lead is deposited beyond the epiphysis of growing end of long bones[8] leading to abnormal development in children (**lead osteopathy**).

  P → Pallor (facial pallor due to vasospasm).

  P→ Palsy—due to degeneration of nerves and atrophy of muscles leads to tingling numbness, weakness, tremors, cramps, etc. and ultimately leads to wrist drop and foot drop due to paralysis of extensor muscles of wrist and foot

---

(**Blue line of gums** is also seen in mercury, copper, silver, iron, bismuth and thallium poisoning).

Treatment: Chronic arsenic poisoning
1. Prevention of exposure
2. BAL/penicillamine
3. Vitamin B complex
4. Supportive

Treatment: Chronic lead poisoning
1. Prevent further exposure
2. Antidote: Calcium versenate—1 gm/day slow IV drip or BAL/penicillamine
3. Potassium iodide (1–2 gm) and potassium citrate remove lead from bones and circulation respectively.[8]
4. **Supportive:** Magnesium sulfate—for constipation
   Atropine sulfate for severe colic
   $NaHCO_3$, vitamin D, calcium diet

PM findings (chronic arsenic poisoning)
1. Dehydration, jaundice, anemia
2. Degenerative changes in thoracic and abdominal organs and nerves
3. Bone marrow aplasia
4. **Keratin/cutaneous changes:** Skin pigmentation, Mee's line in nails, alopecia, bone marrow aplasia

PM findings (chronic lead poisoning)
1. Emaciated
2. Blue lining over gums
3. Alopecia
4. Evidence of anemia
5. Degenerative changes in liver, kidney, heart
6. Bone marrow aplasia

Laboratory investigation
Urine:[8] Arsenic level of >100 microgram/day is suggestive of poisoning. It becomes positive within 6 hrs of poisoning and continuous for about 2 wks.
Hair and nails:[5] Arsenic level of >1 mg/kg body weight indicates acute poisoning, while 0.1–0.5 mg/kg on a hair sample indicates chronic poisoning.

Blood: Basophilic stippling of RBC present

Laboratory investigation
Urine:[6] Presence of coproporphyrin level >0.15 mg/day
Blood:[8] Lead level of >50 microgram per dL.
X-ray shows higher density beyond epiphysis
Blood:[6,13] Basophilic stippling of RBC presents with elevated level of delta amino-laevulinic (ALA) acid in postmortem blood.

Interpretation of arsenic in exhumed body
In dead bodies recovered from graves, there is the possibility that either the arsenic from the body percolates to the soil or arsenic from the soil may imbibe the body. Hence, the presence of arsenic should be interpreted very carefully in exhumed body:
1. Arsenic absorbed during life usually consists of soluble salt forms.[8] The inorganic pentavalent forms of arsenic is absorbed at higher rate than bivalent forms.[14]
2. If arsenic has gone from the body to the soil, then not only the concentration of arsenic will be more in the body, the concentration in soil below the body will be more than the soil on both sides of the body and over the top of the body.

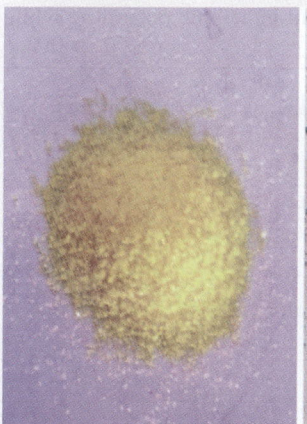
Arsenic trisulfide

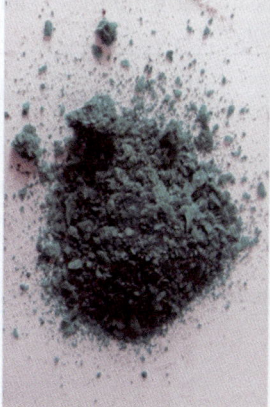
Copper arsenite

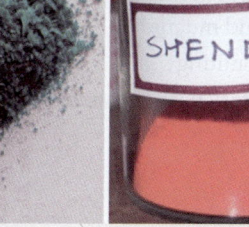
SHENDOOR

Lead tetraoxide

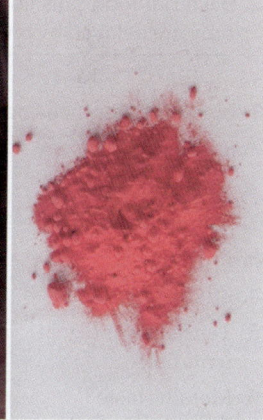
Lead monoxide

Medicolegal aspects:
1. Suicidal: Not preferred due to painful death.
2. Homicidal: Earlier it was the most popular and considered as ideal homicidal poison and signs and symptoms resemble that of cholera. But it has got great disadvantages as it is detected not only in decomposed body but also in the body ash[7,8] and there is also chemical test to detect the poison

Medicolegal aspects:
1. Suicide: Rare—long, painful
2. Homicide: Rare, detection in CA
3. Accidental: Due to chronic exposure, to children
4. Accidental chronic lead poisoning may also occur due to retained bullet in the body after firing.[15–17]
5. Abortifacient: Sometimes used to procure abortion
6. Cattle poison

3. **Accidental due to**
    i. Consumption of contaminated food and drinks,
    ii. Exposure while in agricultural field, or in industries
    iii. **Its abuses**[8]
4. Abortifacient for procuring criminal abortion
5. Cattle poison[18] and as stupefying poison

Preservation of viscera	Preservation of viscera
1. Routine viscera	1. Routine viscera
2. Additional viscera like hair, nails and ends of long bones are also preserved. A serial analysis of hair and nails gives an indication of arsenic toxicity.	2. Additional viscera like nails and ends of long bones are also preserved.

Abuses of arsenic:[8]

a. It is used as **love philter**—it increases the affection towards the giver. In ancient days, the wives used to administer arsenic to their husband to gain attraction of the husband in the wake of unhealthy competition amongst the wives
b. **Aphrodisiac purpose**—it gives a sense of well-being and is used to increase sexual desire
c. It is also used to **improve the dark** complexion
d. **Arsenophagists**[6]—are the person who takes arsenic daily. They can tolerate unbelievable amount of arsenic without much harm. It leads to tolerance and addiction

Differential diagnosis of arsenic poisoning

1. Cholera—the manifestation starts with diarrhea in cholera and vomiting in arsenic poisoning. (Table 7.5 for the differences). The stools are described as 'rice water' in cholera, and bloody rice water in acute arsenic poisoning due to presence of blood in GIT
2. Bacterial food poisoning—vomiting and diarrhoea occur within 15–30 min in arsenic poisoning while they are delayed by few hours in bacterial food poisoning.

Table 7.5: Differences between arsenic poisoning and cholera

Points	Arsenic poisoning	Cholera
1. Start with	Vomiting	Diarrhea
2. Vomitus contains	Blood and mucus	Mucus only, watery
3. Purging	After vomiting	Before vomiting
4. Stool	Rice watery with blood and mucus	Rice watery liquid
5. Tenesmus and anal irritation	Present	Absent
6. Metallic taste	Present	Absent
7. Motive	Present	Absent
8. Restricted to	Individual	Not restricted, affects many
9. Lab test	On CA, arsenic present	On hanging drop-darting motility of bacteria present

MERCURY (QUICK SILVER, PARA)	COPPER (TAMBA)
Pure metallic mercury is not poisonous as it is not absorbed through GIT. Mercury is a liquid metal, heavy, silvery and non-adhesive. Vapors of mercury are toxic and induce severe pneumonitis.[1]	Pure metallic copper is not absorbed through GIT and not poisonous[6]

Absorption, distribution, excretion
- Absorption through GIT. The vapors and salts are also absorbed through RT, vagina (in vaginal douche), and bladder.
- Distributed in liver, spleen, kidney, bone and brain (in phenyl mercuric acetate). Soluble forms get deposited in liver, spleen, kidney, intestines, heart, muscles and lungs.
- Excreted in urine, bile, feces and body secretions.

ACUTE MERCURY POISONING
Clinical features
- **Local:** Skin—corrosion.
- MM of mouth and tongue: Corroded and is greyish-white in color[6]
- Burning sensation, metallic taste, difficulty in speech and swallowing, excessive salivation, thirst with abdominal pain, vomiting, diarrhea with painful defecation and micturition. This is followed by dehydration, muscle cramps, convulsion, collapse, and coma
  - Vomiting contains mucous with altered blood and shreds of mucosa
  - Diarrhea is blood stained with necrosed mucus shreds of colon
- Scanty urine containing blood and albumin
- **General:** Headache, tremor, deafness, scotoma, loss of memory, loss of appetite, fatigue
- **Inhalation of mercury vapors:** Cough, dyspnea, salivation, stomatitis, gingivitis, conjunctivitis.

Treatment
1. **Emesis:** By lukewarm $NaHCO_3$ solution, Ipecacuanha
2. **Stomach wash:**[6] 5–10% sodium formaldehyde sulfoxylate
3. **Demulcent:** Egg albumin, milk, gelatin, etc.
4. Purgatives, high colonic lavage
5. **Antidote:**[10, 12] BAL/penicillamine
6. Supportive:
   Shock/dehydration—IV fluids
   Renal failure—$NaHCO_3$/peritoneal, or hemodialysis
   Exchange tranfusion

Antidote
a. **Physical:** Egg albumin (forms mercuric albuminate), demulcents, charcoal
b. **Chemical:**[6] 5% solution of sodium formaldehyde sulfoxylate with 5% $NaHCO_3$
c. **Pharmacological:** DMPS (2,3-Dimercapto-1-propanesulfonate)—3 mg/kg IV over 5 min, 100 mg TID × 2 wks followed by QID for 6 weeks[2,19] or DMSA (dimercaptosuccinic acid), an analog of BAL has high affinity for mercury.[20]

Absorption, distribution, excretion
- Absorbed through GIT
- Distributed in liver, spleen, and kidney
- Excreted in urine, bile, feces

ACUTE COPPER POISONING
Clinical features
- **Anemia:** Due to increase fragility of RBC causes hemolysis
- Burning sensation, metallic taste, difficulty in speech and swallowing, excessive salivation, thirst with abdominal pain, vomiting, diarrhea with painful defecation and micturition. This is followed by dehydration, muscle cramps, convulsion, collapse, and coma
  - Vomiting is greenish blue—**turns to deep blue with ammonia/NH_4OH.**[6]
  - Diarrhea is greenish blue
- Scanty urine containing blood, albumin
- **Liver damage:** Jaundice

Treatment
1. **Emesis:** There is no use of emetics. (Copper salts are potent emetics.)
2. **Stomach wash:**[6, 12] 1% Pot. ferrocyanide
3. **Demulcent**
4. **Purgatives:** Castor oil
5. **Antidotes:**[10] BAL/penicillamine
6. **Supportive:**
   Diuretics
   Shock/dehydration—IV fluids
   Liver/renal damage—vitamin, AA, hemodialysis[12]
   Exchange transfusion

Antidote
a. **Physical:** Demulcents (forms copper albuminate with proteins)
b. **Chemical:**[6,12] Potassium ferrocyanide (forms insoluble cupric ferrocyanide)
c. **Pharmacological:**[12] BAL followed by penicillamine

PM findings
1. Skin and MM of mouth, tongue, esophagus— corroded and **greyish white**.
2. **Stomach:** Wall—soft, swollen
   MM—desquamated, hemorrhagic, ulcerated, necrosis and greyish white/black
   Contents—altered blood and mucus shreds.
3. **Intestines:** Congested, ulcerated, and sometimes gangrenous.
4. **Kidney:** Swollen, nephritis.
5. **Liver:** Congested, central necrosis and cloudy swelling
6. **Heart:** Sub-endocardial hemorrhages

PM findings
1. MM of mouth, tongue and esophagus—greenish blue lining
2. **Stomach:** Wall—soft, swollen
   MM—desquamated, hemorrhagic, congested, greenish blue lining
   Contents: Greenish blue
3. **Intestines:** Hemorrhages and ulcerations, greenish blue lining
4. Greenish—blue froth at mouth and nostrils.
5. **Liver:** Jaundice

CHRONIC MERCURY POISONING (Hydrargyrism)
It occurs due to:
1. Chronic exposure to people working in industry and laboratory
2. Repeated administration of multiple small doses of medicines containing mercury.
3. Contaminated food, drinks, and sea fish. Mercury is methylated under sea water and consumption of such fish causes chronic poisoning.
   (Minimata disease)[21, 22]

CHRONIC COPPER POISONING
It occurs due to hemocromatosis:
1. Chronic industrial exposure
2. Consumption of vegetables colored with copper sulfate
3. Consumption of contaminated food and drink (stored/cooked in copper utensils—Wilson disease) due to deficiency of ceruloplasmin (<0.2 g/L in 80–95% of cases).[23]

Clinical features
Skin: Contact dermatitis, penetrating ulcers on fingers, nails and knuckles.
GIT and general manifestaion: *Metallic taste,* irritability, fatigability, lack of interest and concentration, loss of weight and appetite, alternate constipation and diarrhea, abdominal colic, *anemia*
Buccal cavity: Suggestive of gingivitis, glossitis, salivation, loosening of teeth
Gums: Blue line, inflammation, ulceration and necrosis
Acrodynia: (due to exposure of methyl mercury)— redness, swelling, vesiculation of palm, soles, fingers and toes with pink coloration **(pink disease—pink and peel).**[22]
Mercuriolentis: Deposition of mercury in lens (brownish discoloration of eye) leading to restricted field of vision
Mercurial erethism, i.e. disturbed personality characterized by irritability, fatigability, lack of interest/concentration, insomnia, anxiety, loss of memory, delusions, hallucinations and tremors **(Hatter's shakes**/glass blower's shakes) affecting fingers, tongue, face, arms and legs
Kidney: Uremia, nephritis

Clinical features
GIT and general manifestation *metallic taste,* irritability, fatigability, lack of interest and concentration, loss of weight and appetite, alternate constipation and diarrhea, abdominal colic, *anemia*
Gums:[6] **Blue lining or greenish blue line (Clapton's line),**[24] unhealthy
Kayser-Fleischer ring:[12] Discoloration of peripheral part of cornea due to deposition of copper.
Muscular weakness and paralysis of limbs and atrophy.
Body secretions—greenish blue
Blood picture altered and presence of premature cells in peripheral blood. Contact dermatitis

Treatment (chronic mercury poisoning)
- Prevent further exposure
- **Antidotes:** BAL
- General/oral hygiene

Treatment (chronic copper poisoning)
- Prevent further exposure
- **Antidotes:** Penicillamine
- General and oral hygiene

PM findings
- **Skin:** Contact dermatitis, penetrating ulcers.
- **Gums:** Blue line, inflammation, ulceration and necrosis
- Signs of acrodynia, mercuriolentis
- Degenerative changes in kidney/liver—necrosis

PM findings
- Gums—blue lining and unhealthy
- Blood pictured altered and presence of prematured cells
- Liver/kidney—degenerative changes

Preservation of viscera
1. Routine viscera
2. **Additional viscera:** Bones, teeth, hair and nails are preserved

Preservation of viscera
1. Routine viscera
2. **Additional viscera:** Bones, teeth, hair and nails are preserved

Medicolegal aspects
1. **Suicidal:** Rare—painful suffering
2. **Homicidal poisoning:** Rare—chemical test
3. **Accidental poisoning** is common and mainly due to:
   i. Excessive use of medicines (diuretics; mercury ointments)
   ii. Consumption of bleaching creams, or **snake-tablet** (mercuric thiocyanate) used in Diwali.
   iii. Consumption of food contaminated with preservative and sea fish—minimata disease[22]
   iv. Chronic industrial or agricultural exposure
4. **Abortifacient:** Sometimes used for criminal abortion

Diagnosis:[12]
   i. Blood mercury level—normal <3 µg/100 mL,
   ii. Urine level—normal <10 µg/100 mL.

Medicolegal aspects
1. **Suicidal:** Mostly but deaths are less due to vomited out of poison
2. **Homicidal poisoning:** Uncommon
3. Accidental poisoning may occur because
   i. Copper salts are used as fungicide
   ii. Also used to retain green color of vegetables
   iii. Contaminated food/drink stored in copper vessels
4. **Abortifacient:** Sometimes used to procure abortion
5. Cattle poison

Diagnosis:
   i. **Low serum ceruloplasmin level**[23]
   ii. Blood copper level[12]: >1.5 µg/100 mL

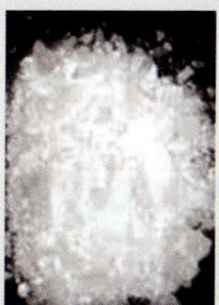 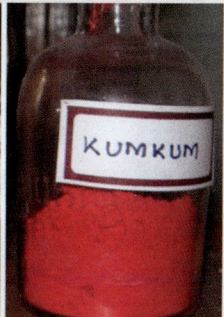 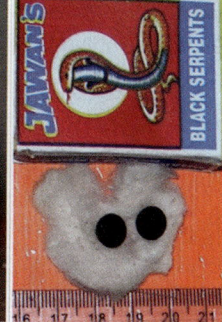 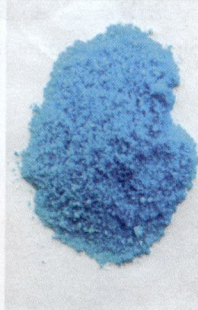

Mercury chloride   Mercury sulfide   Mercury thiocyanate   Copper sulfate

Chemical tests for metallic poisons (*see* Table 3.1)
1. Marsh's test for arsenic
2. Reinsch's test for arsenic, mercury and antimony
3. Gutzeit test for arsenic and antimony
4. **Ammonia test for copper: Test material in TT + few drop of NH_4OH → deep blue precipitate**
5. **Chemical test for iron[6]:** Ammonium sulphide + test material containing ferric/ferrous salt → black precipitate, soluble in dil. HCl.

Autopsy Photo of Metallic Poisons (Courtesy—Dr. Nitin Barmate) *(Figs 7.5 to 7.10)*

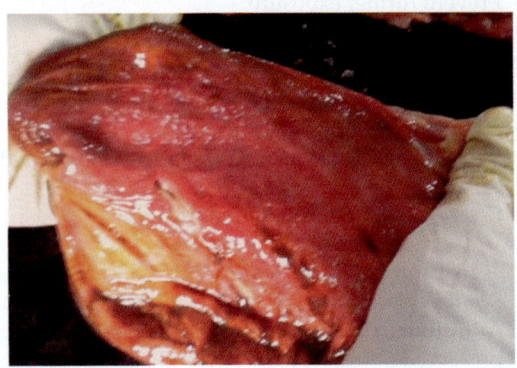

Fig. 7.5: Stomach in sindoor poisoning—mercury

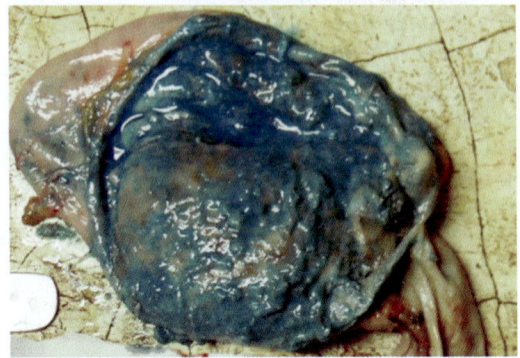

Fig. 7.6: Stomach in paint poisoning

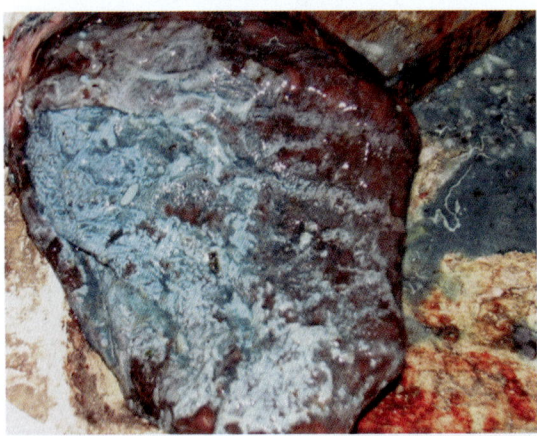

Fig. 7.7: Stomach in copper sulfate poisoning

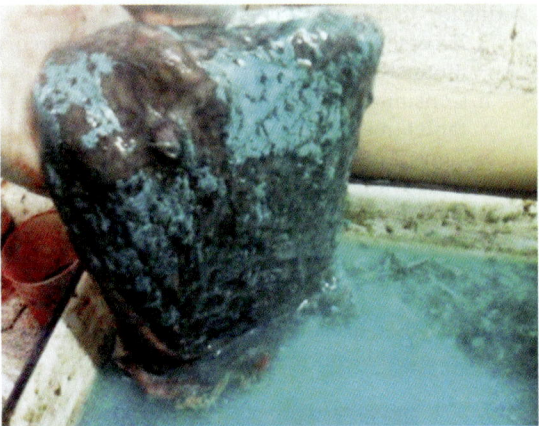

Fig. 7.8: Stomach in copper arsenite poisoning

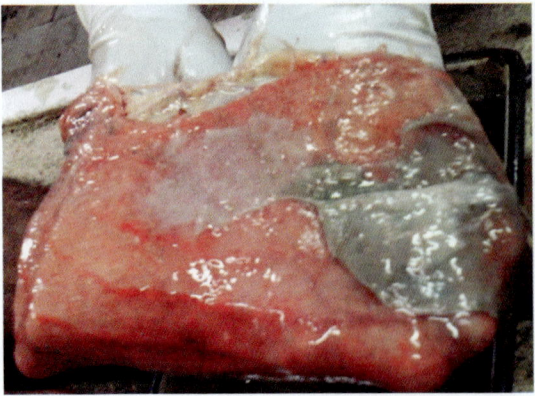

Fig. 7.9: Stomach in lead poisoning

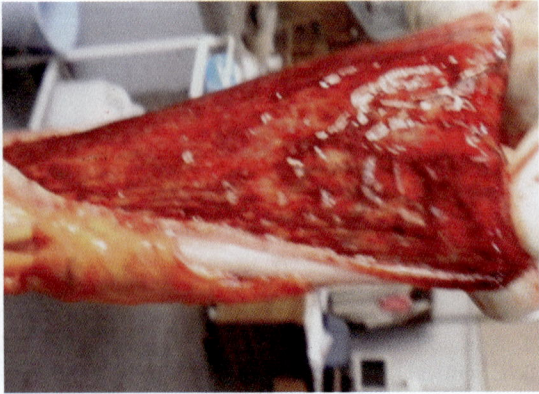

Fig. 7.10: Stomach in metallic poisoning

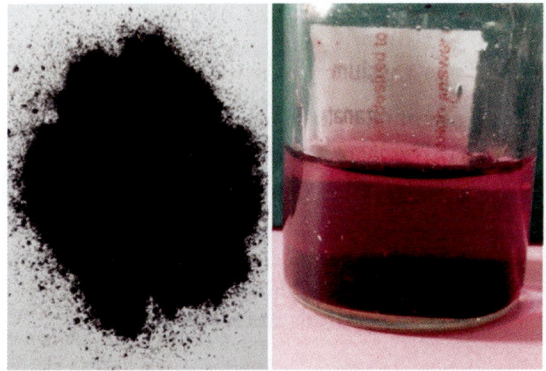

Fig. 7.11: KMnO$_4$ powder and solution

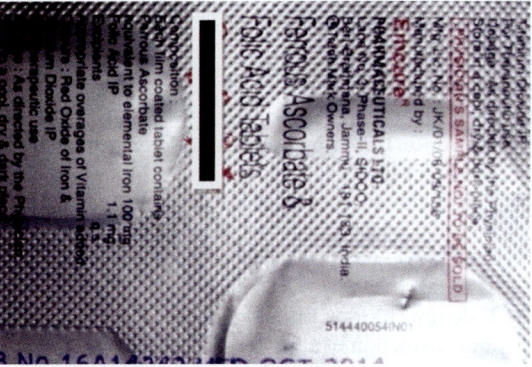

Fig. 7.12: Ferrous tablet

POTASSIUM TOXICITY (HYPERKALEMIA)	IRON TOXICITY
Types: 1. Exogenous toxicity due to: 1. High dose of potassium therapy 2. Poisoning with KMnO$_4$/potassium iodate Endogenous toxicity due to renal failure	*Poisoning is due to iron overload caused by excess:* 1. Consumption of ferrous sulfate tablets 2. IV injection of iron preparation
Fatal dose: 12–15 gm	**Fatal dose:** 10–15 tabs
Toxic compounds:[25,26] Potassium chloride—white crystalline powder; potassium iodide—odorless	1. Ferrous sulfate (green vitriol) 2. Ferric chloride

Clinical features
The administration of oral potassium salts to persons with normal excretory mechanisms rarely causes serious hyperkalemia. It is usually asymptomatic and may be manifested by increased serum pot concentration and ECG changes.
  I. **When taken orally**
    Potassium iodide:[26,27] GIT irritation with liver, kidney, bladder and retinal damage. Also causes serum sickness type of hypersensitivity
    Potassium permanganate: Orally—gastroenteritis, edema of glottis, respiratory distress
  II. **Systemic:** Tingling, numbness and weakness of limbs and fingers and toes with paralysis
  III. **ECG:** Elevation of T-waves
	Clinical features
	Clinically, iron toxicity manifests in four stages.[28]
	Stage I/stage of GI toxicity (0–6 h since ingestion) causes vomiting, hematemesis, abdominal pain and lethargy;
	Stage II/stage of apparent stabilization (6–12 h since ingestion) when symptoms subside;
	Stage III/stage of mitochondrial toxicity and hepatic necrosis (12–48 h since ingestion) where patients may develop acute liver failure, coagulopathy, acute tubular necrosis, metabolic acidosis and shock.
	Stage IV/stage of gastric scarring (4–6 weeks since ingestion) characterized by gastric scarring and pyloric stricture.
	Scanty urine containing bilirubin, bile salts and urobilinogen
	Liver: Jaundice—centrilobular necrosis
	Blood: Increase iron bind with transferrin

Diagnosis of hyperkalemia:[25,26]
  i. Increased serum potassium concentration (6.5–8.0 mEq/L)
  ii. **ECG changes:** Peaking of T-waves, loss of P-wave, depression of S–T segment, and prolongation of the QT interval
	Diagnosis of iron toxicity:
	  i. Blood iron level> 350–500 mcg/dL is indicative of iron toxicity.[29]
	  ii. Administration of desferrioxamine after acute iron intoxication may color the urine a pinkish red, a phenomenon termed *'vin rose'* urine. [30,31]

Treatment	Treatment
<ul><li>Emesis</li><li>Stomach wash</li><li>**Demulcent**</li><li>**Antidote: Calcium chloride**/calcium gluconate (Dose = 1 gm IV)</li><li>Whole bowel irrigation[32] with polyethylene glycol solution when a large number of radio-opaque tablets are seen beyond pylorus.</li><li>**Hemodialysis**</li><li>Calcium chloride infusion, dextrose and insulin and correction of acidosis with $NaHCO_3$ are helpful in controlling the acute, life-threatening cardiac arrhythmias.[33]</li><li>Epinephrine followed by 125 mL of a 4.2% intravenous solution of $NaHCO_3$ results in effective recovery of cardiac irregularity[34]</li></ul>	<ul><li>Emesis</li><li>Stomach wash:</li><li>**Antidote**[10]: Desferroxamine/EDTA/Penicillamine.</li><li>**Deferiprone—50–100 mg/kg orally** daily in 2–4 divided dose.</li><li>Normal saline with whole bowel irrigation[30] polyethylene glycol solution at the rate of 30–40 ml/kg/hr for 4–8 hours.[35]</li><li>Liver transplantation[36] in massive iron ingestion.</li><li>**Symptomatic:** Dialysis and blood transfusion</li></ul>
PM findings	PM findings
<ul><li>GIT—irritation</li><li>Visceral organs—congestion</li></ul>	<ul><li>GIT—irritation</li><li>Pulmonary hemorrhage, petechial hemorrhage</li><li>Liver—centrilobular necrosis[8]</li><li>Kidney—tubular necrosis[8]</li></ul>
Medicolegal aspects	Medicolegal aspects
<ul><li>**Suicidal:** Rare; 20-yr-old nurse has committed suicide by IV pot chloride[34]</li><li>**Homicidal:** Not possible—high dose</li><li>**Accidental:** Mistaken with other</li><li>**Abortifacient**</li></ul>	<ul><li>**Suicidal:** Usually by females</li><li>**Homicidal:** Very rare</li><li>**Accidental:** Overdose, prolonged IV therapy</li><li>**Abortifacient**</li></ul>

IMPORTANT QUESTIONS

1. Enumerate any four inorganic metallic irritants with its uses and toxic compounds. Describe mechanism of action, clinical manifestation, treatment and medicolegal aspect of chronic lead poisoning.

2. Describe action, clinical features, treatment and autopsy findings of arsenic poisoning. Add a note on its medicolegal importance.

3. Describe clinical features, treatment, postmortem findings, and medicolegal aspect of chronic mercury or chronic copper poisoning.

4. Describe clinical features, treatment and postmortem findings of acute poisoning with mercury or copper. Add a note on different chemical tests for metallic poisons.

SPECIFIC LEARNING OBJECTIVES

After reading this chapter, the reader should be able to:

- **Enumerate toxic compounds and fatal dose of different metallic poisons like arsenic, lead, mercury and copper**
- **Recognize the mechanism of action of metallic irritants**
- **Explain clinical manifestation, treatment, postmortem findings in acute arsenic/lead poisoning**
- **Explain clinical manifestation, treatment, postmortem findings and medicolegal aspect in chronic arsenic/lead poisoning**
- **Distinguish between arsenic poisoning and cholera**
- **Explain clinical manifestations, treatment, postmortem findings in acute mercury/copper poisoning**

- **Explain clinical manifestations, treatment, postmortem findings and medicolegal aspect in chronic mercury/copper poisoning**
- **Recognize different chemical tests for metallic poisons**
- **Explain clinical manifestation, treatment, postmortem findings and medicolegal aspects in iron and potassium toxicity**

References

1. Berlin M, Zalups RK, Fowler BA. Mercury. In: Nordberg GF, Fowler BA, Nordberg M, Friberg LT, editors. *Handbook on the Toxicology of Metals*. 3rd edition. chapter 33. Elsevier: New York; 2007.

2. Bernhoft RA. Mercury Toxicity and Treatment: A Review of the Literature. Journal of Environmental and Public Health, 2012; Vol 2012 (Article ID 460508):1–10. doi:10.1155/2012/460508.

3. Hughes MF, Beck BD, Chen Y, Lewis AS, Thomas DJ. Arsenic exposure and toxicology: A historical perspective. Toxicological Sciences. 2011; 123 (2): 305–32. doi:10.1093/toxsci/kfr184. PMC 3179678. PMID 21750349.

4. Naujokas Marisa F, Anderson Beth, Ahsan Habibul, Aposhian H Vasken, Graziano Joseph H, Thompson Claudia, Suk William A. The broad scope of health effects from chronic arsenic exposure: Update on a worldwide public health problem. Environmental Health Perspectives. 2013;121 (3): 295–302. doi:10.1289/ehp.1205875. PMC 3621177. PMID 23458756. For source of arsenic.

5. Ratnaike, RN. Acute and chronic arsenic toxicity. Postgraduate Medical Journal. 2003; 79 (933): 391–6. doi:10.1136/pmj.79.933.391. PMC 1742758. PMID 12897217.

6. Dikshit PC. Textbook of Forensic Medicine and Toxicology. 2nd edn, PEEPEE Publisher and Distributors (P) Ltd. New Delhi. 2014: 482–500.

7. Reddy KSN, Murthy OP. The Essential of Forensic Medicine and Toxicology. 32nd edn, Om Sai graphics: Hyderabad. 2013: 510–20.

8. Nandy A. Principles of Forensic Medicine. New Central Book Agency (P) Ltd: Calcutta, 2nd edn Reprint, 2004: 475–90.

9. Singhal SK. Singhal's Toxicology at a glance. 9th edn, National book depot: Mumbai.2016: 54–63.

10. Tripathi KD. Chelating Agents. In: Essential of Medical Pharmacology. Jaypee Brothers Medical Publishers (P) Ltd: New Delhi, 7th edn, 2014: 905–8.

11. Vij K. Textbook of Forensic Medicine and Toxicology. 3rd edn, 2005. Reed Elsevier India Pvt Limited: New Delhi. 642–61.

12. Pillay VV. Textbook of Forensic Medicine and Toxicology. Paras Medical Publisher: Hyderabad, 17th edn, 2016: 518–37.

13. Hugelmeyer CD, Moorhead JC, Horenblas L, Bayer MJ. Fatal lead encephalopathy following foreign body ingestion: case report. J Emerg Med. 1988; 5: 397–400.

14. Quatrehomme G, Ricq O, Lapalus P, Jacomet Y, Ollier A. Acute arsenic intoxication: forensic and toxicologic aspects (an observation). J Forensic Sci. 1992;37(4):1163–71. [PubMed]

15. DiMaio VJ, DiMaio SM, Garriott JC, Simpson P A fatal case of lead poisoning due to a retained bullet Arn J Forensic Med Pathol. 1983;4:165–9.

16. Linden MA, Manton WI, Stewart RM, Thal ER, Feit H. Lead poisoning from retained bullets: pathogenesis, diagnosis and management. Ann Surg. 1982; 195: 305–13.

17. Garces JBG, Artuz RIM. Lead poisoning due to bullets lodged in the human body. Colomb Med (Cali). 2012; 43(3): 230–4.

18. Dogra TD, Rudra A. Lyon's Medical Jurisprudence and Toxicology. 11th edn, 2007. Delhi Law house: Delhi, 1132–72.

19. Hurlbut KM, Maiorino RM, Mayersohn M, Dart RC, Bruce DC, Aposhian HV. Determination and metabolism of dithiol chelating agents XVI: pharmacokinetics of 2,3-dimercapto-1-propanesulfonate after intravenous administration to human volunteers," *Journal of Pharmacology and Experimental Therapeutics*. 1994; vol. 268, (2): 662– 8.

20. Kosnett MJ. The role of chelation in the treatment of arsenic and mercury poisoning. Journal of Medical Toxicology : Official Journal of the American College of Medical Toxicology. 2013; 9 (4): 347–54. doi:10.1007/s13181-013-0344-5. PMC 3846971. PMID 24178900.

21. Harada M. Minamata Disease: Methylmercury Poisoning in Japan Caused by Environmental Pollution. J Critical Reviews in Toxicology. 1995; 25(1): 1–24.

22. Bose-O'Reilly S, McCarty KM, Steckling N, Lettmeier B. Mercury exposure and children's health. Current Problems in Pediatric and Adolescent Health Care. 2010; 40 (8): 186–215. doi:10.1016/j.cppeds.2010.07.002. PMC 3096006. PMID 20816346. – For Minimata disease.

23. Ala A, Walker AP, Ashkan K, Dooley JS, Schilsky ML. Wilson's disease. Lancet. 2007; 369 (9559): 397–408. doi:10.1016/S0140-6736(07)60196-2. PMID 17276780.

24. Pillay VV. Comprehensive Medical toxicology. 1st edn, Paras Publishing: Hyderabad. 2003: 97–140.

25. Potassium chloride (KCl). In: PubChem. https://pubchem.ncbi.nlm.nih.gov/compound/potassium_chloride

26. Potassium iodide (KI) In: PubChem. https://pubchem.ncbi.nlm.nih.gov/compound/potassium_iodide

27. Gilman AG, Goodman LS, Gilman A. (eds). Goodman and Gilman's The Pharmacological Basis of Therapeutics. 6th ed. New York: Macmillan Publishing Co., Inc. 1980. p. 1414.

28. Baranwal AK, Singhi SC. Acute iron poisoning: management guidelines. Indian Pediatr. 2003; 40(6):534–40.

29. Iron tests. The free dictionary by Falex. Citing: Gale Encyclopedia of Medicine. Copyright 2008. http://medical-dictionary.thefreedictionary.com/Iron+Tests.

30. Schauben JL, Augenstein WL, Cox J, Sato R. Iron poisoning: report of three cases and a review of therapeutic intervention. J Emerg Med. 1990; 8(3):309–19.

31. Kundavaram PP Abhilash, J Jonathan Arul, Divya Bala. Fatal overdose of iron tablets in adults. Indian J Crit Care Med. 2013; 17(5): 311–3. doi: [10.4103/0972-5229.120326].

32. Gunja N. Decontamination and enhanced elimination in sustained-release potassium chloride poisoning. Emerg Med Australasia. 2011;23(6):769–72.doi:10.1111/j.1742-6723.2011.01469.x.

33. Saxena K. Clinical features and management of poisoning due to potassium chloride. Med Toxicol Adverse Drug Exp. 1989;4(6):429–43.

34. Florent Battefort, Emilie Dehours, Baptiste Vallé, Ahmed Hamdaoui, Vincent Bounes, Jean-Louis Ducassé. Suicide Attempt by Intravenous Potassium Self-Poisoning: A Case Report. Case Reports in Emergency Medicine. 2012; Vol 2012, Article ID 323818, 3 pages. http://dx.doi.org/10.1155/2012/323818

35. Bardale R. Principles of Forensic Medicine and Toxicology. 1st edn, Jaypee Brothers Medical Publishers (P) Ltd: New Delhi. 2011: 449–66.

36. Kozaki K, Egawa H, Garcia-Kennedy R, Cox KL, Lindsay J, Esquivel CO. Hepatic failure due to massive iron ingestion successfully treated with liver transplantation. Clin Transplant. 1995 Apr; 9(2):85–7. [PubMed] [Ref list]

Agricultural Poison: Pesticides

Agricultural poisons are the organic irritant poisons that are used in the agricultural field. They are commonly called pesticides. Pesticides are compounds that are used to kill pests, which may be insects, rodents, fungi, nematodes, mites, ticks, molluscus, or unwanted weeds and herbs, which cause much harm to the production and storage of agricultural foods. Pesticides are used as aerial spray mixed with suitable liquid or dust as their vehicle or mixed with soil. When sprayed in air, absorption in the plants occurs through leaves and stems. When mixed with soil, absorption occurs through the roots of the plant without causing any harm to the plants.

When the insect sits on the plant, the poison acts as a contact poison and is absorbed through their exoskeleton or when the insect eats the leaves of the plant, it consumes the poison along with the leaves. But it does not cause any harm to human who consumed the grain, fruits or other part of the plant if used with recommended cautions. But, when it enters in human body due to direct or indirect route, then it causes poisoning. Recently, lot of hue and cry occurs due to death of farmers in Maharashtra due to inhalation of insecticide while spraying on the fields.[1] In these cases, the viscera were found to be negative on toxicological analysis.

World Health Organization (WHO) estimates more than 3 million cases of acute poisoning and 3 lakh deaths globally per year.[2] The incidence of poisoning in India is among the highest in the world. It is estimated that more than 50,000 people die every year from toxic exposure.[3] The commonest cause of poisoning in developing countries is pesticides which includes organophosphates, carbamates, chlorinated hydrocarbons, pyrethroids and aluminium or zinc phosphide.[4] In north India, aluminium phosphide (ALP) is the most common type of poisoning, whereas organophosphorus compounds (OPC) are more common in south India.[5]

Classification of agricultural poisons				
1. Insecticidal	2. Herbicidal	3. Fungicidal	4. Rodenticidal	5. Others
Organophosphorus		Organochlorine	Carbamate	Pyrethroid

1. **Insecticides:** Compounds which kill insects and related species. They are classified into four groups (Tables 8.1 to 8.3) as **Organophosphorus compounds** (Monocrotophos-Nuvacron, Quinolphos, Dimethoate, Chlorpyriphos, Chlorothion, Phorate); **Organochlorine compounds** (Endosulphan, Chlordane, BHC, Lindane, DDT); **Carbamates** (baygon, carbaryl) and **pyrethrines and pyrethroids** (Allethrin, Cypermethrin, Dexamethrin).
2. **Herbicides:** Kill weeds or herbs, e.g.
   - 12% sulphuric acid, potassium cyanide, sodium chlorate, sodium arsenite.
   - Acrolein, dalaphon, paraquat, diquat, atrazine, propazine, simazine, Targa super (Quizolofeb), Glycel (Glyphosate)
3. **Fungicides:** Kill fungi and moulds, e.g. Phenyl mercuric acetate, thiocarbamates, hexachlorbenzene, sodium azide—captan, captafol, bavistin, vitavax, Jatayu (Chlorothalonil), Index (Mycobutanil), Dhanuka (Mancozeb), Benofit (Benomyl).
4. **Rodenticides:** Compounds which kill rats, mice moles and other rodents, e.g.
   - **Inorganic preparations:** Zinc/aluminium phosphide, arsenic, barium carbonate, phosphorus, thallium.
   - **Organic preparations:** Fluroacetate
   - **Convulsant:** Strychnine
   - **Anticoagulants:** Warfarin
   - **Others:** Vacor, cholecalciferol, bromethalin, fluoroacetamide, red squill.
5. **Others:**
   - **Nematicides:** Kill nematodes (i.e. worms), e.g. ethylene dibromide.
   - **Acaricides:** Kill mites, ticks, and spiders. e.g. azobenzene, chlorobenzilate, tedion, and kelthane.
   - **Molluscicides:** Kill molluscs such as snails and slugs, e.g. metaldehyde.
   - **Flowering stimulants,** e.g. Dinitrobenzene-Combiflower

Table 8.1: Agricultural poisons: Organophosphorus compound poisons

Group	Chemical name	Trade/market name of organophosphorus compounds	Clinical features[6]	Treatment
Alkyl	1. Chlorfenvinphos 2. **Chlorpyriphos**	• Birlane, Chlorfenvinphos • Agrofas 20, Blase, Chlorofos 20, Chlorguard, Coroban 20, Durshban, Gilphos, Hyban 20, Pyriban, Ruban 20, Tafaban, Trishul 20 EC, Hilban-20, Sacban-20, Rickcare-50	1. **Muscarinic effect:** **a. Heart-depressed:** Slow pulse, bradycardia, refractive period is increased and conduction is slowed.	1. **Decontamination:** (Remove patient from source of exposure; Remove all clothing; Thorough skin wash with **soap and water;** Eye irrigation with Normal saline or Ringer's solution or tap water.)
	3. **Dimethoate**	• Agrodimet 30, Cygon, Agromet 30 EC, Bangor 30 EC, Corothate, Cropgor 30, Cygon, Devigor, Dimethoate, Dimex, Entogor, Hexagor, Hygro 30, Rogor, Milgor, Paragor, Vikagor, Parrydimate, Ramgor, Rogar, Tagor, Vijaygor,	**b. Blood vessels—dilated:** Fall of BP, flushing **c. Smooth muscle—contracted with sphincter relax:** Abdominal cramps, diarrhea, urinary incontinence, bronchospasm, dyspnea	2. **Stomach wash** with NS/KMnO$_4$ solution 3. **Atropine:**[6] 2 mg IV every 10 min 4. **Oximes:**[6] PAM 1–2 gm in 100 ml normal saline by slow IV infusion
	4. Indoxacarb 5. Malathion	• Awant, Daksha, Dhawa • Agromal, Cython, Finit, Kathion, Licel, Maladan, Malathion, Malazene, Sulmithion, Veg Fru, Malatox	**d. Glands-secretion is increased:** Sweating, salivation, lacrimation, (red tears), with increased tracheobronchial secretion and gastric secretion.	5. **Diazepam for convulsion:**[10] 5–10 mg IV every 5–10 min (max 30 mg). **For children:** 0.2–0.5 mg/kg every 5 min (max 5 mg).
	6. **Monocrotophos**	• Anacron, Azodrin, Biphos, Corophos, Entophos, Guardian, Hycrophos, Macrophos, Microphos, Monocil, Monolik, Monocron, Monokem, HICIL, Monophos, Nuvacron, Poryuphos, Shrimono, Totamonr, Yuromono	**e. Eye—contraction of circular muscle of iris:** Miosis (SLUDGE).[7,8]	Phenobarbital orally to control seizures and myoclonic movements that sometimes persists for several days of poisoning.
	7. **Quinolphos**	• Agroquin, Agroquinol, Anuphos, Bayrusil, Ekalux, Flash, Hyquin, Kilex, Quinal, Quinguard, Shakti 25 EC, Solux, Vikalux, Dhanulux	Salivation Lacrimation, Urination, Dyspnea, Gastrointestinal distress—N, V, AP, D. Extramiosis, sweating, bronchoconstriction)	6. Maintenance of airway and O$_2$ inhalation or artificial respiration. 7. IV fluids.
	8. Temephos/fox 9. Triazophos	• Teme Guard, Abete, Farmicos, Abate 50 EC • Hexban, Hexban 20 EC, Hostatnion, Kranti, Ninza, Sutathion, Tackle, Tricon, Trizer, Trizocel	2. **Nicotinic effect:** **a. Autonomic ganglia:** Stimulates sympathetic and parasympathetic ganglia—tachycardia, hypertension	8. Antibiotics. 9. Prevention of further exposure for a few weeks. 10. Prophylaxis
	10. Others	• HETP, TEPP, OMPA, Demeton, Trichlorfon, Isopestox		
Aryl	1. Diazinon	• Agroziron, Basudin, Bazanon, Ditaf, Suzinon, Zionosul 50		
	2. Methyl parathion 3. **Parathion** 4. Others	• Dhanumar, Paradol, Paradol 2 DP, • Folidol, Kilphos • Paraoxon, Chlorothion,		

(Contd...)

Table 8.1: Agricultural poisons: Organophosphorus compound poisons (Contd...)

Group	Chemical name	Trade/market name of organophosphorus compounds	Clinical features[6]	Treatment
Others	1. Acephate	• Acemil, Agrophate, Asataf, Hythane, Starthene,	**b. Skeletal muscle:** Twitching, fasciculation	
	2. Ethion	• Demite, Dhanunit, Ethion, Ethiosul 50 Force, Mit 50, Miticil, RP-thion, Tafethion, VegFru, Fosmite	3. **CNS-depression:** (It does not penetrate blood–brain barrier and no central effects are seen):	
	3. Fenitrothion	• Accothion, Agrothion, Danathion, Fenicol, Fenitrosul 50, Folithion, Sumithion, Tik 20, Vikathion	Restlessness, headache, dizziness, drowsiness, delirium, tremor, twitching of face and tongue, slurred speech, ataxia, and convulsions	
	4. Fenthion	• Agrocidin, Baytex, Fenthiosul, Lebaycid	**DIAGNOSIS:**[9]	
	5. Formothion	• Anthio	1. **Decrease in RBC and serum cholinesterase** level.	
	6. Glyphosate	• Weed off		
	7. Methyl demeton	• Hexasystox, Hymox, Knock out, Metasystox	2. Urinary P-Nitrophenol test.	
	8. Phenthoate	• Agrofen, Delsan, Elsan, Guard, Phentox	3. Thin layer Chromatography (TLC).	
	9. **Phorate**	• Dragnet, Fortan, Glorat, Luphate, Phoratox, Thimet, Volphor, Veg Fru Foratox, Umet, Starphor-10G	4. Ancillary investigations like increase blood sugar level, leukocytosis, high hematocrit, and anion gap acidosis.	
	10. **Phosphamidon**	• Agromidon 85, Bangdon 85, Cildon, Delphamidon, Dimecron, Directon, Entecron 85, Phamidon, Phosul, Sudon, Vimidon		
	11. Primiphos methyl	• Acetellic		
	12. Thiometon	• Agrothimeton, Ekatin		
	13. Trichlorphon	• Dipterex		

Table 8.2: Agricultural poisons: Organochlorine compound poisons

Group	Chemical name	Trade/market name of organochlorine compounds	Clinical features	Treatment
1. Cyclodienes and related compounds	1. Aldrin	• Agroaldrin, Alcrop, Alditon, Aldrex, Aldrin 30, Mildrin 30, Tarmahit 30, **Endrin**	1. **GIT:** Nausea, vomiting, hyperesthesia / paresthesia of mouth and face, diarrhea	1. Decontamination: (Same measures as described under organophosphate poisoning must be undertaken)
	2. **Endosulphan**	• Agrosulfan, Endohit, Hildon, Hexosulfan, **Thiodan**	2. **CNS:** Headache, vertigo, myoclonus, rapid and dysrhythmic eye movements, mydriasis, weakness, agitation, confusion, and convulsions	2. Stomach wash by activated charcoal.[10]
	3. Heptachlor	• Agrochlor D5, Agrodono, Heptachlor, Heptaf 50, Heptar, Heptox		3. **IV Diazepam for convulsion:**[10] 5–10 mg IV every 5–10 min (max 30 mg). For children: 0.2–0.5 mg/kg every 5 min (max 5 mg). Phenobarbital orally to control seizures and myoclonic movements that sometimes persists for several days of poisoning
	4. Chlordane	• VegFru Heptex, Agrodane 20 EC, Chlordane, Mitox 20 EC, Sudarshan 5 EC, Termex, VegFru Chlortox	3. **Other:** Fever, aspiration, pneumonitis, renal failure	4. **Cholestyramine resin:** 16 gm/day for several days mixed with fruit juice and given orally (4 gm, 6th hourly)[10] before meals. It is a non-absorbable bile acid binding anion exchange resin and is effective in **enhancing the fecal excretion** of organochlorine compounds[11]
2. Benzene hexachloride compounds	1. **BHC** (Benzene hexachloride)	• Agrobenz D10, Agro BHC, Gamazene, Gammexane, Haxaman, Hexidol, Hilbich 50WP, Kargo BHC, Premodol 10EC, Solchlor, Sudarshan, Sulbenz 50	**DIAGNOSIS:**	5. Cold sponging for hyperthermia
	2. Gamma-hexachloro-cyclohexane (**lindane**)	• Agrodane, Bexarid, Emscab, Gab, Gamaric, Gamascab, Lindane 20, Lindex, Scarab, Linsuline, Lintaf, scabex, Scaboma, Rasayan lindane, Ultrascab, Standard lindane.	1. Abdominal X-ray may reveal the presence of certain radiopaque organochlorines.	6. Airway maintenance—monitor pulmonary ventilation
3. DDT and analogues	1. **DDT** (Dichloro-diphenyl-trichloroethane)	• DDT, Sudarshan 50, Didinex 25 EC, Ramdit	2. Organochlorines can be detected in serum, adipose tissue, and urine by gas chromatography	7. Monitor cardiac status for any arrhythmia—continuous ECG
	2. Methoxychlor	• Ranodit, Soltax, Suldit 50, Sunbrand, **Tafarol**, Tafidex		8. **Contraindication:** Do not give **adrenaline or atropine** unless absolutely necessary. Also do not give **oil-based cathertics/demulcent**[10]
4. Toxaphene and related compounds	1. **Toxaphene** 2. Dicofol	• Kelthane		9. **PAM does not play any role in organochlorides poisoning**

Table 8.3: Agricultural poisons: Carbamates and pyrethroids compound poisons

Chemical constituents	Trade/market names	Clinical features	Treatment
Carbamates compounds			
1. Propoxur	• Baygon, Protox bait.	Salivation, lacrimation, sweating, vomiting, diarrhea, slow pulse, low BP, weakness, twitching, convulsions. (Signs and symptoms similar to OP compounds poisoning, but symptoms are less severe and of shorter duration)	1. Remove clothing and thorough skin wash with soap and water
2. Carbendazim	• Bavistin, Carbistin 50, Glizim, Kilex, Carbendazim 50, Spot free, Zen		2. Stomach wash with NS/KMnO$_4$
3. Carbofuron	• Agrofuron 3 G, Carbocil 3, Furadan 3 G, Hexafuran, VegFru, Diafuran		3. **IV atropine 2 mg /15 min (adult) and 0.05 mg/kg/15 min till full atropinization**
4. Methomyl	• Lannate, Duonate		4. IV diazepam 5–10 mg slowly to control convulsions
5. Triallate	• Avadex		5. Maintenance of airway and O$_2$ inhalation or artificial respiration
6. Carbaryl	• Agrovin, Agroyl, Bangvin 50, Caravet, Hexavin, Kevin 50, Kilex Carbaryl, Sevin 50, Sujacarb, Sulfal 50		6. IV fluids
7. Carbaryl + g BHC	• Sevidol		7. Antibiotics
8. Aldicarb	• Temik		8. **Inj. PAM is contraindicated in cases of poisoning with carbamate compounds**[6]
9. Aminocarb	• Metacil		
Pyrethrins and pyrethroids			
1. Allethrin	• Baygon mats, Pynamin forte.	1. **Skin contact:** Dermatitis, blistering	1. **Skin contact** Decontaminate with soap and water Topical application of alpha tocopherol acetate (Vit E) may reduce the severity.[12]
2. D-allethrin	• Baygon knock out aerosol, Baygon power mats, Good night mats, Hit insect repellant.	2. **Eye contact:** Irritation	2. **Eye contact:** Irrigate with normal saline or water for 10–15 min
3. **Cypermethrin**	• Agrocyper, Basathrin, Bilsif, Challanger, Irrigate with normal saline Cilcord,Cybil, Cymbush, Cymet, Cymperm, Cyper, Cannon, Cyperguard, Cyperhit, Cyperin, Cypermethrin sandoz, Cypermil, Cypersul, Cyrux, Gilcyp Tech, Hilcyperin, Ustad, Hypowder, Hyper, Motal, Parathrin, Ralathin, Ramceper, Ripcord, Shakti, Sicerin,Vegfrucott, Starcyprin, Superkiller-25, Tackle	3. **Inhalation:** Increase nasal secretion, sneezing, coughing, dyspnea, sore throat, wheezing	3. **Systemic poisoning: stomach wash with** NS/KMnO$_4$ or activated charcoal
4. Decamethrin	• Decamethrin	4. **Ingestion:** Hypersecretion, nausea, vomiting, salivation, paresthesia, vertigo, fasciculation, hyperthermia, altered mental status, cramp, spasm, convulsions, coma	4. Oxygen and ventilator support
5. Deltamethrin	• Decis, Hexit, K-Othrin		5. Bronchodilator for bronchospasm
6. Fenvalerate	• Agrofen, Caovalerate, Fencidin, Fenhit, Fenkill, Fenval, Fighter, Gilfen, Parafen, Starfen, Sumicidin, Sumitox, Trumpcard.		6. Diazepam for convulsions
7. Fluvalinate	• Marvik		7. **Do not give oil-based cathertics/demulcent. Atropine is given only if needed for hyper-secretion and pulmonary edema**
8. Permethrin	• Ambush, Lee, Permaseet, Permethrin, Pounce		8. **Oximes (PAM): No role in T/t**
9. Pyrethrum	• Tortoise mosquito coil		9. Adrenaline and antihistaminic for allergic reaction
10. Alpha methrin	• Alpha guard, Farssa, Axis		10. **Mats and coils:** Wait and watch, symptomatic treatment

ORGANOPHOSPHATES	ORGANOCHLORINES
Organophosphorus compounds are deadly toxic to human beings and also most effective as insecticidal agents. Hence, they are most popular and most widely used insecticides in India. They are broadly classified into two main groups: a. Alkyl group—**chloropyriphos, dimethoate,** indoxacarb, malathion, **monocrotophos (nuvacron), quinolphos, temefox,** triazophos b. Aryl group—parathion, methyl parathion, **diazinon, chlorothion** c. Others—**phorate**, methyl demeton, phosphamidon	Organochlorine (OC) pesticides used successfully in controlling a number of diseases, such as malaria and typhus, were banned or restricted after the 1960s in most of the technologically advanced countries.[13] But due to low cost and need against various pests, they are among the widely used pesticides in developing countries of Asia.[14,15] There are 4 distinct categories of these pesticides: 1. DDT and analogues—e.g. **DDT** (dichloro-diphenyltrichloroethane), and methoxychlor 2. Benzene hexachloride group—e.g. benzenehexachloride (**BHC**), and gamma-hexachloro-cyclohexane (**lindane**) 3. Cyclodienes and related compounds—e.g. aldrin, dieldrin, **endosulfan (thiodan), endrin**, isobenzan, chlordane, heptachlor. 4. Toxaphene compounds—e.g. toxaphene
Physical appearance These compounds are available as dusts, granules, or liquids. Some products need to be diluted with water before use, and some are burnt to make smoke that kills insects. Kerosene and turpentine oil is used as a solvent	**Physical appearance** These compounds are available as dusting powders, wet powders, emulsions, granules, and solutions. They are insoluble in water but soluble in kerosene, benzene, chloroform and ethyl alcohol. DDT is a white crystalline, slightly volatile solid having a faint smell.
Uses Mainly used in agricultural field as insecticide.	**Uses** 1. Insecticide at home (and in gardens agricultural fields), used to kill mosquitoes, flies, fleas and cockroaches. 2. Gamma benzene hexachloride is used in the treatment of scabies and head lice. It is available as topical ointment, cream, or lotion
Fatal dose[16] • **Highly toxic:** Parathion/systox: 15 to 30 mg **Phosdrin/pestox:** 200 mg; **TEPP:** 5 gm • **Moderately toxic:** Diazinon—10 to 25 gm • **Mildly toxic:** Chlorthion, malathion, dipterex –25 to 60 gm	**Fatal dose**[16] • **DDT, lindane:** 15 to 30 gm • **Chlordane:** 5–7 gm • **Aldrin, dieldrin, endrin:** 2 to 5 gm
Fatal period: 30 min to 3 hours	**Fatal period:** Within 24 hours

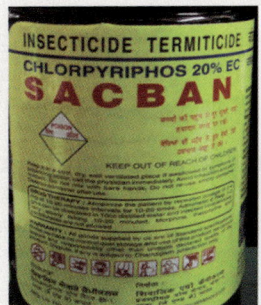 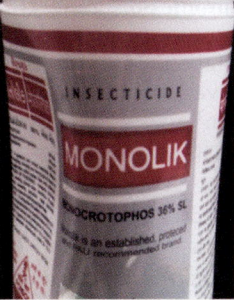 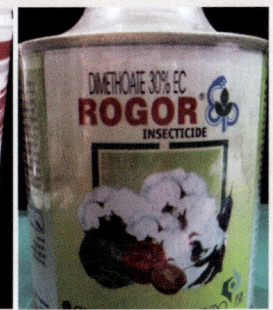 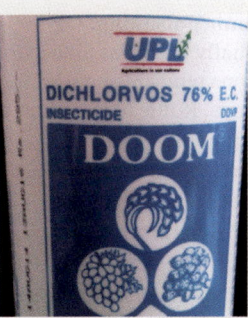

Absorption, fate, excretion:[16] OP
- Absorbed through mucosa of GIT, RT, and through skin and through direct injection
- Parathion is first stored in the body fat and is slowly released in the circulation. It is metabolized first to paraoxon and then to par-anitrophenol, which is excreted through urine
- Malathion is metabolized in liver by esterase and is excreted through urine

Absorption, fate, excretion:[16] OC
- Absorbed through mucosa of GIT, RT, and through skin and through direct injection either as such or when mixed with kerosene or other solvent.
- Most of the hydrocarbons are metabolised slowly and deposited mainly in the body fat and also in liver, kidneys and brain for prolonged periods. They are excreted through urine, milk, and feces

Action

$$\text{Acetylcholine} \xrightarrow[\text{enzyme}]{\text{ACh-esterase}} \text{Acetic acid + choline}$$

1. On ANS: **OP inhibits** the **acetylcholinesterase** enzyme[17] by phosphorylation of serine moiety at myoneural junction and synapses of ganglion. **As a result, there is decrease in the level of serum cholinesterase enzyme and an accumulation of acetylcholine** at nerve ending producing parasympathomimetic action. The action is both muscarinic (postganglionic) and nicotinic (preganglionic)
2. On CNS, the action is depression

Action

1. DDT and like substance affect the sodium channel and sodium conductance across the neuronal membrane especially of the axon[18]
2. They also alter the metabolism of serotonin, norepinephrine, and acetylcholine
3. The cyclodienes[18] and lindane appear to inhibit the GABA-mediated chloride channels in the CNS
4. CNS stimulant and death by overstimulation

Clinical features (Table 8.1)
Acute poisoning: Poisoning may occur through ingestion, inhalation, or absorption through skin.
  A. **ANS:** Parasympathomimetic action:
  1. Muscarinic effects*—nausea, vomiting, diarrhea, abdominal pain, colic, salivation, lacrimation **(increased tears which may be red due to porphyrin),** called chromo-lachyrorrhea,[19] profuse sweating, **Constriction of pupils,** bronchoconstriction (with increased bronchial secretion, wheezing and dyspnea, cough, pulmonary edema), garlicky smell in breath, muscle weakness, slow pulse, bradycardia, hypotension, and urinary incontinence*
  2. Nicotinic effects—fasciculation, weakness, hypertension, tachycardia, and paralysis.
  B. **CNS effects:** CNS depression

Clinical features (Table 8.2)
Acute poisoning
1. **GIT:** Nausea, vomiting, diarrhea, hyperesthesia or paresthesia of the mouth and face with peculiar smell
2. **CNS:** Confusion, headache, dizziness, vertigo, tremor, twitching, convulsion, myoclonus, rapid and dysrhythmic eye movements, **dilatation of pupils, weakness, and agitation**
3. **Other systems:** Fever, aspiration pneumonitis, renal failure

---

* Often summarized in the mnemonic (**DUMBELS**—**D**iarrhea, **U**rination, **M**iosis, **B**ronchospasm, **E**mesis, **L**acrimation, **S**alivation) or **SLUDGE**[7,8]—**S**alivation, **L**acrimation, **U**rination, **D**yspnea, **G**IT distress (N, V, AP, D), **E**xtramiosis, profuse sweating, muscle weakness, slow pulse, fall in HR and BP, and bronchoconstriction

Chronic poisoning: OP

It usually occurs as an occupational hazard in persons who are engaged in pesticide spraying of crops. Route of exposure is usually inhalation or contamination of skin

Following are the main features:

1. **Polyneuropathy:** Paresthesias, muscle cramps, weakness, gait disorders
2. **CNS effects:** Drowsiness, confusion, irritability, anxiety, psychiatric manifestations

Chronic poisoning: OC

It occurs due to long-term exposure to some of these compounds results in cumulative toxicity. There may be vague neurological symptoms and toxic rash in the skin[16]

There may be irritability, fatigability, lack of interest and concentration, loss of weight/appetite, tremor, ataxia, abnormal mental changes, oligospermia

There is increased tendency to leukemias, thrombocytopenic purpura and aplastic anemia. Cancer is known to be associated with use of different OCs.[20]

Diagnosis (Tables 8.1 and 8.2)

1. In the diagnosis of organophosphate poisoning, history and clinical manifestation play an important role along with decreased in serum cholinesterase enzyme level. Every effort should be made to extract information regarding name, type, or trade name of consumed poison from every possible source (patient, relatives, and friends). This information is beneficial for treatment purpose.

2. Decrease in red cell and serum cholinesterase level:[9] For the purpose of estimation of cholinesterase level, blood should be collected only in heparinized tubes and frozen. At autopsy,[21] 5 ml of blood is collected directly from the heart in plain bulb and centrifuge at 3000 RPM for 15 min. Supernatant fluid is collected in separate plastic tube and stored at 2–7°C. Serum cholinesterase level is measured by colorimetric method by using kit.[21]

   a. If the RBC cholinesterase level is less than 50% of normal, it indicates organophosphate toxicity. However, a very low cholinesterase level does not always correlate with clinical illness. False decrease of RBC cholinesterase level is seen in pernicious anemia, hemoglobinopathies, anti-malarial treatment, and blood collected in oxalate tubes

   b. Decrease of plasma cholinesterase level less than 50% of normal is a less reliable indicator of organophosphate toxicity, but is easier to assay and more commonly done. Plasma cholinesterase activity is depressed in cirrhosis, neoplasia, malnutrition, and infections

3. **Urinary P-nitrophenol test:**[9] P-nitrophenol is a metabolite of some organophosphates (e.g. parathion, ethion), and is excreted in the urine. The test can also be done on vomitus or stomach contents.

   Procedure: Steam distill 10 ml of urine (or vomitus or stomach contents). Add NaOH (2 pellets) and heat on a water bath for 10 minutes. Production of yellow color indicates the presence of p-nitrophenol.

Treatment (Tables 8.1 and 8.2)

Treatment for organophosphates

a. **Atropine:** It blocks the muscarinic manifestations of organophosphates but does not reverse nicotinic action; and higher dose is required to antagonize the central effects.[6]

   Dose:[6] 2 mg IV every 10 minutes till dryness of mouth or other signs of atropinization appears (up to 200 mg in a day). Continued treatment with maintenance dose for 1–2 weeks.

b. **Cholinesterase reactivators (Oximes):**[6] Oximes are used to restore neuromuscular transmission only in case of organophosphate anti-ChE poisoning. Pralidoxime (pyridine-2-aldoxime methiodide; 2-PAM) has a positive charged quaternary nitrogen attaches to the anionic site of the enzymes which remains unoccupied in the presence of organophosphate inhibitors. It is available in 500 mg PAM tabs for oral use; inj PAM-A of 500 mg in 20 ml for IV use.

   Dose:[6] 1–2 gm in 100 ml of normal saline given slow IV infusion (20–40 mg/kg in children), repeated according to the need (max 12 gm in first 24 hours). Or another regime is 30 mg/kg IV loading dose followed by 8–10 mg/kg/hr continuous infusion till recovery.

c. **Prevention of further exposure:** Patient should not be re-exposed for at least a few weeks

d. **Prophylaxis:** Use protective clothes; spraying against direction of wind flow and move backward; No smoking, eating, drinking at workplace; spraying not >2 hr/day for >6 days/week[16]; intermittent medical check up; proper washing of hands and face after spraying; immune-compromised/ill/injured person should avoid spraying.

Table 8.4: Atropine and oximes in the treatment of different groups of insecticidal poisoning

Groups	Atropine	Oximes
Organophosphorus (OP)	Antidote	Antidote
Organochlorines (OC)	Do not give	No role in treatment
Carbamates	Antidote	Contraindicated
Pyrethroids	Given only if needed	No role in treatment

In OC:[10] Do not give **epinephrine or atropine unless absolutely necessary**, because of the enhanced myocardial irritability induced by chlorinated hydrocompound, which predispose to ventricular fibrillation. Do not give **oil-based cathartics/demulcent** as they enhance absorption.

PM findings
1. Characteristic odor (garlicky) near mouth
2. Frothing at mouth and nose—blood stained
3. Cyanosis of extremities
4. **Constricted pupils**
5. It resists decomposition and can be easily detected even in putrefied bodies
6. Stomach—garlicky or kerosene/turpentine like odor of solvent and content, mucosa-congested, hemorrhagic
7. Pulmonary and cerebral edema
8. Froth in the respiratory tract
9. Visceral organs are congested

PM findings
1. Characteristic odor (chlorinated/pungent)
2. Discharge of bloodstained froth from nose and mouth
3. Cyanosis and s/o asphyxia
4. **Dilatation of pupils**
5. Detected even in putrefied bodies
6. Stomach—chlorinated or kerosene/turpentine smell of solvent and content, mucosa-congested, hemorrhagic
7. Lungs—congested, edematous, subpleural hemorrhagic spots
8. Froth in the respiratory tract
9. Visceral organs are congested, brain—edema.
10. Liver, kidneys, adrenal—fatty degeneration

A useful postmortem finding in insecticidal poisoning case infested with flies at mortuary is that some of these flies after settling on decomposed body may subsequently die and found on the body.

In death during spraying of insecticide in the field, the nasal swab, blood and lung should be preserved for toxicological analysis. The insecticide poison may not be detected in routine viscera in such case and chemical analyser's report is negative.

ML aspects
1. **Suicidal:** Common in India both rural and urban areas
2. **Homicidal:** Not occur due to detectable smell of solvent. However, a few cases have been reported
3. **Accidental:** Mainly to manufacturer, packers, sprayers in the fields, and also due to contaminated food grains

ML aspects
1. **Suicidal:** Common, more in rural areas
2. **Homicidal:** Very rare where the smell of kerosene is masked by alcohol
3. **Accidental:** Usually in children, and one who handle the poison

Stomach in Insecticidal Poisoning (Courtesy—Dr. Barmate/Dr. Tumram) (Figs 8.1 to 8.6)

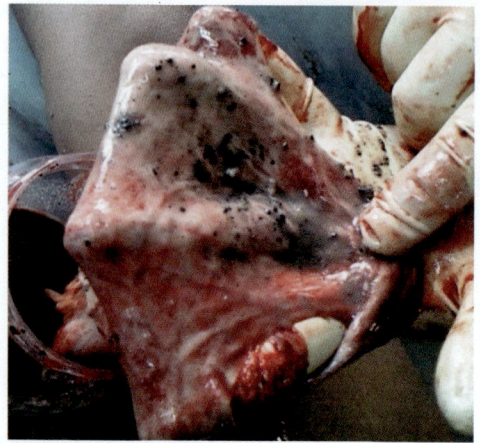

Fig. 8.1: Phorate poisoning (OP)

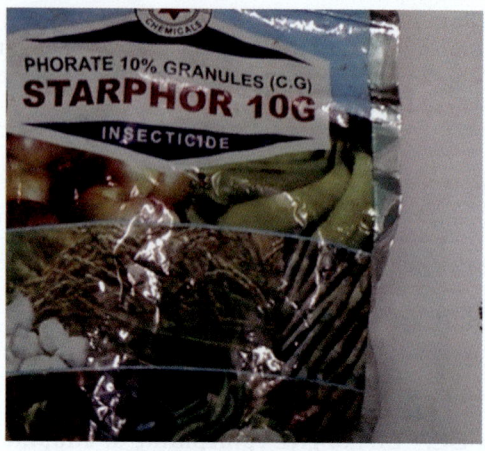

Fig. 8.2: Phorate granules

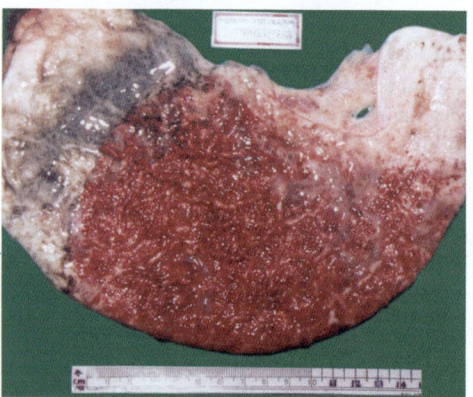

Fig. 8.3: Monocrotophos—Nuvacron poisoning (OP)

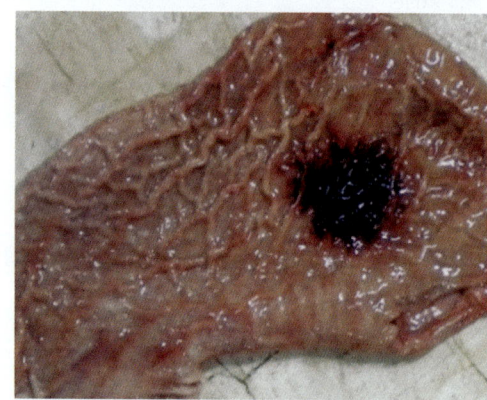

Fig. 8.4: Dimethoate—Rogar poisoning (OP)

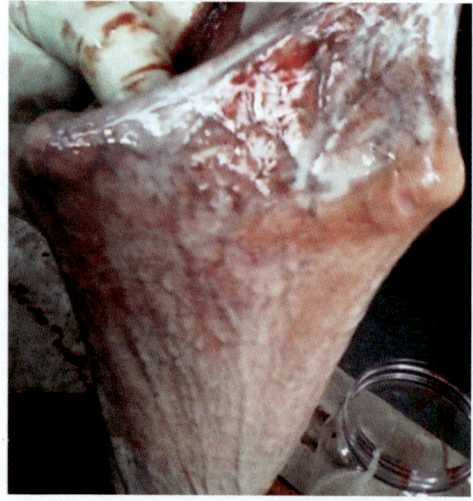

Fig. 8.5: Endrin poisoning (OC)

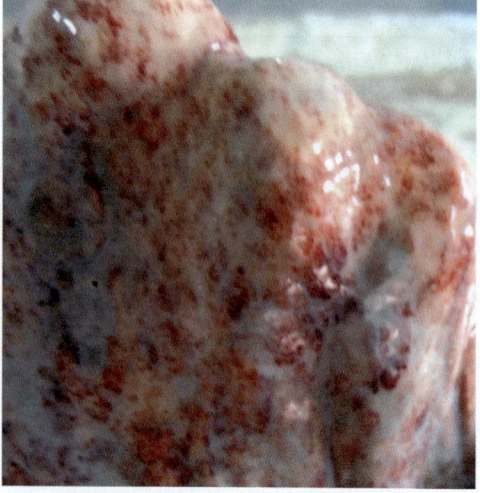

Fig. 8.6: Endosulphan—thiodan poisoning

CARBAMATES	PYRETHRINS AND PYRETHROIDS
They are as popular as organophosphates in their role as insecticides and share a number of similarities	Pyrethrins are active extracts of the Chrysanthemum plant (*Chrysanthemum cinerariaefolium*), and include pyrethrum and piperonyl butoxide. Most mammals are resistant since they can rapidly metabolize and detoxify these agents.
Properties They are available as liquids, sprays, dusts and powders	**Properties** They are available as liquids, sprays, dusts, powders, mats, and coils
Uses Apart from insecticidal use, these are used to kill insect and ants in household spray	**Uses** These compounds are used as insect repellants and insecticides in household sprays, mosquito coils, and mats They are also used to prevent pest infestation in granaries and in agriculture as pesticides
Fatal dose • Highly toxic: Carbaryl, carbofuran, methomyl, propoxur. • Moderately/slightly toxic: Aldicarb, carbendazim, triallate **Fatal period:** Uncertain	**Fatal dose** • Pyrethrum has an LD50 of over 1 gm/kg. • Most cases of toxicity are actually the result of allergic reactions **Fatal period:** Uncertain
Action Carbamates (like organophosphates) are inhibitors of acetylcholinesterase, but carbamylate the serine moiety at the active site instead of phosphorylation.[9] This binding is of reversible type and so the clinical features are less severe and of shorter duration.	**Action** Pyrethroids prolong the inactivation of the sodium channel by binding to it in the open state. Type II agents are more potent in this regard, and also act by inhibiting GABA-mediated inhibitory chloride channels
Clinical features: • The clinical manifestations of carbamate poisoning are very **similar to organophosphate poisoning but symptoms are less severe and of shorter duration** • Salivation, lacrimation, sweating, vomiting, diarrhea, slow pulse, low BP, weakness, twitching, convulsion	**Clinical features:**[12] 1. **Skin contact:** Dermatitis, blistering 2. **Eye contact:** Irritation 3. **Inhalation:** Rhinorrhoea, sore throat, wheezing, dyspnea 4. **Ingestion:** Increased salivation, nausea, vomiting, abdominal pain, mouth ulceration, dysphagia. 5. **Systemic effects:** Headache, dizziness, fatigue, palpitation, chest tightness, vertigo, fasciculation, hyperthermia, altered mental status, convulsion, coma.
Diagnosis 1. Blood cholinesterase **level is decreased** 2. X-ray may reveal the presence of certain radiopaque carbamates 3. Carbamates can be detected in serum, adipose tissue and urine by gas chromatography	**Diagnosis** 1. Blood cholinesterase **levels are normal** 2. ECG may demonstrate ST-T changes, sinus tachycardia, and ventricular premature beats 3. Thin layer chromatography

Treatment (Table 8.3):	Treatment (Table 8.3):
• Inj. PAM is contraindicated in cases of poisoning with carbamate compounds • But, IV atropine is useful	• Inj. PAM—no role in treatment. • Atropine is given only if needed for hyper-secretion and pulmonary edema

In carbamate poisoning treatment: An important differentiating point from organophosphates is that oximes are generally not recommended, while atropine can be given. *Pralidoxime is ineffective as an antidote to carbamate anti-ChEs (carbaryl, propoxur, physostigmine, neostigmine) in which case the anionic site of the enzyme is not free to provide attachment to it. It is rather* **contraindicated** *in carbamate poisoning, as it does not reactivate carbamylated enzyme, but it has weak anti-ChE activity of its own.*[6] Oximes given in carbamate poisoning leads to the production of carbamylated oximes which may be more potent acetylcholinesterase inhibitor than carbaryl itself.[9]

PM findings	PM findings
1. Characteristic odor (peculiar or kerosene like) near mouth	1. Characteristic odor (garlicky or kerosene like) near mouth
2. Blood stained frothing at mouth and nose	2. Blood stained frothing at mouth and nose
3. Cyanosis of extremities	3. Cyanosis of extremities
4. **Stomach:** Mucosa congestion with kerosene-like odor of contents	4. Stomach: Mucosa congestion with characteristic odor of contents
5. Pulmonary and cerebral edema	5. Pulmonary and cerebral edema
6. Froth in the respiratory tract	6. Froth in the respiratory tract
7. Generalized visceral congestion	7. Generalized visceral congestion

ML aspects	ML aspects
1. Suicidal: Usually	1. Suicidal: May occur
2. Accidental: Common	2. Accidental: Common in children due to consumption of mats and coils

Carbamate and Pyrethroids (Figs 8.7 to 8.13)

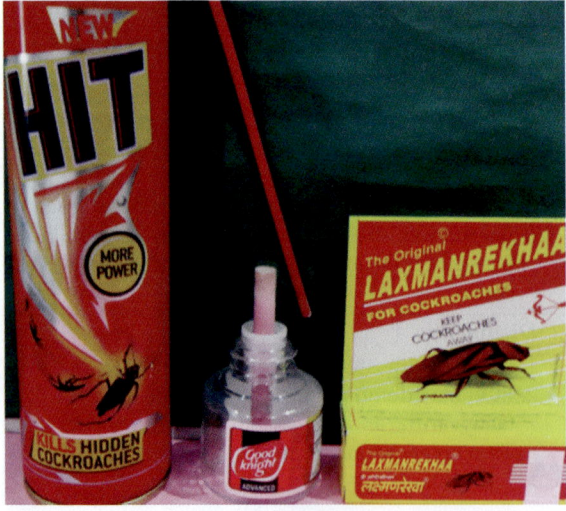

Fig. 8.7: Cypermethrin/allethrin

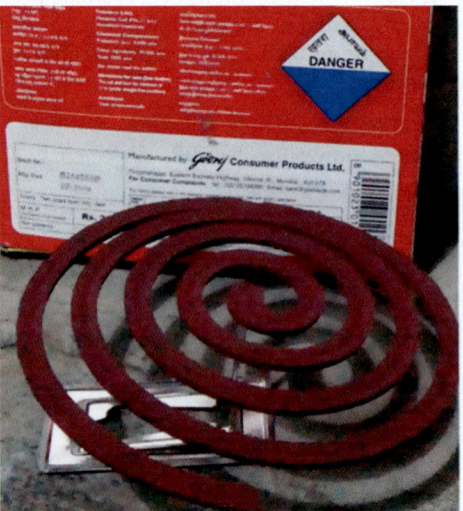

Fig. 8.8: Pyrethrum

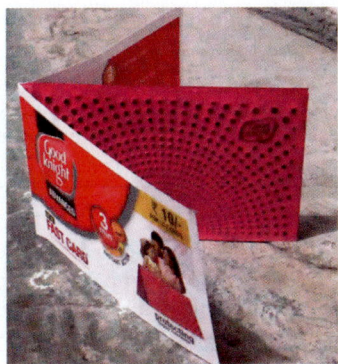

Fig. 8.9: Transfluthrin

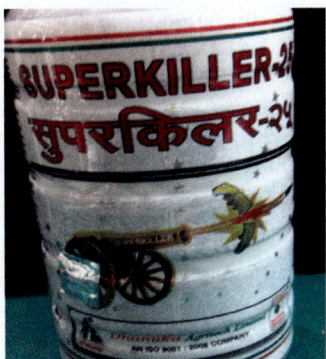

Fig. 8.10: Cypermethrin

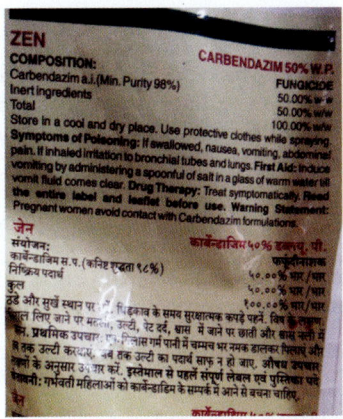

Fig. 8.11: Carbendazim (carbamates)

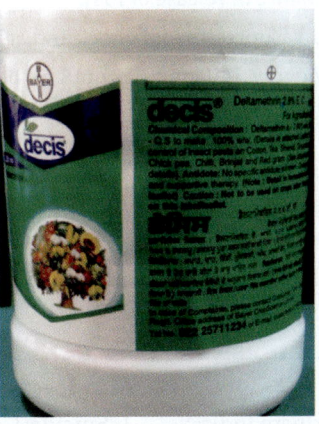

Fig. 8.12: Deltamethrin

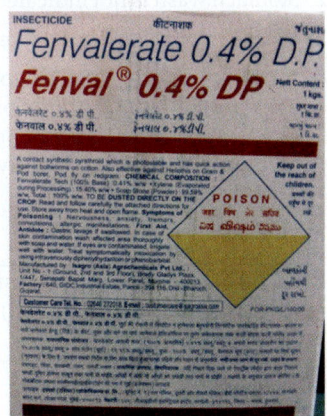

Fig. 8.13: Fenvalerate

Rodenticidal Agents (Figs 8.16 and 8.17)

ALUMINIUM PHOSPHIDE	ZINC PHOSPHIDE
Preparations: Alphos, Celphos, Phosfume, Phostoxin, Phosphotek, Quickphos, etc.	**Preparations:** Synphos, Ratol, Sudharshan
They are available as greenish grey tablets of aluminium phosphide urea and ammonium carbonate. They have **garlic smell**. On exposure to air, it releases phosphine,[9] ammonia and carbon dioxide $AlP + 3H_2O \rightarrow Al(OH)_3 + PH_3$	It is a steel grey, crystalline powder with **fishy smell**. It also releases phosphine. It is used as fumigant to control insects and rodents $ZnP + 3H_2O \rightarrow Zn(OH)_3 + PH_3$
Action: It acts by blocking the cytochrome C oxidase enzyme and inhibiting oxidative phosphorylation which eventually leads to cell death.[22,23]	
Fatal dose: One tablet (3 gm) **Fatal period:** 12–24 hours	**Fatal dose:** 5 gm **Fatal period:** 24 hours

Uses: For protecting stored grain (rice tablet)[23], rodenticidal

- It is used as fumigant to control insects and rodents (rodenticidal)

Clinical features:[22,24] Nausea, vomiting, diarrhea, epigastric pain, dizziness, restlessness, cyanosis, rapid respiration, with garlicky/fishy odor breath, dyspnea, tachycardia, cardiac arrhythmia, peripheral circulatory failure, convulsion, coma. Death is due to circulatory failure.

Diagnosis:

Garlicky odor, ECG changes (sinus tachycardia, ST-T wave changes, bradycardia, heart block), Silver Nitrate test:[9,25] When a patient is asked to breath in and out through a piece of filter paper impregnated with 0.1N silver nitrate solution for 5–10 min, then the filter paper turns black due to the presence of phosphine in the breath which reduces silver nitrate to silver. This test is also positive for hydrogen sulphide.

Treatment:[9,22]

1. Fresh air.

2. Stomach wash is not indicated—chance of release of PH_3.

3. IV fluids, sodium bicarbonate and vasopressors for shock and acidosis.

4. Additionally, 1 mg of glucagon IV every 5–10 minutes until his blood pressure becomes control followed by 4 mg/hr slow IV infusion. Subsequently, digoxin (0.5 mg), magnesium sulfate (1 gm), calcium gluconate (1 gm), hydrocortisone (200 mg) given every 6 hourly with vit C (1000 mg), vit E (400 unit IM) and N-acetylcysteine 140 mg/kg orally as a loading dose followed by 70 mg/kg orally every 4–6 hrly for 4–5 days.[9,22]

5. Hemodialysis.

PM findings: Garlicky/fishy smell in the stomach with mucosal haemorrhage (Figs 8.14 and Fig 8.15), visceral organs—congested; Liver and kidneys—necrotic changes; pulmonary edema, toxic myocarditis

ML aspects	ML aspects
1. Suicide: Common, usually in Northern India[24]	**1. Suicide:** Commonly in young age.
2. Homicidal: Not used.	**2. Homicidal:** Not used
3. Accidental: Rare, usually in children.	**3. Accidental:** Rare, usually in children.

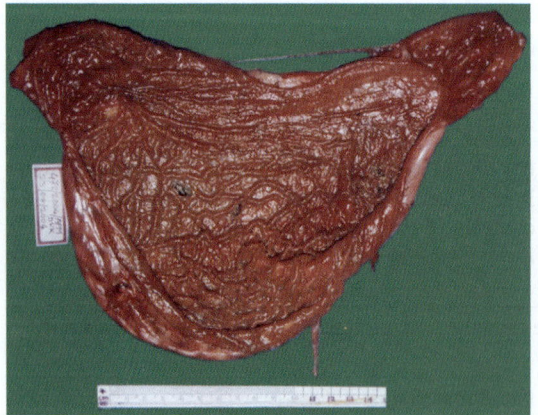

Fig. 8.14: Stomach in zinc phosphide poisoning

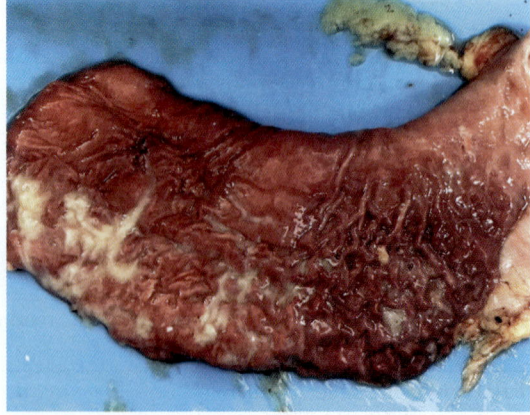

Fig. 8.15: Stomach in aluminium phosphide poisoning

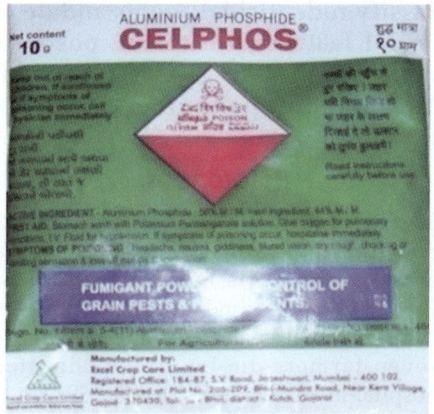

Fig. 8.16: Aluminium phosphide

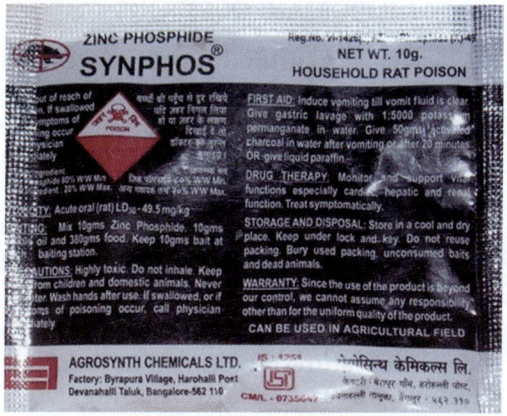

Fig. 8.17: Zinc phosphide

Other Pesticides: Fungicidal and Herbicidal *(Figs 8.18 to 8.22)*

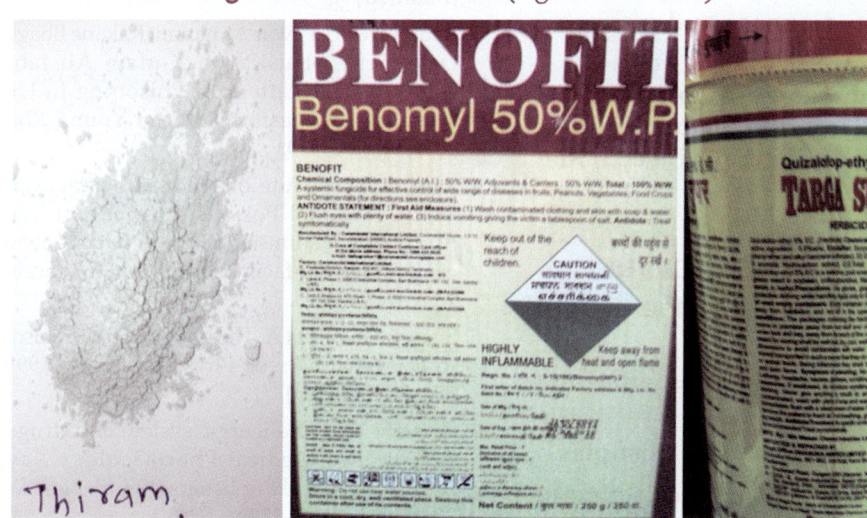

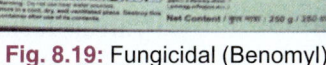

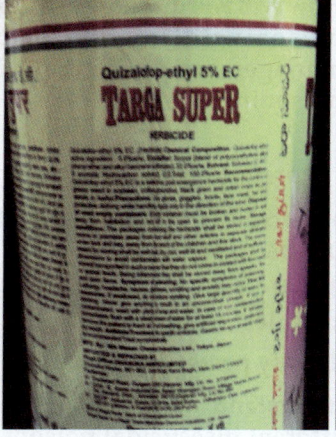

Fig. 8.18: Fungicidal (Devithiram)

Fig. 8.19: Fungicidal (Benomyl)

Fig. 8.20: Herbicidal (Quizolofeb)

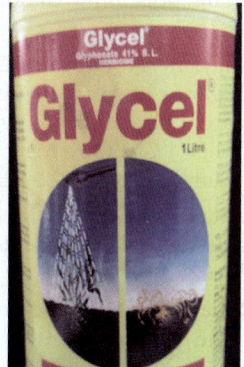

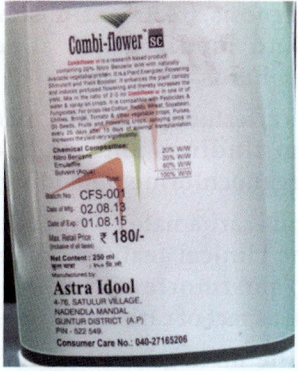

Fig. 8.21: Herbicidal (Glyphosphate)

Fig. 8.22: Flowering stimulant (Nitrobenzene)

IMPORTANT QUESTIONS

1. Classify agricultural poisons. Describe mechanism of action, clinical features, treatment, laboratory diagnosis and autopsy findings of organophosphorus poisoning.

2. Classify pesticides. Describe clinical features, treatment and autopsy findings of organochlorine poisoning.

3. Classify insecticidal poisons. Describe clinical features, treatment and autopsy findings of carbamate poisoning.

4. Classify rodenticidal agents. Describe clinical manifestation, treatment and medicolegal aspect of rodenticidal poisoning.

5. How will you diagnose and manage a case of baygon poisoning?

6. How will you diagnose a case of insecticidal poisoning? Describe in brief about management of different insecticidal poisoning.

SPECIFIC LEARNING OBJECTIVES

After reading this chapter, the reader should be able to:

- Classify insecticidal poisons with their examples

- Classify pesticides with their examples

- Understand the mechanism of action of different insecticidal poisons

- Enumerate different organophosphorus compounds and describe the clinical features, diagnosis, treatment, postmortem findings and medicolegal aspect of organophosphorus poisoning

- Explain clinical features, diagnosis, treatment, postmortem findings and medicolegal aspect of organochlorine poisoning

- Enlist various carbamate compounds and describe the clinical features, diagnosis, treatment, postmortem findings and medicolegal aspect of carbamate poisoning

- Delineate the management of different insecticidal poisoning

- Classify rodenticidal agents and describe clinical features, treatment, postmortem findings and medicolegal aspect of aluminium/ zinc phosphide poisoning

References

1. Seven farmers die, hundreds admitted to hospital in Yavatmal district after inhaling insecticide spray. The Indian Express. Dated 23/Feb/2019. https://indianexpress.com /article/cities/mumbai/maharashtra-insecticide-spray-seven-farmers-die-hundreds-admitted-to-hospital-in-yavatmal-district-4866394/

2. Thundiyil JG, Stober J, Besbelli N, Pronczuk J. Acute pesticide poisoning: a proposed classification tool. Bull World Health Organ 2008;86:205–9. [PubMed]

3. Raut Asawari, Pawar Atmaram, Kakane Bhagwan, Dave Priti, Shaj Kavya, Gulam Ali Jabeen. Toxicological Pattern of Poisoning in Urban Hospitals of Western India. J Young Pharm, 2017; 9(3):315–20.

4. All India Institute of Medical Sciences, New Delhi. National Poisons Information Centre. http://www.aiims.edu/en/departments-and-centers/central-facilities.html?id=167 (accessed 18 August 2016).

5. Siwach SB, Gupta A. The profile of acute poisoning in Haryana. J Assoc Physicians India.1995;13: 756–9. [PubMed]

6. Tripathi KD. Cholinergic system and drugs. In: Essential of Medical Pharmacology. Jaypee Brothers Medical Publishers (P) Ltd: New Delhi, 7th edn, 2014:99–112.

7. Organophosphate poisoning: diagnosis and treatment. https://www.openanesthesia.org/organophosphate_poisoning_diagnosis_and_treatment/

8. Peter JV, Sudarsan TI, Moran JL. Clinical features of organophosphate poisoning: A review of different classification systems and approaches. Indian J Crit Care Med. 2014 Nov; 18(11): 735–45. doi: [10.4103/0972–5229.144017]

9. Pillay VV. Textbook of Forensic Medicine and Toxicology. Paras Medical Publisher: Hyderabad, 17th edn, 2016: 602–17.

10. Reigart JR, Roberts JR. Organochlorines. In: Recognition and Management of Pesticide Poisonings. 6th Ed., 2013. Published by: Office of Pesticide Programs, US Environmental Protection

Agency, Washington. Pg: 63–9. https://www2.epa.gov/pesticide-worker-safety

11. Cohn WJ, Boylan JJ, Blanke RV, Fariss MW, Howell JR, Guzelian PS. Treatment of chlordecone (Kepone) toxicity with cholestyramine. Results of a controlled clinical trial. N Engl J Med. Feb 2 1978;298(5):243–8.

12. Bradberry SM, Cage SA, Proudfoot AT, Vale JA. Poisoning due to pyrethroids. Toxicol Rev. 2005;24(2):93–106.

13. Aktar MW, Sengupta D, Chowdhury A. Impact of pesticides use in agriculture: their benefits and hazards. Interdiscip Toxicol. 2009 Mar; 2(1): 1–12. doi: [10.2478/v10102-009-0001-7]

14. FAO. Proceedings of the Asia Regional Workshop. Bangkok: Regional Office for Asia and the Pacific; 2005.

15. Gupta PK. Pesticide exposure—Indian scene. Toxicology. 2004;198:83–90. [PubMed]

16. Nandy A. Principles of Forensic Medicine. New Central Book Agency (P) Ltd: Calcutta, 2nd edn Reprint, 2004:491–7.

17. Lotti M. Clinical toxicology of anticholinesterase agents in humans. In: Krieger R, editor. Handbook of pesticide toxicology. Volume 2. Agents. 2 edn. Academic Press; San Diego: 2001. pp. 1043–85.

18. J R Coats. Mechanisms of toxic action and structure activity relationships for Organochlorine and synthetic pyrethroid insecticides. Environmental Health Perspectives. 1990;87:255–62.doi: 10.1289/ehp.9087255.

19. Dikshit PC. Textbook of Forensic Medicine and Toxicology. 2nd edn, PEEPEE Publisher and Distributors (P) Ltd. New Delhi. 2014:587–96

20. Zorawar Singh, Jasminder Kaur, Ravneet Kaur, Swarndeep Singh Hundal.Toxic Effects of Organochlorine Pesticides: A Review. American Journal of BioScience. 2016;4(3–1)11–8.

21. Kukde HV, Ambade VN, Batra AK, Keoliya AN. Significance of serum cholinesterase level in organophosphorus poisoning. Medicolegal update 2012; 12(2):70–4.

22. Oghabian Z, Mehrpour O. Treatment of Aluminium Phosphide Poisoning with a Combination of Intravenous Glucagon, Digoxin and Antioxidant Agents. Sultan Qaboos Univ Med J. 2016 Aug; 16(3): e352–5. doi: [10.18295/squmj.2016.16.03.015]

23. Mehrpour O, Singh S. Rice tablet poisoning: a major concern in Iranian population. Hum Exp Toxicol. 2010 Aug; 29(8):701–2. [PubMed] [Ref list]

24. Gurjar M, Baronia AK, Azim A, Sharma K. Managing aluminum phosphide poisonings. J Emerg Trauma Shock. 2011 Jul; 4(3):378–84. [PubMed] [Ref list]

25. Bardale R. Principles of Forensic Medicine and Toxicology. 1st edn, Jaypee Brothers Medical Publishers (P) Ltd: New Delhi. 2011: 490–9.

Plant and Vegetable Irritants

These are the organic irritants derived from poisonous plant and vegetables. There are various plants/vegetables that are poisonous/toxic to human beings. The study of plant poison which produces toxic effect on human is called phytotoxicology and its poison is referred to as phytotoxins.[1] Based on their toxic effects, poisonous plants are classified as:

1. Gastrointestinal irritant: Abrus, ricin, etc.
2. Neurotoxin: Opium, datura, cannabis, nux vomica.
3. Cardiotoxic: Aconite, olender, quinine, tobacco.
4. Contact poison: Poison ivy, sumac, mango, cashewnut.
5. Airborne allergic: *Acer negundo* (box elder).

Some of the plants whose toxic part on ingestion causes gastrointestinal irritation are only included in this chapter. Vegetable irritants are *Abrus precatorius, Ricinus communis, Croton tiglium, Semicarpus anacardium,* Calotropis, *Plumbago rosea*, Capsicum.

Toxalbumin[2] is the toxic protein present in some of the vegetable irritants. The action resembles the action of bacterial toxin, e.g. Ricin, Abrin, Crotin, Snake venom.

It is antigenic in nature and capable of producing specific antibodies when injected into the body. It causes agglutination, haemolysis and cell destruction.[2,3]

Abrus precatorius	Ricinus communis	Croton tiglium
Synonyms: Rati, Gunj, Kunch, Crab eyes, Precatorius beans, Lucky beans	**Synonyms:** Castor, Arandi	**Synonyms:** Croton, Jamalgota
Toxic parts: Seeds. **Seeds:** Small beautiful, glossy bright red/brownish/faint yellow with black head, and weigh 102 mg	**Toxic parts:** Seeds. **Seeds:** Small/big (2 varieties) brownish oval glossy seeds with yellowish marking	**Toxic parts:** All part of plant (max. conc. in oil and seeds) **Seeds:** Small dark brown oval matt/dull dusty seeds
Uses 1. Decoration purpose 2. To weigh gold by goldsmith 3. Have hair promoting factor 4. Antifertility effects 5. Leaves used in paan masala	**Uses** 1. Purgatives 2. Ayurvedic medicine—for arthritis 3. Bland oil 4. Cream for sole crack	**Uses** 1. Strong purgatives 2. Ayurvedic medicine—for arthritis 3. For creating comedy scenes
Active principle: Abrin	**Active principle:** Ricin castor oil—nontoxic	**Active principle:** Crotin, crotonoside croton oil—highly toxic
Action **Local:** Irritation CVS depressant Viper bite like action[4] injected	**Action** Local: Irritation CVS depressant Viper bite like action[4] injected	**Action** **Local:** Irritation CVS depressant

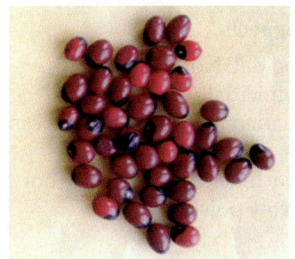

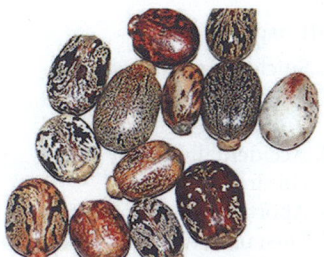

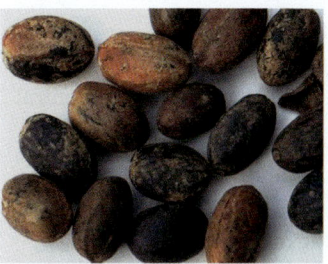

Fig. 9.1: Seeds of Abrus (red and pink variety)

Fig. 9.2: Seeds of Ricinus

Fig. 9.3: Seeds of Croton

Abrus precatorius	*Ricinus communis*	*Croton tiglium*
Fatal dose: 1–2 seeds **Fatal period:** 12 hrs to 3 days	6–8 seeds 12 hrs to 3 days	6–8 seeds 12 hrs to 3 days

Clinical features
1. Local
  a. At the site of injection by *sui*—local severe reaction in the form of inflammation, edema, swelling, oozing, necrosis with evidence of hemolysis (viper bite like)[5]
  b. Conjunctivitis
	Clinical features
	1. Local
	  a. At the site of injection—local severe reaction in the form of inflammation, edema, swelling, oozing, necrosis with evidence of hemolysis (viper bite like).
	  b. Conjunctivitis
		Clinical features
		1. Local: At the site of contact of oil to skin—erythema and blister formation
		
		–

2. Burning pain in mouth/throat, difficulty in speech and deglutition, increase salivation, abdominal pain, nausea, vomiting, diarrhea, dizziness, dyspnea, dilatation of pupil, flushing of face, cold calmy skin, rapid pulse, fall in BP, with muscular weakness, cramps, tremor, convulsion, collapse, coma		
Treatment 1. Local: Wash with soap water, application of bland ointment. 2. Stomach wash 3. Demulcent 4. Supportive 5. Correction of fluids and electrolyte imbalance/circulation[2,6] 6. Antiabrin[2]	**Treatment** 1. Local: Wash with soap water, application of bland ointment. 2. Stomach wash with activated charcoal[6] 3. Demulcent 4. Supportive 5. Correction of fluids and electrolyte imbalance/circulation[2,6,7]	**Treatment** 1. Local: Wash with soap water, application of bland ointment. 2. Stomach wash 3. Demulcent 4. Supportive 5. Maintenance of circulation[2]
PM findings Not specific 1. Local reaction with presence of spike/sui/sutari 2. GIT—inflamed, hemorrhagic, crushed seeds may be present 3. Organs—congested, petechial hemorrhage present	**PM findings** Not specific 1. Local reaction with presence of injection mark 2. GIT—inflamed, hemorrhagic, crushed seeds may be present 3. Organs—congested, petechial hemorrhage present	**PM findings** Not specific 1. Local reaction at the site of contact with oil 2. GIT—inflamed, hemorrhagic, crushed seeds may be present 3. Organs—congested, petechial hemorrhage present

ML aspects	**ML aspects**	**ML aspects**
1. Suicidal: Often used	1. Suicidal: In villages	1. Suicidal: Not common
2. Homicidal: Through parentral route using *sui*.	2. Homicidal: Rare, through umbrella gun[7]	2. Homicidal: Very rare
3. Accidental: Children are attracted towards the seeds	3. Accidental: Usually in children	3. Accidental: Mistaken with castor oil
4. Abortifacient	4. Abortifacient	4. Abortifacient: Using oil, root
5. Arrow poison	5. Dust used to malingerers to produce conjunctivitis	5. Arrow poison
6. Cattle poison		
7. Dust used to malingerers to produce conjunctivitis		

Preparation of *Sui/Sutari* from *Abrus precatorius* seeds

It is prepared by crushing the seeds of Abrus along with datura seeds and opium[2,6] to make it in a powder form, from which paste is formed. *Sui* (needles) of size 1.5 cm × 1 cm is prepared from the paste. These *suis* are then dried and used to kill cattle by keeping it in front of the bamboo stick used to push cattle and also used for homicide purpose by keeping it in between the finger and then slapped over cheek or other parts of body.

Semicarpus anacardium	**Calotropis**	**Plumbago rosea**
Synonyms Marking/dhobi nut, bhela, bhilwan, biba	**Synonyms:** Rui Gigantae—Akand: *Purple* flower Procera—Madar: *White* flower	**Synonyms** Lal chitra
Toxic parts All parts of plant (max. conc. in juice, seeds) Seeds: Black large heart-shaped seeds.	**Toxic parts** All parts of plant (max. conc. in juice, stem, leaves) Seeds: Datura like seeds with cotton fibers at one point in the spindle/crescent-shaped fruit having purple or white flowers	**Toxic parts** All parts of plant (max. conc. in root)
Uses 1. Abdominal pain 2. Ayurvedic medicines 3. Marking over the clothes (brownish-yellow oily juice yields from the pericarp of seeds turns black on exposure to air,[2] so used to write identification number over clothes)	**Uses** 1. Depilatory agent 2. Ayurvedic medicines—by quack 3. Keeps snakes away from area. 4. Flower used for worshipping God (Lord Hanuman/Shiva)	**Use** Ayurvedic medicines—quack
Active principle Semicarpol, Bhilawanol	**Active principle** Calotropin, calotoxin uscharin,[2] gigantin	**Active principle** Plumbagin
Action Local: Irritation CVS depressant	**Action** Local: Irritation CVS depressant	**Action** Local: Irritation CVS depressant
Fatal dose: 6–8 seeds **Fatal period:** 12 hrs to 3 days	**Fatal dose:** Uncertain **Fatal period:** 12 hrs to 3 days	**Fatal dose:** Uncertain **Fatal period:** 12 hrs to 3 days
Clinical features 1. Local: Contact of juice to skin—bruise like painful lesion with marginal small blister called **"Branding"**, the lesion may itch and may ulcerate	**Clinical features** 1. Local: Contact of juice to skin—irritation of skin with blister formation which excoriates later[2]	**Clinical features** 1. Local: Contact of juice to skin—irritation of skin with blister formation which excoriates later[4]

2. Burning pain in mouth/throat, difficulty in speech and deglutition, increase salivation, abdominal pain, nausea, vomiting, diarrhea, dizziness, dyspnea, dilatation of pupil, flushing of face, cold calmy skin, rapid pulse, fall in BP, with muscular weakness, cramps, tremor, convulsion, collapse, coma

Treatment	**Treatment**	**Treatment**
1. Local: Wash with soap water, application of bland ointment	1. Local: Wash with soap water, application of bland ointment	1. Local: Wash with soap water, application of bland ointment
2. Stomach wash	2. Stomach wash	2. Stomach wash
3. Demulcent	3. Demulcent	3. Demulcent
4. Supportive	4. Supportive	4. Supportive
PM findings: Not specific	**PM findings:** Not specific	**PM findings:** Not specific
1. Local reaction	1. Local reaction	1. Local reaction
2. GIT—inflamed, hemorrhagic, crushed seeds may be present	2. GIT—inflamed, hemorrhagic, crushed leaves/stem may be present	2. GIT—inflamed, hemorrhagic, crushed root may be present
3. Organs—congested, petechial hemorrhage present	3. Organs—congested, petechial hemorrhage present	3. Organs—congested, petechial hemorrhage present
ML aspects	**ML aspects**	**ML aspects**
1. Suicidal: Rare	1. Suicidal: Rare	1. Suicidal: Rare
2. Homicidal: Rare	2. Homicidal: Rare	2. Homicidal: Rare
3. Accidental: By mistake, quack medicine	3. Accidental: By mistake, quack medicine	3. Accidental: By mistake, quack medicine
4. Abortifacient	4. Abortifacient: By juice	4. Abortifacient—by root
5. Arrow poison—not used	5. Arrow poison—used	5. Arrow poison—not used
6. Cattle poison—not used	6. Cattle poison—used	6. Cattle poison—used
7. False charge[2]: Juice split on the body to cause injury and make a false charge of assault against enemy	7. False charge: Juice split on the body to cause injury and make a false charge of assault against enemy	7. False charge: Juice split on the body to cause injury and make a false charge of assault against enemy

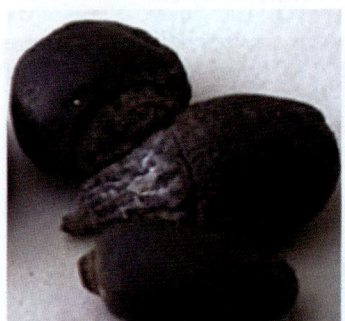

Fig. 9.4: Seeds of Semicarpus

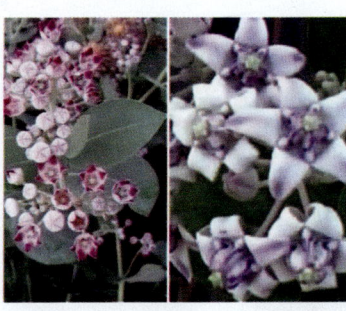

C. gigantae   *C. procera*

Fig. 9.5: Flowers of Calotropis

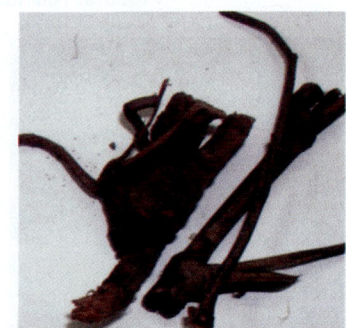

Fig. 9.6: Roots of Plumbago

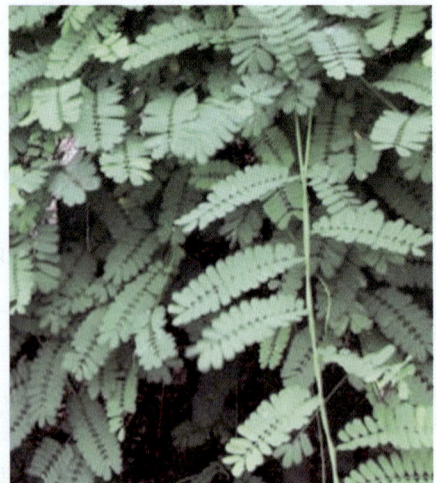

Fig. 9.7: *Abrus precatorius*

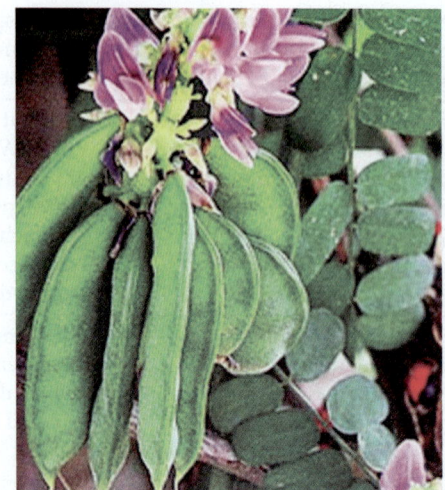

Fig. 9.8: Beans of Abrus with seeds

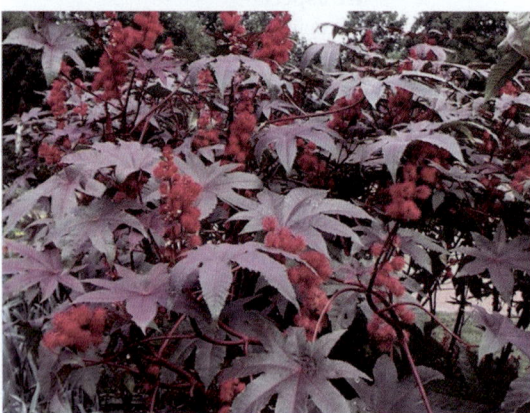

Fig. 9.9: Ricinus

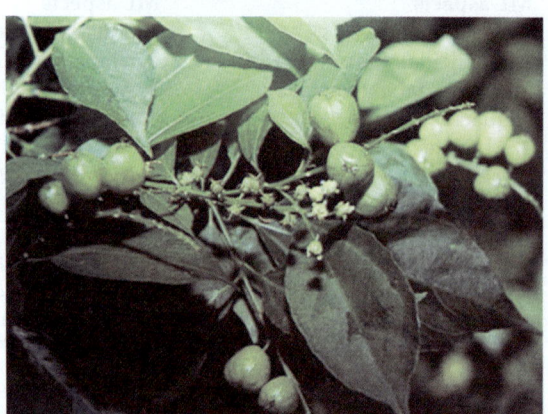

Fig. 9.10: *Croton tiglium*

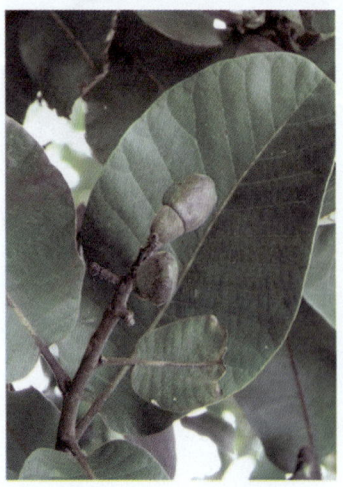

Fig. 9.11: Semicarpus

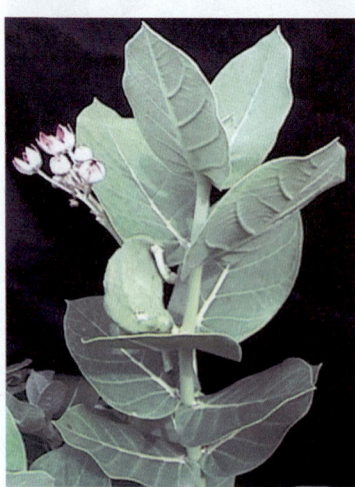

Fig. 9.12: Calotropis

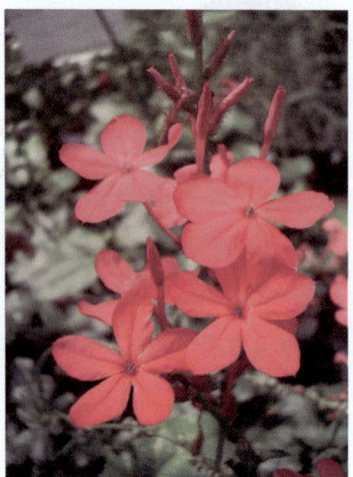

Fig. 9.13: Plumbago

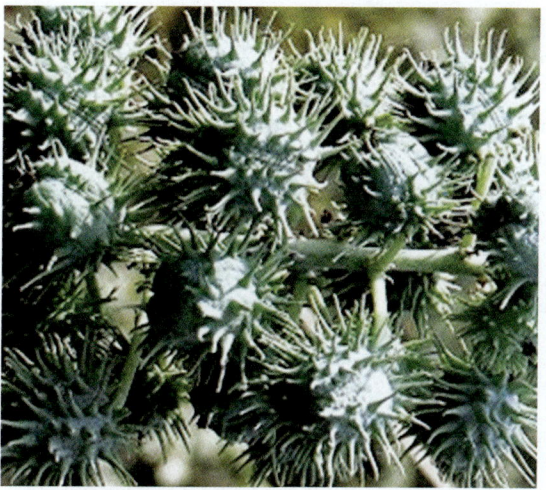

Fig. 9.14: Fruit of Ricinus (castor fruit)

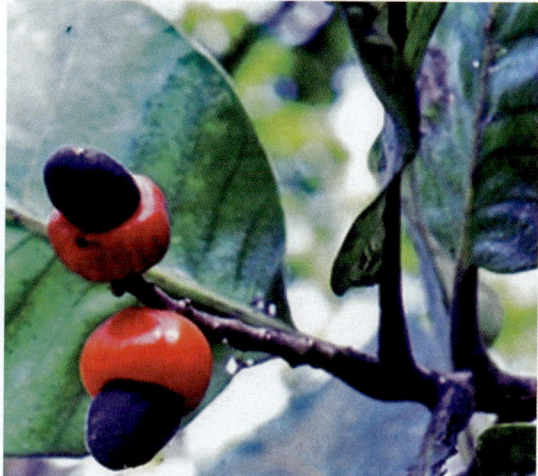

Fig. 9.15: Fruit of Semicarpus

Capsicum annum (CHILLI)

Active Principle

Capsicin, capsaicin fruit, seeds and dust cause irritation

Signs and Symptoms

- Burning, irritation, redness and swelling of mouth/throat, increase salivation, increase perspiration, watering from eyes and nose, abdominal pain, burning sensation during defecation
- Death is unusual except in neonates.

Treatment

- When swallowed—curd, bulky food and demulcent.
- Applied to skin/eyes—wash with water, xylocaine ointment

Medicolegal Aspects

1. Powder is thrown in the eyes either to snatch money/articles or to escape arrest after crime
2. It is used to kill unwanted newborn baby
3. It is applied in eyes/nose/anus/vagina/ or injury to extract confession
4. It is applied in the vagina for giving punishment for infidelity
5. **Hyderabadi goli:** It is the paste of chilli powder used to push in the rectum for torture and confession.

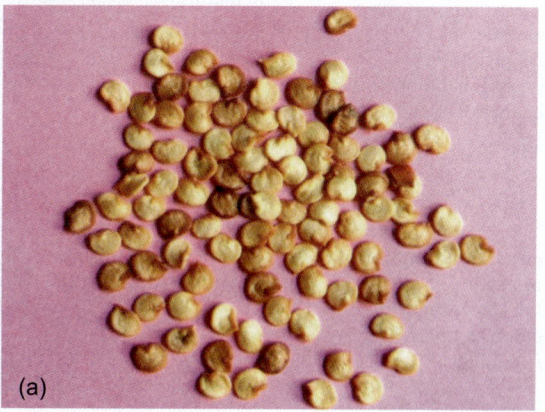

(a)

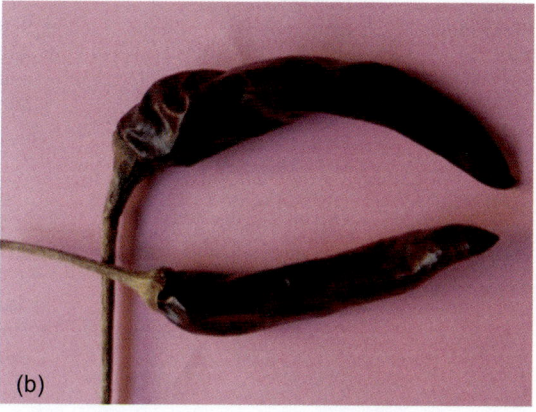

(b)

Figs 9.16a and b: Chilli seeds and fruit

Table 9.1: Phyto-toxicology of vegetable irritants

Name	1. Aloe	2. Anacardium occidentale	3. Chrysanthemum cinerariaefolium
Synonyms:	Aloe vera, Ghritakumari,	Cashewnut	Pyrethrum
General:	Bitter taste	Bitter taste.	Acrid bitter taste
Active principle:	Dried juice contains glycoside and barbaloin	Cardol present in the pericarp of the fruit	Pyrethrin I and II, Cinerin I and II present in the flowers
Clinical feature:	Abdominal pain, vomiting, diarrhea, inflammation of kidneys, kidneys increase intestinal movement and cause congestion of pelvic organs	Contact dermatitis with redness and urticaria-like lesion	Acrid bitter taste, numbness of tongue/mouth, with nausea, vomiting, diarrhea. Headache, restlessness, tremor, muscle weakness and respiratory failure.
Treatment:	Symptomatic.	• Wash the part with soap water. • Symptomatic	• Prevention of exposure. • Symptomatic. • Artificial respiration and oxygen inhalation
PM findings:	Nonspecific	Nonspecific	Nonspecific
ML aspect:	• **Abortifacient:** Procure abortion—quackery use	• **Accidental:**[2] to workers who collect and process the fruit for extraction of nuts • **Abortifacient:** Quack	• **Accidental:**[2] Exposure and inhalation of pollen grain leading to allergic reaction. • Suicidal—unusual. • Homicidal—unusual

Name	4. Cytrullus colocynthis	5. Eucalyptus globulus	6. Pinus palustris
Synonyms:	Bitter apple, colocynth, makal, indrayan	Nilgiri oil	Turpentine
General:	–	Used in Ayurvedic medicines	–
Active principle:	Colocynthin-fruits	Cinehole—a volatile oil in stem and leaves	d and l-pinene
Clinical feature:	Abdominal pain, diarrhea (blood tinged), increase body temperature, circulatory collapse	• Dyspnea, cyanosis, excitement, ataxia, convulsion, circulatory collapse	• Abdominal pain vomiting, diarrhea. When inhaled—RT irritant. Excitement, confusion, coma, oliguria, hematuria
Treatment:	Symptomatic	• Symptomatic. • Artificial respiration and oxygen inhalation. • Maintenance of circulation	• Stomach wash. • Symptomatic
PM findings:	Nonspecific GIT—irritation Kidneys—inflammation Organs—congested	Nonspecific	Nonspecific
ML aspect:	• **Accidental:** By mistake. • Abortifacient	• **Accidental:** Consumption of oil by mistake • **Suicidal:** Uncommon • **Homicidal:** Not possible due to the smell	• **Accidental:** By mistake • **Suicidal:** Occasionally

Table 9.2: Active principle and clinical features of other vegetable irritants

Name	Synonyms	Active principle	Clinical features
1. *Mangifera indica*	Mango	Resinous exudate	Irritation, contact dermatitis
2. *Nephrolipis rosaltata*	Fern	Filicin	–
3. Narcissus	Daffodil	Lycorine- bulb	Abdominal pain, nausea, vomiting, titanic convulsion
4. Poison Oak	Sumac	–	Skin irritation causes rash and dermatitis
5. *Aristolocia indica*	–	Aristolocin	Contact dermatitis, respiratory paralysis, hemorrhagic nephritis, GIT irritation
6. *Rhus toxicodendron*	Poison Ivy	3-pentadecyl-catechol	Contact dermatitis
7. Indian Wintergreen	(Jav)	Methyl salicylate	–
8. Pherulanarthex	(Asafoetida, hing)	–	Digestive stimulant, psychogenic and neurogenic action
9. *Eugenia caryophyllus*	(Cloves, lavang)	Tannin, caryophyllin	
10. *Colchicum leutium*	(Hirah tutigu)	Colchicine	–

Table 9.3: Toxic substance and active principles in poisonous plants[4–6, 8]

Toxic substance	Active principles	Plants	Type of poison
Toxalbumin	Abrin	*Abrus precatorius*	Vegetable irritant
	Ricin	*Ricinus communis*	Vegetable irritant
	Crotin	*Croton tiglium*	Vegetable irritant
	Curcin	*Jatropha curcas*	Vegetable irritant
Glycosides	Calotropin, calotoxin	*Calotropis*	Vegetable irritant
	Crotonoside	*Croton tiglium*	Vegetable irritant
	Plumbagin	*Plumbago rosea*	Vegetable irritant
	Cerberin, thevetin, thevotoxin	*Cerbera thevetia/odallam*	Cardiac poison
	Nerin, oleandrin	*Nerium odorum*	Cardiac poison
	Digoxin, digitalin	*Digitalis purpura*	Cardiac poison
Alkaloids	Capsaisin	*Capsicum annum*	Vegetable irritant
	Atropine, hyoscine	Datura	Deliriant
	Aconitine	*Aconitum ferox/napellus*	Cardiac poison
	Nicotine, nicotianin	*Nicotiana tabacum*	Cardiac poison
	Strychnine, brucin	*Strychnos nux vomica*	Spinal poison
	Curarine	*Chondrodendron tomentosum* (Curare)	Peripheral nerve poison
	Morphine, codeine, thebaine	*Papaver somniferum*	Somniferous poison
	Cocaine	*Erythroxylum coca*	Deliriant poison
	Conine	*Conium maculatum*	Peripheral poison
	Berberine, protopine	*Argemone mexicana*	Food poisoning
Glucoside	Abralin	*Abrus precatorius*	Vegetable irritant
Resins	Cannabinol (THC)	*Cannabis sativa*	Deliriant poison
Juice/oils	Semicarpol, bhilawanol	*Semicarpus annacardium*	Vegetable irritant
Plant acid	Oxalic acid	Spinach	–

IMPORTANT QUESTIONS

1. Enumerate vegetable irritants with their uses. Describe clinical manifestation, treatment and medicolegal aspects in case of consumption of seeds of *Abrus precatorius*. Add a note on preparation of sui from these seeds.

2. What is the difference in the seeds of crotin and castor? Write clinical features and management of their poisoning.

3. Enumerate roadside poisons. Write clinical features and medicolegal importance of poisoning with *Semicarpus anacardium*.

4. Enumerate active principle of any four vegetable irritants. Write clinical feature, treatment and medicolegal aspect of Calotropis poisoning.

5. Write difference between seeds of datura and capsicum. Write medicolegal aspect of chilli powder. Describe the fruit of datura and castor.

SPECIFIC LEARNING OBJECTIVES

After reading this chapter, the reader should be able to:

- Classify poisonous plants with their examples
- Enumerate different vegetable irritants
- Enlist toxic parts, uses, fatal dose, fatal period and active principle of different vegetable irritants
- Explain clinical features, treatment, post-mortem findings and medicolegal aspect of different vegetable irritant poisoning

- Define toxalbumin with examples and describe the method for preparation of needles (sui) from *Abrus precatorius* seeds.
- Enlist different toxic substances and principles in poisonous plants

References

1. Phytotoxicology. https://www. britannica. com/science/phytotoxicology. Plant poisons (Phytotoxins). https://www.britannica.com/science/poison-biochemistry/Types-of-poison#ref28140. Assessed on 2/12/2018.

2. Nandy A. Principles of Forensic Medicine. New Central Book Agency (P) Ltd: Calcutta, 2nd edn Reprint, 2004: 498–505.

3. Singhal SK. Singhal's Toxicology at a glance. 9th edn, National book depot: Mumbai.2016: 66–71.

4. Dikshit PC. Textbook of Forensic Medicine and Toxicology. 2nd edn, PEEPEE Publisher and Distributors (P) Ltd. New Delhi. 2014: 501–8.

5. Bardale R. Principles of Forensic Medicine and Toxicology. 1st edn, Jaypee Brothers Medical Publishers (P) Ltd: New Delhi. 2011: 467–76.

6. Pillay VV. Textbook of Forensic Medicine and Toxicology. Paras Medical Publisher: Hyderabad, 17th edn, 2016: 538–49.

7. Rashmi Aggarwal, Hemant Aggarwal, Pradeep Kumar Chugh. Medical management of ricin poisoning. Journal of Medical & Allied Sciences. 2017; 7(2): 82–6.

8. Reddy KSN, Murthy OP. The Essential of Forensic Medicine and Toxicology. 32nd edn, Om Sai Graphics: Hyderabad. 2013:503–97.

Animal Irritants

Animal irritants include snakes, scorpions, bees, wasps, cantharides, spider, etc. which cause venomous bite or stings. **Envenomation**[1] is the process by which venom is injected by the bite or sting of a venomous animal. Venom refers to injection of toxin through bite or sting. Poison refers to toxin that has to be ingested or swallowed for causing deleterious effect. Snakes may be venomous and non-venomous. But still poisonous and non-poisonous snakes have been commonly referred in practice. It has been estimated that five million snakebite cases occur worldwide every year, causing about 100,000 deaths. In India, nearly 200,000 fall prey to snakebite per year and 35,000–50,000 of them die every year.[2]

SNAKES (OPHIDIA)

Snakes belong to class reptilia, order squamata and suborder serpentes. Snakes are found all over the world except Antarctica region and in Ireland, Iceland and New Zealand.[3] In the world, there are about 3000 species of snakes, 600 are venomous[4] (WHO) and only half of these are capable of inflicting a lethal bite. India has over 250 species of snakes out of which about 50 species are venomous.[5] The common poisonous snakes in India are Cobra, Krait, Russell's viper, Saw-scaled viper and Sea snakes. Deaths due to snakebites are mainly accidental in nature.

GENERAL CHARACTERISTICS

1. Snakes have an elongated body and a short tail that is the part behind vent, and has no limbs. Vent is an opening in the rear part of the body for intestine and genitourinary system.
2. The body is covered with scales.
3. On the head, there are 2 eyes, 2 nostrils, but no external ear.
4. Tongue is forked and serves as a sense organ.
5. They are cold blooded creatures with carnivorous habits. They use sharp teeth and strong muscles to catch the prey. The mouth is easily distensible allowing it to swallow even large animals as a whole.
6. Teeth are thin, directed backwards and the upper marginal teeth are modified and are known as fangs. Fangs can be replaced in 3–6 weeks when broken. The fangs are solid in non-poisonous and grooved/canalized in poisonous snakes for transport of venom from the poison glands, i.e. modified parotid salivary glands, to which they are connected through ducts.
7. In poisonous snakes, parotid glands are situated below and behind the eyes, one on each side secreting toxic saliva and acts as poison glands. Fangs of elapids/sea snakes are short, fixed and grooved, and that of vipers are long, movable and canalized.
8. During the process of bite, the glands are pressed and venom is squeezed and channeled through the grooves or canal of the fangs.
9. Some are viviparous (gives birth to young ones in vipers) and some are oviparous (lays eggs, e.g. cobra, pythons, water snakes).

Classification of Snakes

On the Basis of their Families[6]

1. Colubridae: African boomslang, twig snake
2. Elapidae: Cobra and krait (commonly called elapids), coral snakes, all Australian venomous snakes.
3. Hydrophiidae: Sea snakes.
4. Viperidae: Vipers
5. Atractaspididae: Mole vipers or adders.

On the Basis of Venom

1. Elapids—neurotoxic
2. Vipers—vasculotoxic
3. Sea snakes—myotoxic

Snakes may be:

1. Poisonous/venomous
2. Non poisonous/non-venomous

Common Poisonous Snakes in India

1. Cobra: King/common cobra (Table 10.2)
2. Krait: Common/banded
3. Viper: Pit/Russell's/Saw-scaled
4. Sea snakes: Banded sea snakes, amphibian sea snakes

Common Non-poisonous Snakes in India[7]

1. Rat snake (Dhaman)
2. Vine snake
3. Bronze back tree snake

4. Banded kukri
5. Sand boa

The non-poisonous snakes, which may resemble poisonous snake are as follows:

Non-poisonous snakes	Poisonous snakes
Rat snake	Common cobra
Common cat	Saw-scaled viper
Banded kukri	Banded krait
Sand boa	Russell's viper
Common wolf	Common krait

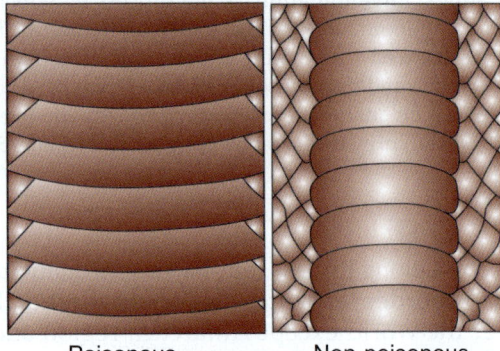

Poisonous   Non-poisonous

Fig. 10.1: Belly scales

Differences Between Poisonous and Non-poisonous Snakes

Table 10.1 shows the differentiating features between poisonous and non-poisonous snakes.

Table 10.1: Differences between poisonous and non-poisonous snakes

Features		Poisonous snakes	Non-poisonous snakes
1. Belly scales:	Size (Fig. 10.1)	Large	Small
	Distribution	Cover entire breadth	Never cover entire breadth
2. Head:	Size	Usually small (pit, cobra, krait)	Usually large
	Scales (Fig. 10.2)	Usually small except cobras	Usually large
3. Teeth		At least one pair of teeth in upper jaw is modified to form fangs	All teeth are uniformly small, attached to short maxillary bone
4. Fangs		Present and canalized/grooved	Absent
5. Tails		Abruptly tapering tail, rounded	Gradually tapering long tail
6. Habits		Usually nocturnal	May be nocturnal or diurnal
7. Physical features		Stout, dull colour	Slender, bright-coloured
8. Bite marks (Fig. 10.18)		Usually two fang marks present	Semicircular set of teeth mark present

Table 10.2: Differences between king cobra and common cobra

Common cobra	King cobra
5–6 feet length	8–18 feet length
Black, brown or cream color	Usually jet black color
Habitat near human dwelling	Found in hills and dense forest
Spectacle mark present on hood	No spectacle mark on hood

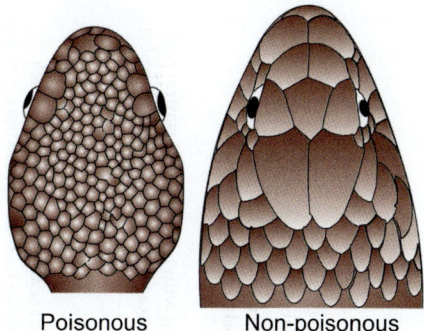

Poisonous   Non-poisonous

Fig. 10.2: Head scales

Features of Poisonous Snakes in India
(Tables 10.4 and 10.5)

1. **Cobra:** It is usually black of about 5–6 feet. It has a hood with one or two spectacle marks on its dorsal surface. The third supralabial is large and touches the eye. **It prefers barren land near human habitate.**

2. **King-cobra:** It is usually jet black color of about 6–18 feet. It has a hood without having any mark. It **prefers dense forests.**

3. **Common Krait:** It is usually steel-black, 3–5 feet. There are four infralabial shields on head of which 4th is largest. The central rows of scales on back are large and hexagonal. **It prefers agricultural area and near the houses.**

4. **Banded krait:** It is 5–7 feet and has alternate black and yellow bands on the body.

5. **Pit viper:** It is usually green or yellow of about 1–3 feet. It has a green pit between eye and nostril. It is found in hills.

6. **Russell's viper:** It is usually light brown of about 4–5 feet. Head is triangular and has white **V-shaped mark with its apex pointing forwards**.

7. **Saw-scaled viper or echis carinata:** It is usually brown of about 1–1.5 feet. Head is triangular with **white mark resembling an arrow or foot of a bird.** The ridges in the middle of each scale are like a saw, hence the name saw-scaled viper.

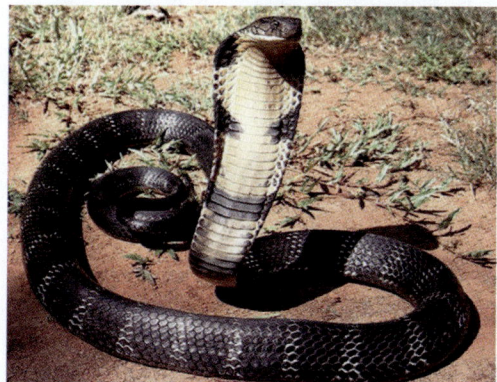

Fig. 10.3: King-cobra (no spectacle mark on hood)

Table 10.3: Differences between cobras and vipers

Features	Cobras	Vipers
1. Body	Long and cylindrical	Short and stout
2. Head	Small with hood seldom broader than body Same width as neck	Large and triangular Broader than body Wider than neck
3. Upper jaw	Has 2 fangs (~4–6 mm) and other teeth	Has only 2 fangs (12–15 mm)
4. Fangs	Short, fixed, grooved	Long, movable, canalized
5. Venom	Neurotoxic	Hemotoxic (vasculotoxic)
6. Eyes	Round pupil	Vertical pupil
7. Tail	Round	Tapered
8. Parity	Oviparous	Viviparous

Table 10.4: Characteristic features of common poisonous snakes in India—Cobra and Krait

Snakes	Common cobra	King-cobra	Common krait	Banded krait
Synonyms	Nag, Gokhurra	NagRaja, Daras	Maniyar (Maharashtra), Kawariya (Punj.), Chitti (Cal.), Kalotaro (Guj)	–
Found in	All over India, Sri Lanka, Burma	Hills and forest of S. India, Odisha, Assam, Himalaya	All over India, and near dwelling house	–
Length	5–6 feet	8–18 feet	3–5 feet	5–7 feet
Colour	Usually black or cream to black to brown	Usually jet black or brownish black, greenish, yellow	Usually steel black with single or double narrow band across their back all over up to tip of tail	Alternate jet black and yellow bands across its back
Head shape and mark	Flat with hood present with one or two dark round spots surrounded by an eclipse c/s 'spectacle mark' on dorsal aspect	Flat with hood present with no 'spectacle mark' on dorsal aspect	Oval with one enlarged central row of hexagonal scales on dorsal aspect	Oval with one enlarged central row of hexagonal scales on dorsal aspect
Head scales	Head scales are large with 3rd supralabial touches the eye and nasal shields	Head scales are large with 3rd supralabial touches the eye and nasal shields	Head scales are small	Head scales are small with black mark on its neck spreading up to the eyes
Pupils	Round	Round	Round	Round
Ventral aspect of mouth	• Ventral aspect of hood bears 3 dark bands on central part and a white band in an area where hood touches the body • Tiny triangular shield between 4th and 5th infralabial shield	• Ventral aspect of hood bears 3 dark bands on central part and a white band in an area where hood touches the body • Tiny triangular shield between 4th and 5th infralabial shield	• Ventral aspect of mouth has only 4 infralabials and 4th infralabial is the largest	• Ventral aspect of mouth has only 4 infralabials and 4th infralabial is the largest
Belly scales	Cover the entire width	Cover the entire width	Cover the entire width	Cover the entire width
Tail	Scales are entirely present proximally but divided in the distal ends	Scales are entirely present proximally but divided in the distal ends	Scales are entirely present and not divided	Scales are entirely present and not divided
Toxin	Neurotoxin	Neurotoxin	Neurotoxin	Neurotoxin
Fatal dose	15 mg	15 mg	1 mg	10 mg
Fatal period	20 mins to 6 hours	20 mins to 6 hours	20 mins to 6 hours	20 mins to 6 hours

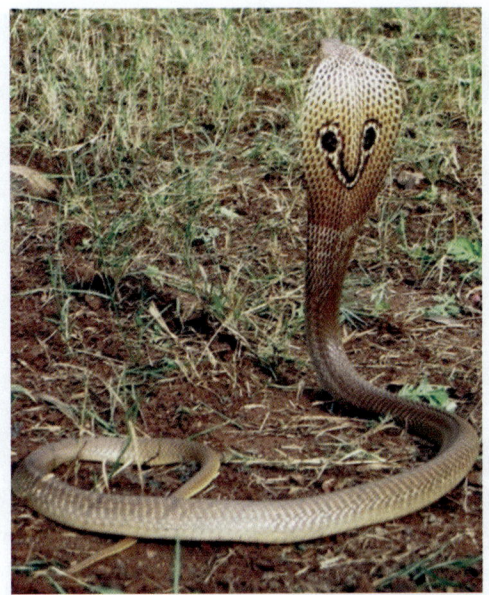

Fig. 10.4: Common cobra with spectacle mark

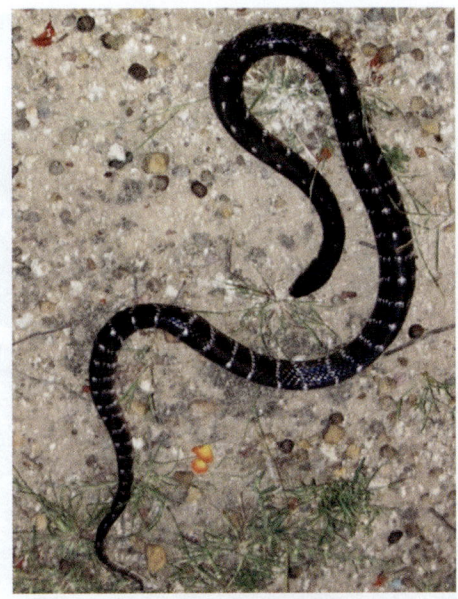

Fig. 10.5: Common krait (*Courtesy*: Shrikant Uike)

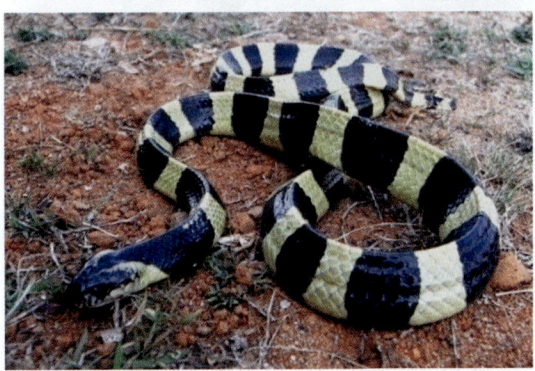

Fig 10.6: Banded krait (*Courtesy*: Shrikant Uike)

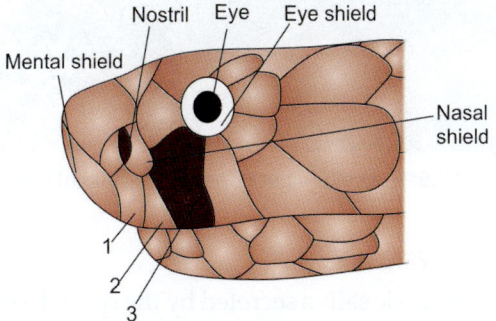

Fig. 10.7: Cobra head scales—large scales and 3rd labial touches the eye and nasal shields

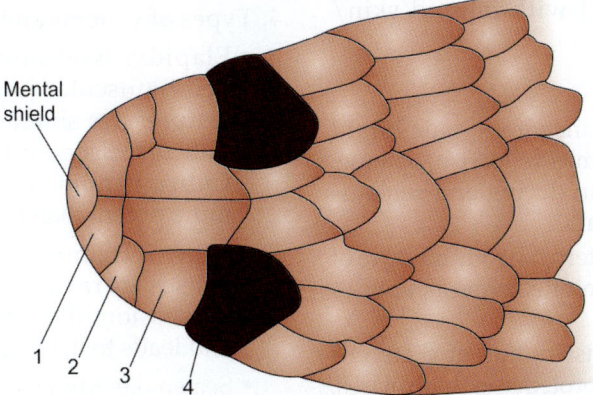

Fig. 10.8: Krait head—4th infralabial is largest (view from below)

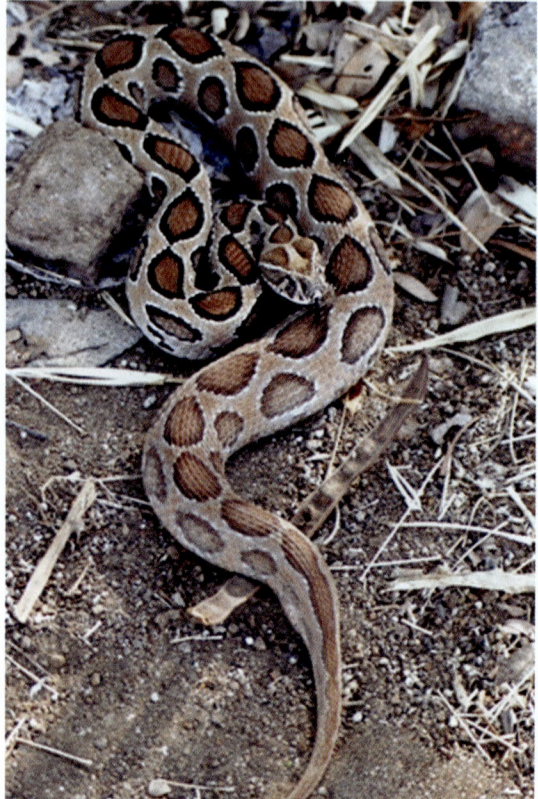

Fig. 10.9: Russell's viper (*Courtesy*: Shrikant Uike)

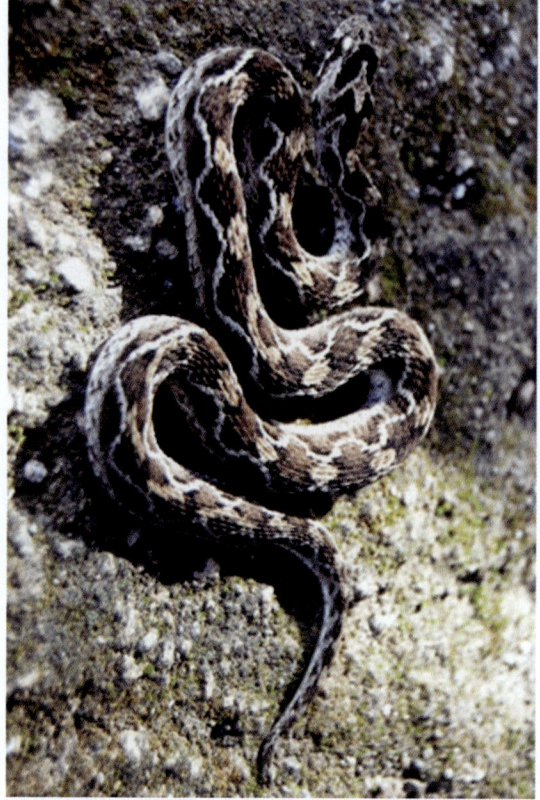

Fig. 10.10: Saw-scaled viper

SNAKE VENOM

It is the toxic saliva secreted by the specialized salivary glands. The snake venom on ingestion is non-poisonous since it can be digested. Envenomation (poisoning) occurs only due to direct snakebite or when the venom is injected or on contact with injured skin/mucosa.[8]

Features

1. **Physical:** Clear, transparent, pale liquid when fresh. It becomes yellowish, opaque, granular powder on drying and remains active for many years.
2. **Chemical:** It is a heterogeneous mixture of proteins in the form of enzymes, peptides and polypeptides.
3. **Enzymes:** The constituents of different snakes venoms are proteinases, hydrolases, transaminase, hyaluronidase, phos-

pholipase A, B, C and D, ribonuclease, deoxyribonuclease, phosphomonoesterase, phosphodiesterases, 5-nucleotidase, ATPase, alkaline phosphatase, acid phosphatase, cholinesterases, coagulases, agglutinins, fibrinolysin, hemolysin, etc.

4. **Types of venoms and action**
   - **Elapids:** Neurotoxin. It blocks the neuromuscular junction.[9] Neurotoxic features are similar to d-tubocurarine leading to flaccidity of muscles. However, **Cobra** venom is almost 15–40 times more potent than tubocurarine.
   - **Vipers:** Hemolytic and hemotoxic. It causes intravascular hemolysis and depression of coagulation mechanism and leads to hemorrhage and necrosis.
   - **Sea snake:** Myotoxic. It leads to muscle pain, myoglobinuria and hyperkalemia.[9]

Table 10.5: Characteristic features of common poisonous snakes in India —Vipers

Snakes	Pit viper	Russell viper	Saw-scaled viper
Synonyms	–	Ghonus (Marathi), Kander (Hindi), Chital (Gujarati), Daboia	Phoorsa
Found in	Hilly area	Throughout India in the plains	–
Length	2–4 feet	4–5 feet, heavy body with narrow neck	1–1.5 feet
Colour	Usually green or **yellow** with pit between eye and nostril	Buff or light brown and pitless with 3 longitudinal regular chain-like pattern or rows on the back	Brownish or brownish grey
Head shape and mark	Triangular, heavy with deep **depression 'pit'** on each side between eye and nostril	Triangular, heavy with **white V-shaped mark** with its apex pointing forward	Triangular, heavy with **white mark resembling a bird's foot-print or an arrow**
Head scales	Smaller	Smaller	Smaller
Pupils	Vertical	Vertical	Vertical
Body	Flat and broad	Roundish, smooth	Broad and rough having **serrated ridge** and **continuous wavy line along** each flank of the back
Other peculiar	–	Snake produces **terrible hissing sound** when about to attack	Snakes produce peculiar **rustling sound while moving**
Belly scales	Cover the entire width	Cover the entire width and broad	Cover the entire width and broad
Tail	Scales are divided throughout	Scales are divided throughout	Scales are divided throughout
Toxin	Vasculotoxic	Vasculotoxic	Vasculotoxic
Fatal dose	100 mg	40 mg	8 mg
Fatal period	2–4 days	2–4 days	2–4 days

Tail of poisonous snakes

Cobra: Scales are divided distally

Viper: Scales are divided throughout the tail

Krait: Scales are not divided

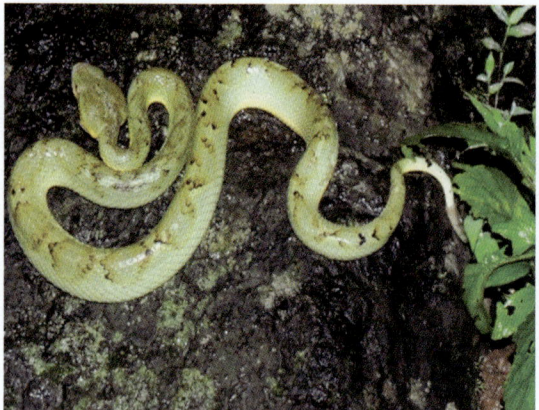

Fig. 10.11: Pit viper

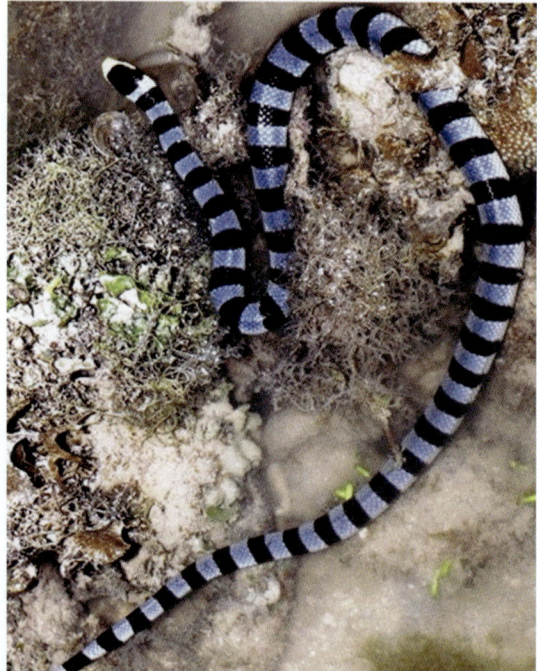

Fig. 10.12: Belcher's sea snake

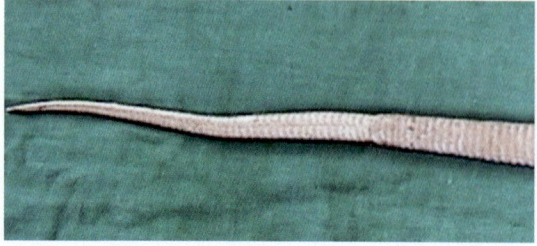

Fig. 10.13: **Poisonous snake:** Viper-Belly scales complete and tail scales are divided throughout

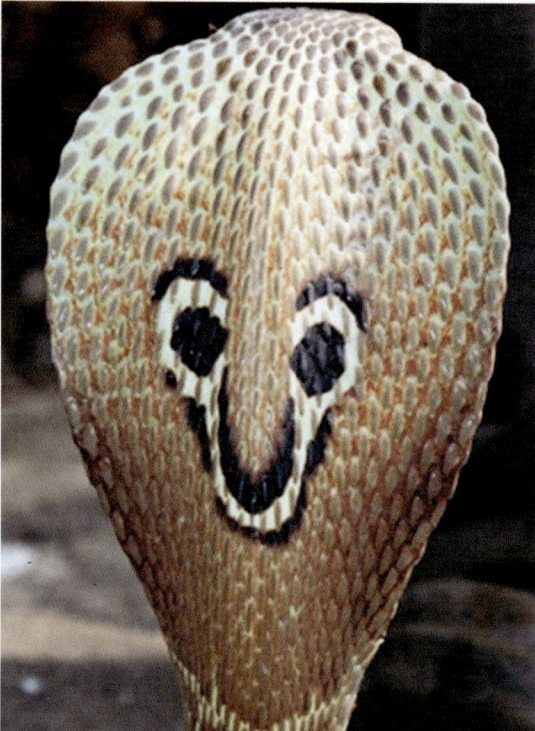

Fig. 10.14: Dorsal aspect of hood of common cobra

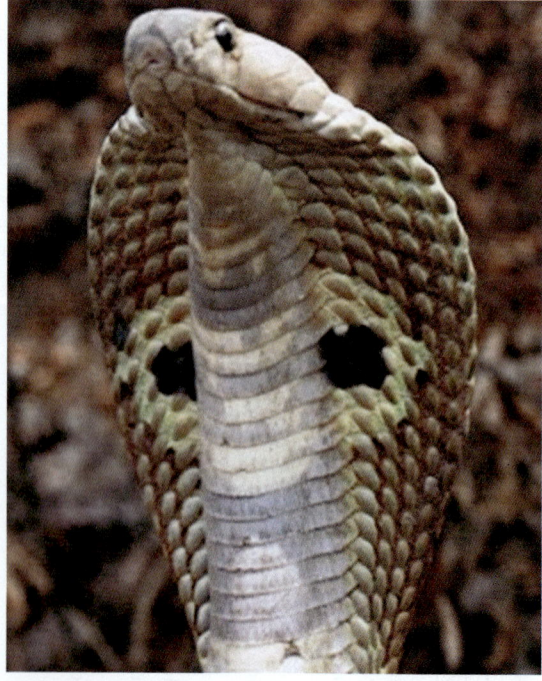

Fig. 10.15: Ventral aspect of hood of common cobra

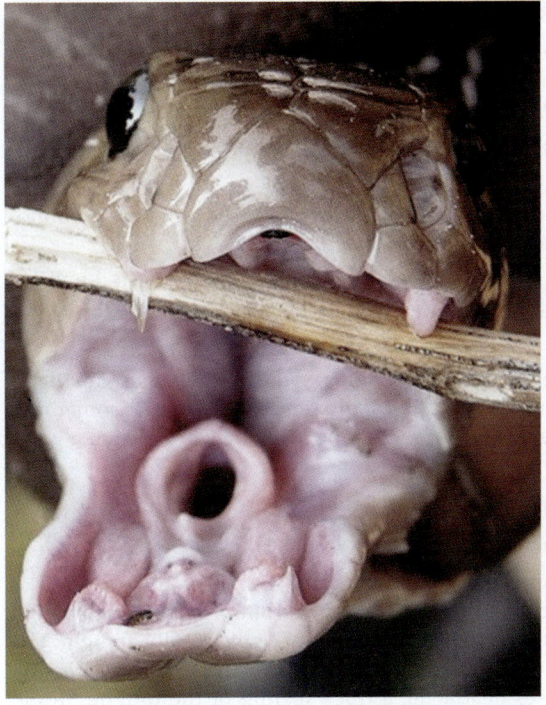

Fig. 10.16: Fangs of cobra

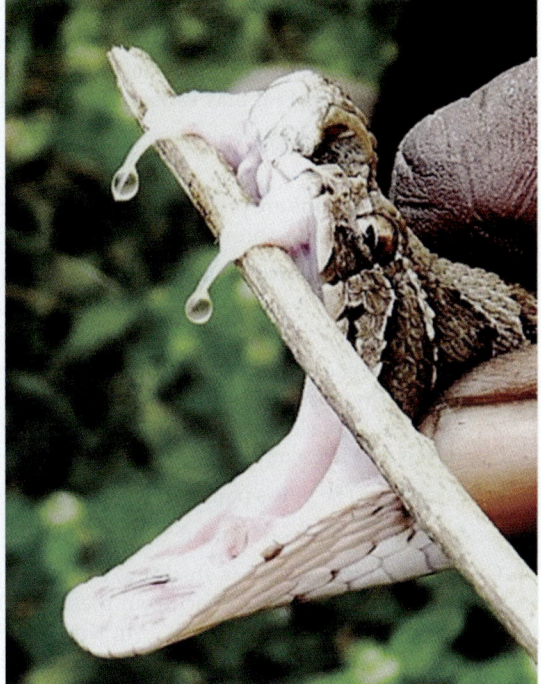

Fig. 10.17: Fangs of viper

5. The action of different constituents of snake venom is as follows:

- Hyaluronidase: Spread venom.
- Hemolysin: Lysis of RBC.
- Phospholipase: Hemolysis.
- Proteases: Dissolution of blood vessels.
- Proteolytic enzymes: Digestion and destruction of tissue proteins.
- Leukolysin: Lysis of WBC.
- Cytolysin: Damage of internal viscera.
- Rhabdomyolysin: Necrosis of muscles.
- Fibrinolysin: Breakdown of fibrin/clot.

6. Absorption:[10–12] The neurotoxins of elapids and sea snakes are absorbed rapidly into the bloodstream (therefore causing rapid systemic effects), whereas the much larger molecules of viper venom are taken up more slowly through the lymphatics (causing severe local effects). Most venoms do not cross blood–brain barrier.

7. Fatal dose, fatal period and amount of venom injected per bite:[13]

Snakes	Fatal dose (of dried venom)	Amount injected per bite
Cobra	12–15 mg	200–250 mg
Krait	5–6 mg	20–25 mg
Russell's viper	15–20 mg	150–200 mg
Saw-scaled viper	8 mg	5 mg

Fatal period

Colubridae: 1/2 hr to 24 hr.

Viperidae: 1 to 4 days.

CLINICAL FEATURES OF NON-POISONOUS SNAKEBITES

- Fear and apprehension; sweating.
- Feeble pulse, hypotension, syncope, rapid and shallow breathing.
- Bite area may show multiple teeth marks.

SIGNS AND SYMPTOMS OF POISONOUS SNAKEBITES

1. **Psychological trauma:** Fright is the most common symptom following snakebite due to enhanced systemic absorption of venom. It develops almost rapidly and may produce psychological shock and cause sudden death. Fear may cause transient pallor, sweating and vomiting

2. **Dry bites:** In at least 20% of pit viper bites and a greater percentage of elapid and sea snakebites, no venom is injected.[12]

3. **Local manifestations** are present in the form of one or more fang (bite) marks seen as punctured wound. Local features are more prominent in vipers as compared to elapids bites.

   a. **Elapids:** There is **burning with triple response** (i.e. redness, swelling, and inflammation) at the site of bite. Thus, there is mild pain with local swelling and blistering. In Krait, usually do not have any local reaction.[12]

   b. **Vipers: Intense pain with radiation** and tenderness followed by **edema, swelling, cyanosis, oozing of blood, ecchymosis, hemorrhagic bullae and serum-filled vesicles/ blisters,**[6] **cellulitis** and sometimes significant tissue loss with features of necrosis/gangrene.[13] If there is no swelling 2 hours after a viper bite, it is safe to assume that there has been no envenoming.[14]

   c. **Sea snakes:** The bite is painful but soon becomes painless. It takes 2 hours to produce signs.

   Secondary infection may occur due to bacterial flora in the oral cavity of the snakes.[15]

4. **General features:** There is flushing, dyspnea, palpitation, sweating, and tightness in chest due to sympathetic overactivity. Apart from these, **in elapids bites**, there may be vomiting, hypersalivation, blurring of vision and 'gooseflesh'.[12] **In Krait**, the bite may be unnoticed as it occurs usually at night. The patient wakes up with vomiting and cramping abdominal pain followed by diarrhea[12] (predominantly ANS involvement). **Sea snake** envenomation causes headache, a thick feeling of the tongue, thirst, sweating and vomiting.[12]

5. **Systemic manifestation:**[6, 12] Systemic manifestation depends upon the type of venom predominantly present like neurotoxic (cobras and kraits), hemorrhagic (vipers) and myotoxic (sea snakes).

   a. **Elapids:**

   Neurotoxicity: In elapids, paralysis is first detectable as ptosis and external ophthalmoplegia appearing within 15 min of bite along with difficulty in speech and deglutition, salivation and frothing from mouth. This is followed by respiratory paralysis, muscle weakness and pain, staggering, spreading paralysis (ascending from lower limbs), convulsions and death. With **Krait bite**, the s/s is less rapid and there is no convulsion, nausea and frothing but there is more drowsiness.

   Cardiotoxicity: Cause direct myocardial damage leading to arrhythmias, tachy/bradycardia, hypotension.

   b. **Vipers:**

   Clotting defects and hemolysis: Hemostatic abnormalities are characteristic of envenoming by viperidae. Bleeding from multiple sites including gums, nose, GIT (hematemesis, malena), urinary tract, injection sites, skin (multiple petechiae and purpura), conjunctivae, and internal organs particularly kidneys. There is intravascular hemolysis leading to hemoglobinuria and hypotension and intracranial hemorrhage.

   Nephrotoxicity: Renal failure secondary to ischemia.

   Shock: Due to fright and hypovolemia, and hemorrhage into adrenals/pituitary.

   c. **Sea snakes:**

   Myotoxicity: Myotoxin causes myalgia, myopathy and rhabdomyolysis (leading to myoglobinuria—due to muscle necrosis), vomiting, collapse, muscular pain, muscle stiffness, hyperkalemia (increased K^+) and increased serum transaminase levels.

Table 10.6: Difference in clinical manifestation of colubrine bite and viperine bite

Features	Colubrine bite (cobra) (Neurotoxicity)	Viperine bite (viper) (Hemotoxicity)
1. Onset of symptoms	Early—within 5–10 min	Longer—within 10–20 min
2. Feeling of intoxication	Marked	Not marked
3. Drooping of eyelids (ptosis)	Present	Not observed
4. Involvement of tongue/larynx	Paralyzed	No effect
5. Salivation	Drooling of saliva from mouth	Absent
6. Speech and deglutition	Lost	No effect
7. Pupils	Normal	Dilated, not reacting to light
8. Gait	Staggering	Not so, but s/o general paralysis
9. Blood coagulability	Not affected	Completely deranged
10. Hemorrhagic features	Not present or less marked	Most important feature
11. Death	Due to respiratory paralysis	Pulmonary thrombosis or toxic action on heart, blood, kidneys.
12. Development of gangrene	Early, wet type	Slow, dry type

DIAGNOSIS OF SNAKEBITE POISONING (IN OPHITOXEMIA—POISONING BY SNAKE VENOM)

Diagnosis depends on

1. **Fang marks:** Usually two fang marks are seen in the form of punctured wound, separated from each other by about 1 to 4 cm.
2. **Identification of snakes:** Refer to Tables 10.4 and 10.5.
3. **Laboratory methods:** Lab diagnosis is poor but are useful for monitoring, prognosis and determining stages of intervention:
   a. Blood changes: Like anemia, leukocytosis and thrombocytopenia and hypofibrinogenemia.
   b. Peripheral smear: Shows evidence of hemolysis, particularly in viperine bites.
   c. Deranged coagulant activity: Prolonged clotting time and prothrombin time.
   d. Immunodiagnosis: Consists of:
      i. ELISA: To identify the species based on antigens in the venom. These tests are expensive and not freely available and hence are of limited value.
      ii. Radioimmunoassay (RIA).
      iii. Immunodiffusion.
      iv. Countercurrent immunoelectrophoresis.

4. **Metabolic changes:** Like hyperkalemia and hypoxemia with respiratory acidosis, especially with neuroparalysis.

5. **Urine changes:** Hematuria, proteinuria, hemoglobinuria or myoglobinuria.

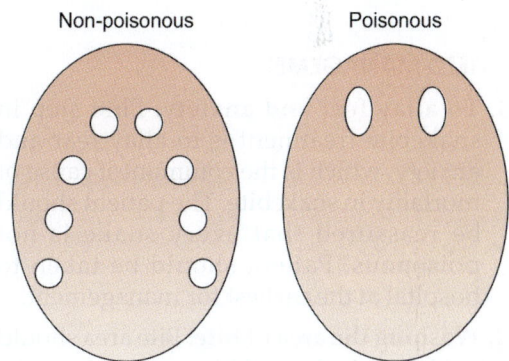

Non-poisonous   Poisonous

Fig. 10.18: Fang marks of snakes

TREATMENT

In non-poisonous snakes

a. Allay fear and anxiety.
b. Console patient that not all snakes are poisonous.

In poisonous snakes, treatment includes

a. Field management
b. Hospital management

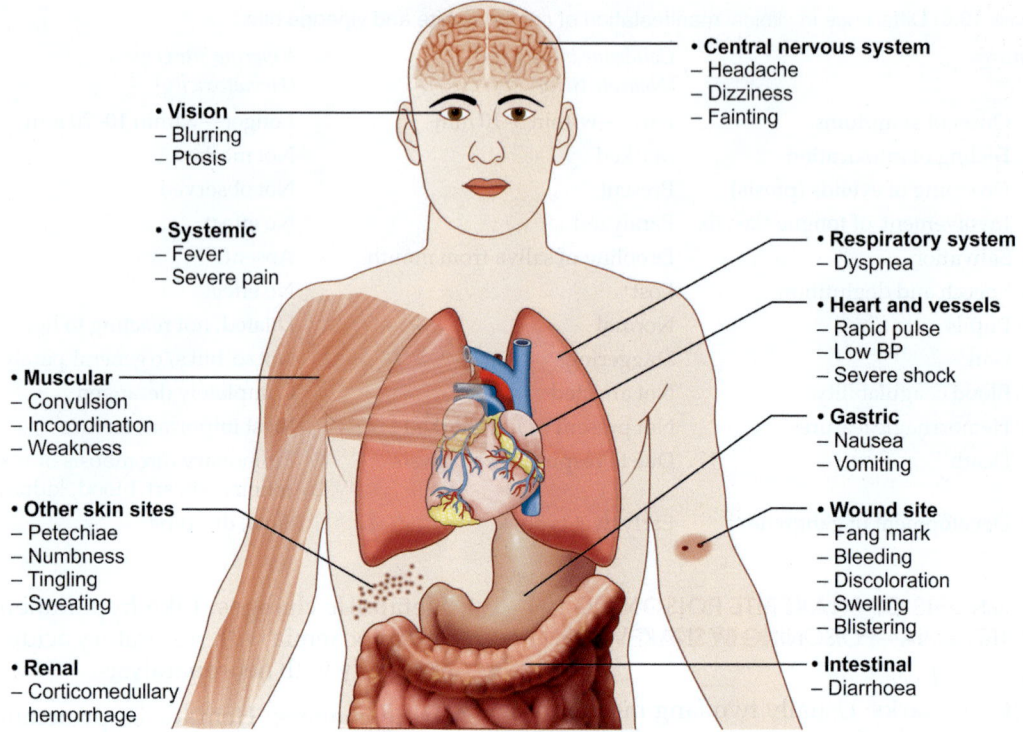

• **Central nervous system**
  – Headache
  – Dizziness
  – Fainting

• **Vision**
  – Blurring
  – Ptosis

• **Systemic**
  – Fever
  – Severe pain

• **Respiratory system**
  – Dyspnea

• **Heart and vessels**
  – Rapid pulse
  – Low BP
  – Severe shock

• **Muscular**
  – Convulsion
  – Incoordination
  – Weakness

• **Gastric**
  – Nausea
  – Vomiting

• **Other skin sites**
  – Petechiae
  – Numbness
  – Tingling
  – Sweating

• **Wound site**
  – Fang mark
  – Bleeding
  – Discoloration
  – Swelling
  – Blistering

• **Renal**
  – Corticomedullary hemorrhage

• **Intestinal**
  – Diarrhoea

Fig. 10.19: General manifestations of snakebite

A. FIELD MANAGEMENT

1. **To allay fear and anxiety:** First step in snakebite treatment is to allay fear and anxiety, which is the commonest cause of mortality in snakebite. The patient should be reassured that every snake is not poisonous. Patient should be taken to hospital at the earliest for management.

2. **Washing the area of bite:** Bite area should not be washed as rubbing or touching the area will help the venom to spread more rapidly. Moreover, traces of venom that are left on the skin can be used to identify the snakes (where such facilities are available) and type of anti-venom that should be used.

3. **Avoid incision and sucking:**[6] There is no benefit in cutting or sucking the bite as the venom is deeply injected and or absorbed. Rather avoid incising or cooling bite site, as neurotoxin may be rapidly absorbed through it.

4. **Pressure immobilization technique:** Immobilization is the most effective first aid. It greatly restricts absorption and circulation of these venoms (particularly neurotoxic in elapids/sea snakebites[6]) which tends to cause lesser local tissue effects than viper bites. It prevents spread of venom and relieves pain.

   Apply firm bandage/broad tourniquet **proximal to the site of bite** (if on extremity, preferably on a single bone) to minimise the spread of the venom. The pressure of tourniquet should be **tight enough to occlude the lymphatics and venous flow but not the arterial flow,**[12] **so as to permit a finger to slip under it.** The tourniquet should be released for 20–30 sec. every 15 min to avoid gangrene. In viper bite, the torniquet should not be applied as the procoagulant enzymes present in viper venom cause the blood to clot. When such torniquet is released, the clot will rapidly enter the circulation and cause embolism and death.[13] Moreover, application of bandages/tourniquet to limit venom spread is ineffective and may cause greater local tissue damage, particularly due to necrotic venom.[6]

B. HOSPITAL MANAGEMENT[6]

Victim should be closely monitored while a history is obtained quickly and rapid through physical examination is performed.

- Evaluation of progression of local envenomation by marking the level of swelling in the bitten extremity every 15 minutes (after positioned the limb at ~ heart level and release of tourniquet).
- Evaluation of local and systemic hemorrhage by hypotension.
- Evaluate the degree of hemolysis/thrombocytopenia/renal or hepatic function by whole blood clotting time (for 20 min[12]) and urine testing for blood or myoglobin, every 6 hourly until clinical stability is achieved.
  1. Fluid resuscitation with isotonic saline (20–40 ml/kg IV) should be initiated if there is any evidence of hemodynamic instability. If fail to respond, then 5% albumin (10–20 ml/kg) may be given.
  2. Antivenom administration
  3. Vasopressor (e.g. dopamine) should be added.
  4. Tetanus immunization
  5. Prophylactic antibiotics
  6. Pain control with acetaminophen or narcotic analgesic.
  7. Wound care once coagulation has been restored.
  8. Neurotoxicity from the elapid bites may be harder to reverse with antivenom and further doses of antivenom is not beneficial. In such cases, victim may be maintained on mechanical ventilator until recovery (takes days or weeks).[6]
- Patient with clear evidence of neurotoxicity after snakebite (e.g. ptosis) should receive:
  a. Pretreatment with atropines—0.6 mg IV (children—0.02 mg/kg)
  b. Acetylcholinesterase inhibitors like Edrophonium—10 mg IV (children – 0.2 mg/kg) OR Neostigmine—1.5–2 mg IM (children 0.025–0.08 mg/kg)
- If improvement is evident within 5 min, then continue neostigmine 0.5 mg IV/SC every 30 minutes as needed along with continuous IV infusion of atropine over 8 hours. Neostigmine is given to prevent respiratory paralysis.[16]
- Maintain airway with endotracheal intubation, if required.

Specific Therapy: Antivenom Serum or Antivenene

Preparation: It is prepared by injecting the snake venom into horse and extracting the antibodies in the serum. **Antivenoms or Antivenins** may be **monovalent** (species specific, not available in India) or **polyvalent** (effective against cobra, krait, pitless viper). This serum is freeze dried (lyophilised) and is available as granular powder. It is reconstituted by adding 10 ml of diluents supplied along with serum.

Indications:[6] Antisnake venom (ASV) should be used cautiously because of its hypersensitivity reactions, but should be given irrespective of the sensitivity.

1. For Viperids bites and cytotoxic elapids: Any evidence of systemic envenomation (like coma, hypotension, shock, bleeding, DIC, ARF, etc. and laboratory abnormalities) and significant progressive local findings (swelling crossing a joint or involving more than half the affected limb).
2. For neurotoxic elapids: First sign of any e/o neurotoxicity (like ptosis-cranial nerve dysfunction) or peripheral neuropathy.

Dose: Firstly, sensitivity test is done (if time and condition of the patient permits) by giving 0.1 ml reconstituted serum intradermally on one forearm. Control with 0.1 ml saline in opposite forearm.

- **If a person is sensitive,** i.e. +ve test (appearance of erythema or wheal > 10 mm within 30 minutes), then desensitise with 0.01 ml of 1:100 solution and increase the concentration gradually at intervals of 15 minutes, till 1.0 ml SC can be given 2 hourly; **under cover of adrenaline, antihistaminic, and corticosteroids.** Some recommended[6] pretreatment with **IV antihistamines** (e.g. diphenhydramine, 1 mg/kg to a maximum of 100 mg and cimetidine, 5–10 mg/kg) or even **epinephrine** (0.01 mg/kg IM up to 0.3 mg) or **glucocorticoids** (for serum sickness) like oral prednisone 1–2 mg/kg daily until all findings resolve and then tapered over 1–2 weeks.

- **If not sensitive, conventionally:**
  a. For elapid (neurotoxic) bite—100 ml ASV (10 vials) dissolved in DNS/normal saline in IV drip for 1 hour, followed by 100 ml ASV slowly over 6 hours
  b. For viper (hemotoxic) bite—100 ml ASV (10 vials) dissolved in DNS/normal saline in IV drip for 1 hour. Then after 6 hours, whole blood clotting time is done. If clotting time is more than 20 min, then 50 ml ASV is repeated; and if less than 20 minutes, then there is no need of further dose. The antivenom should be continued until the victim shows definite improvement like stabilized vital signs, reduced pain and restored coagulation.[6]

Types

  a. Polyvalent Antisnake Venom Serum[17] (**ASV serum**—prepared in Haffkine's Institute, Bombay) is given 20 ml IV prepared by dissolving powdered serum in distilled water, administered at the earliest, but may be helpful even after 6–7 days after bite. It is repeated at 1–6 hourly interval till symptoms of envenomation disappear (up to 300 ml in viper bites and more in cobra).[17] Local injection is useful in vipers to avoid local gangrene.[17]
  b. Polyvalent antivenene (prepared at Kasauli) may be used as a substitute, if ASV serum is not available or patient is very sensitive.

Despite widespread use of antivenom, there are virtually no clinical trials to determine the ideal dose.

PM FINDINGS

a. Colubrine Snakebite

- Two puncture marks of fangs: ½ inch deep with oozing of serum and blister and necrosis at the site of bite (Figs 10.20 and 10.21).
- Blood is fluid with dark red color.
- Froth in mouth/nostrils.
- Signs of asphyxia present.
- Histology:[13] Nervous tissue shows changes in Nissl's granules, fragmentation and swelling of nuclei. Cells of medulla show acute granular degeneration.

b. Viperine Snakebite

- Two puncture marks of fangs: 1 inch deep with oozing of fluid blood and swelling, inflammation, discolouration, extravasation of blood or cellulites. On cut section underlying soft tissue edema, hemorrhage and oozing of fluid blood present (marked local features) (Figs 10.22 and 10.23).
- Blood is fluid with dark red color.
- Evidence of hemorrhage in GIT, RT, UT and petechial hemorrhage in pleura, pericardium, *lungs, and kidneys. Hemorrhage present* over endocardium, IV septum, papillary muscle.
- Visceral organs are congested.

MEDICOLEGAL ASPECTS

1. **Accidental:** Snakebite is usually accidental.[18] Annually about 2 lakh people are bitten by snakes and 50,000 die.[2] It is also seen in snake charmers.

2. **Suicidal:** Rarely except by Cleopatra.[19]

3. **Homicidal:** Rarely and mostly by indirect method or for giving punishment in ancient period. One case of contract killing by direct snakebite has also been reported.[8]

4. Cattle poisoning by placing snakes and banana in an earthen pot and irritating snakes by firing it. The cobra bites the banana. Fruit is then taken out and smeared into a rag to be injected into rectum of the animal by bamboo stick.

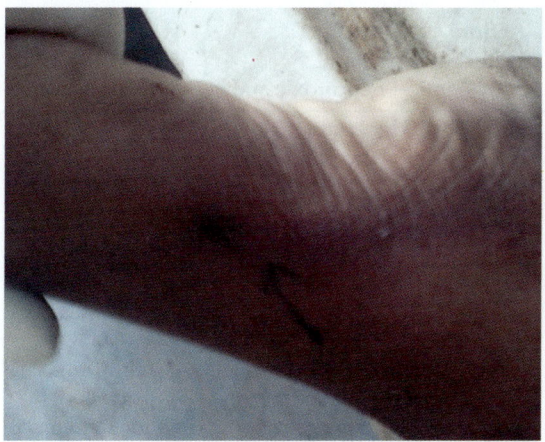

Fig. 10.20: Cobra bite mark

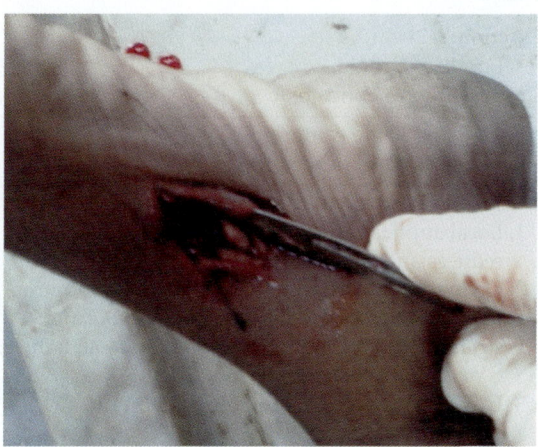

Fig. 10.21: Hemorrhage on cut section

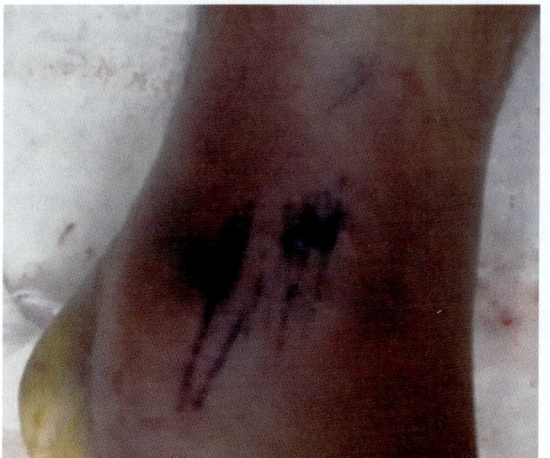

Fig. 10.22: Viper bite marks

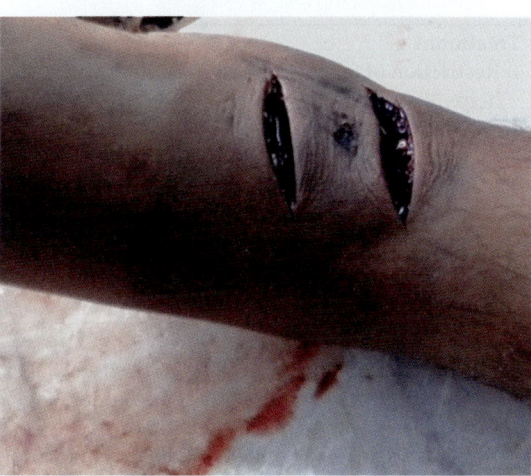

Fig. 10.23: Extensive hemorrhage on cut section

CANTHARIDES (SPANISH FLY—NOT SEEN IN INDIA)	SCORPIONS
It is an insect about 1.5 cm long, shining greenish in appearance[18]	Scorpions are long, fleshy, five segmented, eight legged, and have a tail. The end part of the tail has two poison glands and a sting. The scorpion when agitated injects the venom by pressing its sting leaving behind the broken tip of sting in the tissue on the body of victim.[18] Color varies from light yellow to black.
Uses 1. As counterirritant and in other medicinal preparation 2. Aphrodisiac	–
Active principle—cantheridin	Active principle—scorpion venom is a toxalbumin (a proteinous substance) consist of neurotoxin and hemolysin

Action:[18] • Locally—irritant • Systemic—nephrotoxic	**Action:** • Locally—irritant • Systemic—neurotoxic and hematotoxic actions
Fatal dose: 30 mg cantheridin **Fatal dose:** 12–24 hrs	**Fatal dose:** Uncertain **Fatal period:** Uncertain
Clinical features[18] 1. Local application to skin causes burning pain, redness and vesiculation/blister formation 2. On ingestion—burning pain in throat, abdominal pain, vomiting, blood tinged mucus stool and straining during motion followed by renal failure, CV collapse, convulsion, coma, death. 3. Urine—scanty containing blood, albumin	**Clinical features** 1. Local manifestations—(more severe than snakes)—bite is usually associated with little swelling, severe pain, paresthesia and hyperesthesia, accentuated by tapping on the affected area (tap test).[6] 2. Systemic manifestations—nausea, vomiting, restlessness, blurred vision, convulsions, cyanosis with perspiration, salivation, and nasal secretion, slurred speech. 3. Small quantity of the venom is injected—hence mortality is negligible
Treatment 1. Restriction of fat as it dissolves cantheridin and helps absorption 2. Stomach wash 3. Plenty of water to drink 4. Demulcent drinks 5. Symptomatic	**Treatment** 1. Immobilization and application of tourniquet proximal to bite 2. Wash the wound with water or $KMnO_4$ 3. Ice packs, analgesic and antihistaminics[6] 4. Anti-inflammatory. 5. Local infiltration of anaesthetics to lessen pain. 6. Antivenin.[6,18] 7. IV calcium gluconate to control swelling 8. IV glucose, saline and hydrocortisone
PM findings • S/o irritation in mouth/esophagus/stomach • Stomach: Wall—swollen; Mucosa—hemorrhagic; Contains—particles of exoskeleton of insect • Visceral organs—congested with hemorrhagic spots present • Urinary bladder—reddish urine due to hemorrhagic mucosa. Kidneys—hemorrhagic	**PM findings** • **Local:** At site of scorpion bite—swelling, edema, underlying tissue haemorrhagic • Visceral organs congested
Medicolegal aspects 1. **Accidental:** During medicinal use for counterirritant or for aphrodisiac use 2. **Suicidal/homicidal:** Rare 3. **Abortifacient** 4. **Aphrodisiac:** To increase sexual desire	**Medicolegal aspects** 1. Poisoning is accidental 2. Spraying DDT kills scorpions
BEES	**WASPS, HORNET**
It causes manifestation by stinging	It causes manifestation by stinging
Venom 1. Biogenic amines: Histamine, 5-hydroxytryptamine, acetylcholine 2. Enzymes: Phospholipase A, hyaluronidase, cardiotoxin 3. Toxic peptides: Mellitin, apamin, mast cell degranulating peptides	**Venom** 1. Biogenic amines: Histamine, 5-hydroxytryptamin, acetylcholine 2. Enzymes: Phospholipase A, hyaluronidase, cardiotoxin 3. Toxic peptides/other: Kinin/antigen-5, acid phosphatase

Clinical features
Local: Stinging causes local pain, redness, swelling
Systemic effect: S/o collapse with sweating, fall of BP, nausea, vomiting, bronchospasm, tingling sensation, flushing, dizziness, syncope, urticaria, glottis edema, angioedema, renal failure, hemolysis with hematoglobinuria

Treatment
1. Remove honeybee/wasps sting embedded in the skin.
2. Wash the bite site with **bicarbonate in bee sting** and with **vinegar in wasp's sting** followed by application of ice packs to reduce spread.
3. Elevation of affected site with administration of analgesic, antihistaminic and local calamine cream.
4. Epinephrine HCl: 0.3 mg SC for anaphylaxis
5. Glucocorticoids IM in severe reaction[6]
6. Artificial respiration + O_2 inhalation.
7. Antihistaminic cream locally

ML aspect: It is almost always accidental	**ML aspect:** It is almost always accidental	
BLACK SPIDER	**BROWN SPIDER**	**RED ANTS**
Black spider bite is toxic	Bite inject hemolysin and norepinephrine[18]	Red ants bite injects alkaloid, solenopsin A (has hemolytic and phytotoxic actions)[18]
Clinical manifestation 1. Local: Pain and cramps which extends upward 2. Systemic: Increase BP, nausea, vomiting, respiratory difficulty	**Clinical manifestation** 1. Local: Painful ulceration at the site of bite 2. Systemic: Nausea, vomiting, fever, hematuria, albuminuria, arthralgia[18]	**Clinical manifestation** 1. Local: Urticarial lesion followed by pustulation 2. Systemic: Increased BP, retrosternal pain, respiratory difficulty[18]
Treatment 1. Sedatives 2. Ca gluconate 3. Neostigmine + atropine sulphate (0.5 mg each) 4. Curariform drug	**Treatment** 1. Symptomatic	**Treatment** 1. Adrenaline 2. Antihistaminic
ML aspect: Accidental	**ML aspect:** Accidental	**ML aspect:** Accidental

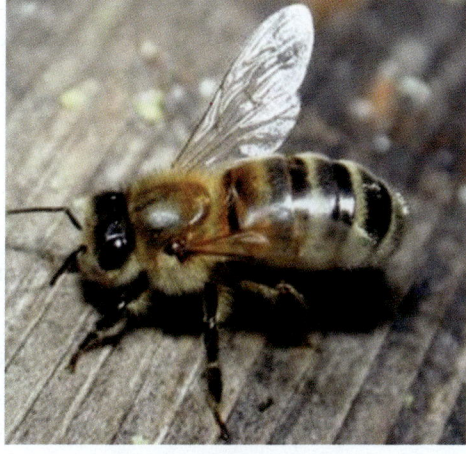

Fig. 10.24: Honeybee

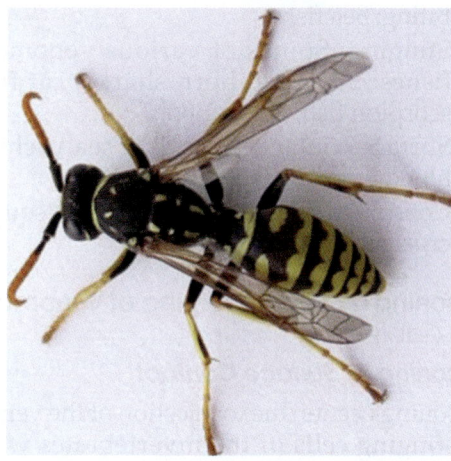

Fig. 10.25: Wasps

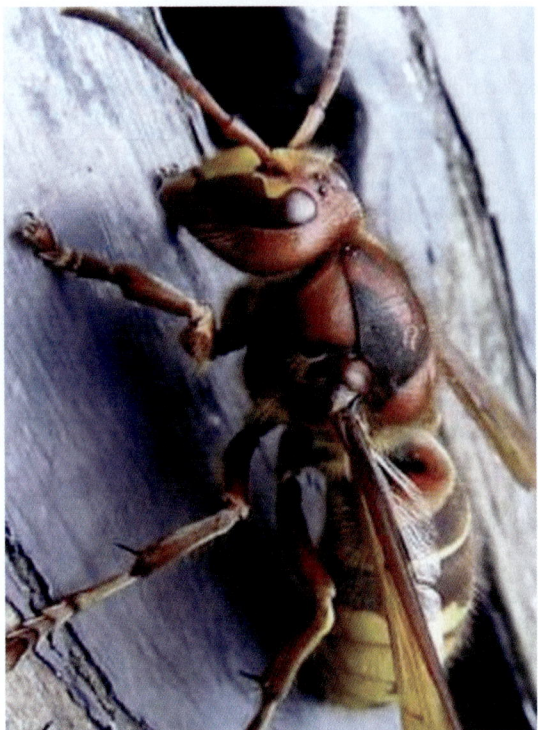

Fig. 10.26: Giant Indian hornet

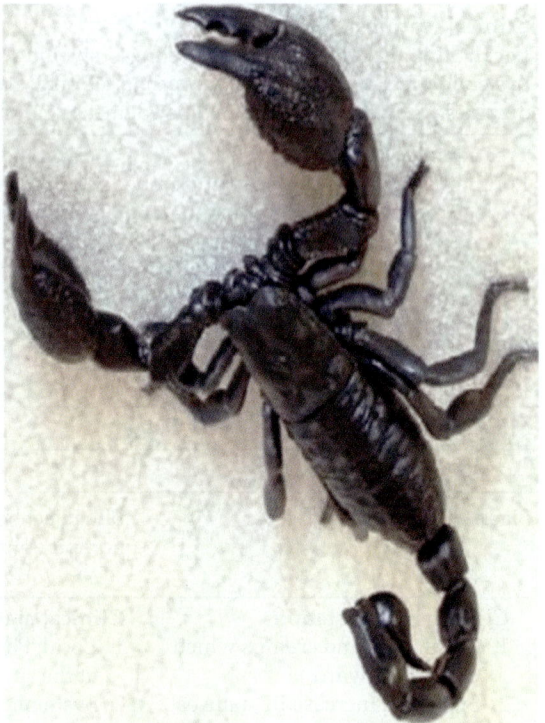

Fig. 10.27: Black scorpion

VENOMOUS AQUATIC ANIMALS

Some of the venomous aquatic animals are
  a. Vertebrates: Sea snakes, venomous fishes.
  b. Invertebrates: Shells, mussels, squids, crustaceans, jelly fish.

Poisoning by venomous aquatic animals occurs due to:
  a. Biting: Sea fish.
  b. Stinging: Spines of various venomous fishes: Stingray, horn sharks, cat fish, scorpion fish, weever fish.
  c. Surface contact: Jelly fish, sea urchins, blood worm, bristle worm.
  d. Consumed as food: Shells, mussels, squids, crustaceans (*see* Chapter 22).

Poisoning by Biting/Stinging of Venomous Fish (Table 10.7)

Poisoning by Surface Contact

Poisoning occurs due to injection of the venom by stinging cells of the invertebrates when they come into contact with the skin of person.

1. Jelly fish like Portuguese man of war/sea anaemone: Venom contains 5-HT, urocanyl-choline.[18]
2. Molluses or mussels (conch shells, squid, octopus): Venom apparatus cause punctures on the skin and inject venom.
3. Sea urchins: Venomous spines covering their body surface.
4. Bristle worm
5. Blood worm: Bites and inject toxic substances.

Clinical Manifestation: In Poisoning by Surface Contact

Local: Pain, swelling, redness.

Systemic: Nausea, vomiting, muscular cramps, paralysis, convulsion, collapse, coma, respiratory distress and death.

Treatment of Poisoning by Aquatic Animals

1. Washing the area of bite with plain warm water, $MgSO_4$ solution, alcohol or alkaline solution or 1% povidone iodine solution.

Table 10.7: Venomous fishes[18]

Venomous fishes	Sting/spines	Venom gland/venom	Local manifestation	Systemic manifestation
1. Stingray:	Sting is present in the dorsal aspect of tail.	Venom is secreted from ventro-lateral glandular tissue. It causes vasoconstriction and inhibits contraction and dilatation of heart	**Bite:** Intense, sharp, shooting, spasmodic or throbbing pain. There is swelling and necrosis of marginal area	Nausea, vomiting, diarrhea, faintness, vertigo, drowsiness, sweating, fall of BP, arrhythmia and muscular paralysis (flaccid/spastic)
2. Horn-sharks:	It has 2 dorsal spines at anterior margins of two dorsal fins. The spines are grooved	Venom is secreted from glandular cell	**Sting:** Immediate, intense, stabbing pain with swelling, redness	Death due to shock
3. Cat fish:	Have 3 stings, one dorsal in front of anterior dorsal fin and 2 pectoral stings one in each side in front of pectoral fins	Venomous glands are axillary glands for pectoral stings and glandular structure at base of dorsal sting. The venom is neurotoxic and haemotoxic	**Sting:** Intense pain may lead to shock and death. Secondary infection occurs and takes time to heal	Respiratory distress
4. Scorpion fish:	Have 12 dorsal spines, 3 anal spines and 2 pelvic spines with associated venom glands	Venom is neurotoxic, haemotoxic and cardiotoxic	**Stinging:** Intense pain + swelling, warm, bluish area surrounding red zone	Nausea, vomiting, convulsion, delirium, fever, pain in joints, respiratory distress and cardiac failure
5. Zebra fish and stone fish:	Have 13 dorsal spines, 3 anal spines and 2 pelvic spines with associated venom glands	–	**Stinging:** Intense pain with swelling	Nausea, vomiting, convulsion, delirium, fever, pain in joints, respiratory distress and cardiac failure
6. Weever fish:	Have 5–7 dorsal spines and 2 opercular spines with associated venom glands	The venom is neurotoxic and cardiotoxic	**Stinging:** Extreme pain with tingling and numbness. Area is firstly ischemic and then becomes red and swollen	Nausea, vomiting, convulsion, headache, chill, fever, palpitation, bradycardia, cardiac failure, respiratory distress, ankylosis

2. Analgesic like opiates to relieve pain
3. Application of antihistaminic cream locally.
4. Antibiotics to prevent secondary infection due to bite.
5. Symptomatic
6. Tetanus immunization.

ML Aspect of Poisoning by Aquatic Animals

1. Accidental.
2. Poisoning occurs in divers.

IMPORTANT QUESTIONS

1. **Classify snakes with examples. Describe clinical manifestation and treatment of ophitoxemia (snakebite poisoning). Write difference between cobra and viper.**

2. **Write difference between venomous and non-venomous snakes. Describe clinical features and management in case of cobra bite.**

3. **Describe clinical features and management in case of viper bite. Describe postmortem findings and medicolegal aspect of ophitoxemia.**

4. **Write difference in clinical manifestation of Colubrine bite and Viperine bite. Describe laboratory diagnosis of ophitoxemia. Add a note of anti-snake venom.**

SPECIFIC LEARNING OBJECTIVES

After reading this chapter, the reader should be able to:

- **Define envenomation and venom**
- **Classify snakes on the basis of their families and on the basis of venom**
- **Enlist common poisonous (venomous) and non-poisonous (non-venomous) snakes in India**
- **Differentiate between poisonous and non-poisonous snakes**
- **Identify common poisonous snakes in India from its peculiar features and to differentiate the belly and tail scales of Cobra, Krait and Viper**
- **Distinguish between king cobra and common cobra**

- **Distinguish between cobras and vipers**
- **Explain the features of snake venom**
- **Explain clinical features of snakebite poisoning—envenomation (cobra, viper, krait and sea snakes)**
- **Compare clinical manifestations of colubrine bite and viperine bite**
- **Diagnose ophitoxemia (snake bite poisoning)**
- **Understand the management in snakebite poisoning**
- **Summarize antisnake venom with respect to indications, types and doses in colubrine bite and viperine bite**
- **Explain clinical features and treatment in scorpion bite, bee bite and wasp bite**

References

1. Weinstein Scott, Dart RC, Staples A, White J. Envenomations: An overview of clinical Toxinology for the primary care physician. American Family Physician. 2009; 80 (8): 793–802.

2. David AW, Guidelines for the clinical management of snake bites in the South East Asia region. New Delhi: World Health Organization, Regional office for South East Asia, 2005:1–67.

3. Roland Bauchot, ed. (1994). Snakes: A Natural History. New York: Sterling Publishing Co., Inc. p. 220. ISBN 1-4027-3181-7.

4. World Health Organization. http://apps.who.int/bloodproducts/snakeantivenoms/database/default.htm

5. Sarangi A, Jena I, Sahoo H, Das JP. A profile of snake bite poisoning with special reference to haematological, renal, neurological and electrocardiographic abnormalities. J Assoc Physicians India. 1977 Aug; 25(8):555–60.

6. Longo DL, Fauci AS, Kasper DL, Hauser SL, Jameson JL, Loscalzo J. (edi). Disorder caused by venomous snake bites and marine animal exposures. In: **Harrison's Principles** of Internal Medicine. McGraw Hill Companies: New York. 18th edn. (vol 2), 2012:3566–83.

7. Bardale R. Principles of Forensic Medicine and Toxicology. 1st edn, Jaypee Brothers Medical Publishers (P) Ltd: New Delhi. 2011:477–87.

8. Ambade VN, Borkar JL, Meshram SK. Homicide by direct snake bite: a case of contract killing. Med Sci Law. 2012; 52:40–3.

9. Singhal SK. Singhal's Toxicology at a glance. 9th edn, National book depot:Mumbai.2016:62–6.

10. Reid HA, Theakston RBG. The management of snakebite. Bull of WHO 1983; 61(6):885–95.

11. Grenvik AKE, Ayers SM, Holbrook PR, Shoemaker WC (editors). Injuries by venomous and poisonous animals. In: Textbook of Critical Care 4th ed 2000: 224–33 [Ref list]

12. Mehta SR, Sashindran VK. Clinical Features And Management Of Snake Bite. Med J Armed Forces India. 2002 Jul; 58(3):247–9. doi: [10.1016/S0377-1237(02)80140-X]

13. Dikshit PC. Textbook of Forensic Medicine and Toxicology. 2nd edn, PEEPEE Publisher and Distributors (P) Ltd. New Delhi. 2014:509–22.

14. Weatherall DJ, Ledingham JGG, Warrell DA, editors. 3rd ed. I. Oxford Medical Publications; 1996. Injuries, envenoming, poisoning, and allergic reactions caused by animals; pp. 1126–39. (Oxford Textbook of Medicine). [Ref list]

15. Malani Ajit, Keoliya Ajay. Snake Bite-Bacterial Flora and Role of Antibiotics. Medico-Legal Update. 2016; 16(2):6–11. Article DOI: 10.5958/ 0974-1283.2016.00049.9

16. Tripathi KD. Cholinergic system and drugs. In: Essential of Medical Pharmacology. Jaypee Brothers Medical Publishers (P) Ltd: New Delhi, 7th edn, 2014:99–112 (110).

17. Tripathi KD. Vaccines and Sera. In: Essential of Medical Pharmacology. Jaypee Brothers Medical Publisher (P) Ltd: New Delhi, 7th edn, 2014:919– 27.

18. Nandy A. Principles of Forensic Medicine. New Central Book Agency (P) Ltd: Calcutta, 2nd edn Reprint, 2004:506–16.

19. Aggrawal A. Homicides with snakes: a distinct possibility and its medicolegal ramifications. Anil Aggrawal's Internet J Forensic Med Toxicol. 2003; 4:1–8.

Somniferous Poison: Opium and its Alkaloids

Somniferous poison/drugs: These are the sleep inducing drugs obtained or derived from the *Papaver somniferum* plant. It includes opium and their alkaloids. Opium is a dark brown resinous material and has a peculiar smell and bitter taste. It is obtained by giving incision to the unripe fruit (poppy capsule) of *Papaver somniferum* (poppy plant). It is the milky exude which on exposed to air becomes dark brown or black crude opium commonly called **"Afim"**.

Plant: *Papaver somniferum* is a herb growing up to a length of 1 meter. Flowers are large purple white or white in color. Each plant bears 5–10 fruits (poppy capsules) containing numerous small poppy seeds. The plant is a native of Turkey and is cultivated worldwide under Government control. In India, it is cultivated and distributed in Ghaziabad, Uttar Pradesh under Government supervision and also in Rajasthan and Madhya Pradesh. Opium has 20 alkaloids of which morphine is most important. A dried poppy capsule contains little narcotine.[1]

Types of opiates and active principle: It has alkaloids classified as:[2]

1. **Natural:** It has two groups:
   a. Phenanthrene: Morphine, codeine and thebaine.
   b. Benzyl isoquinolene: Papaverine, noscapine/narcotine and narcine.
2. **Semisynthetic opiates:** Diacetyl morphine (heroin), dehydromorphine, oxymorphone, hydromorphone, hydrocodone, oxycodone, N-allyl-normorphin (nalorphine).
3. **Synthetic opiates:** Pethidine, fentanyl tramadol, methadone hydroxypethidine.

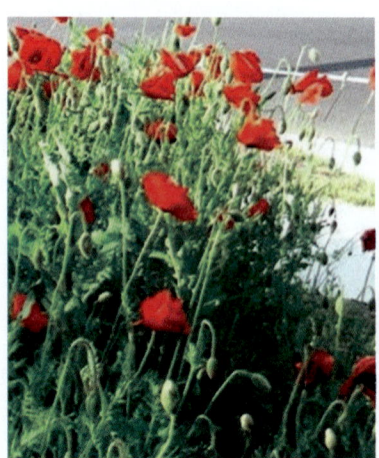
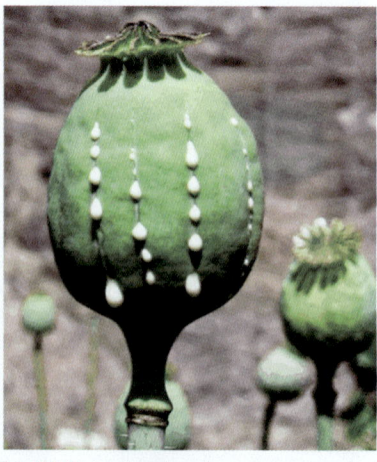
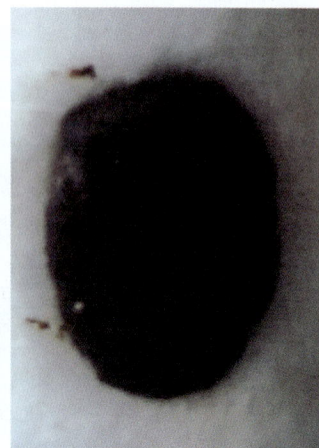

Fig. 11.1: Poppy plant   **Fig. 11.2:** Incised unripe poppy capsules   **Fig. 11.3:** Afim-crude

Uses

1. Morphine and codeine have maximum use as analgesic and cough depressant respectively.
2. Poppy seeds (khas-khas) are used in different food preparations.
3. Heroin is used as cough suppressant and is a drug of addiction.
4. Pethidine is used as analgesics. A single dose of pethidine may make an individual addict.
5. Morphine being respiratory depressant, is contraindicated in head injury and is a drug of addition.
6. Apomorphine, prepared from morphine is used as an emetic.

Mechanism of Action

- It causes CNS depression and narcosis (analgesic + hypnosis).
- It depresses all centres (in cortex and medulla—respiratory and cough) except vomiting centre, occulomotor centre and sweating (vagus).[1]

Fatal dose: Opium—2 gm, morphine—100–200 mg, codeine—500 mg, heroin—50 mg, pethidine—1 gm, methadon—100 mg.

Fatal period: 6–12 hours.

Absorption, Fate and Excretion

- It is absorbed through mucous membrane of GIT. When smoked, it is absorbed through lungs.
- Metabolised in liver.
- Excreted through kidneys, bile, milk, saliva and also through stomach and intestine.

SIGNS AND SYMPTOMS

Poisoning occurs due to ingestion of opium or its alkaloids or injection of morphine. In Tehran (Iran), 41.54% of the poisoning deaths were due to opioid alone followed by other drugs and organophosphates.[3] There are 3 stages of opium poisoning:[1,4,5]

Stage I: Stage of Excitation and Euphoria

- There is excitement, increased sense of well-being, increased mental activity, flushing of face, increased pulse hallucinations and convulsion.
- But soon there is restlessness, anxiety, dizziness, nausea and dysphoria.

Stage II: Stage of Depression or Stupor

Headache, giddiness, drowsiness, dizziness, disorientation, ataxia, lack of interest/concentration, uneasy feeling, contracted pupils, cyanosed face and generalized itching.

Stage III: Stage of Narcosis/Coma

- Muscles relaxed, reflexes are lost, pinpoint pupils
- There is hypotension, Cheyne-Stokes breathing, sweating, hypothermia (due to reduction in oxygen consumption, low metabolic activity and failure of heart regulating mechanism), cyanosis and froth at mouth and nose (due to pulmonary edema[6]) with progressive **respiratory depression**.
- Pulse is slow, and skin is moist, cold, clammy, and pale. Face is flushed, conjunctiva suffused.
- There is constipation due to constriction of smooth muscles of the sphincter. Emptying of stomach is delayed.
- There is oliguria, hyperglycemia, glycosuria and renal failure.
- There is uneasiness, sleep, coma and death.

DIAGNOSIS OF OPIUM POISONING

The triad[5] of following features strongly suggests opium poisoning:

- **Coma,**
- **Pinpoint pupils,**
- **Depressed respiration**, along with
- **Typical opium smell (raw flesh)**
- Cyanosis
- Froth at mouth and nostrils
- Cheyne-Stokes breathing
- Slow pulse, bradycardia
- Moist cold skin and hypothermia.

DIFFERENTIAL DIAGNOSIS

- Alcoholic intoxication, barbiturate/carbolic acid/CO poisoning
- Cerebral malaria/encephalitis/meningitis,
- Epileptic coma, hysterical coma, cerebrovascular accidents (IC hemorrhage with compression of the brain)
- Heat stroke
- Uremia, diabetic coma

TREATMENT

1. Stomach wash with 1 : 5000 dilution of $KMnO_4$. About 200 ml of the solution is left in the stomach after last wash to neutralize morphine, which is resecreted in the stomach after absorption even if morphine has been injected.[2]
2. Enema and purgatives: 20 gm $MgSO_4$
3. Antidote: **Naloxone** (is an opioid antagonist): 0.4–0.8 mg IV every 2–3 minutes till respiration improves[2] and dilatation of pupil. Naltrexone—long acting pre-opioid antagonist can be given three times a week at the dose of 100–150 mg orally.[7] Newer antidote is Nalmefene 0.1 mg IV followed by 0.5 mg IV. Methadone is used in chronic poisoning. However, opioid antagonists can precipitate acute withdrawal symptoms in chronic opioid users.[8]
4. Safeguarding respiration:
   - Bronchial suction to make airway free from secretion.
   - Artificial respiration and O_2 inhalation
   - Endotracheal intubation to ensure free air passage.
5. Stimulants: Methyl amphetamine HCl—10–20 mg, acts as stimulant to different system. Coramine as cardiorespiratory stimulant.
6. Supportive:
   - Antibiotic to prevent pulmonary infection.
   - Correction of fluid and electrolyte imbalance.
   - Benzodiazepines for convulsion.

POSTMORTEM FINDINGS

External

- Face congested with deep cyanosis over lips, ear lobules and nailbeds.
- Black postmortem lividity.
- Froth at mouth and nostrils.
- Smell of opium (raw flesh) present.
- Features of drug addiction—injection marks with pigmented and scar formation and tattooing.

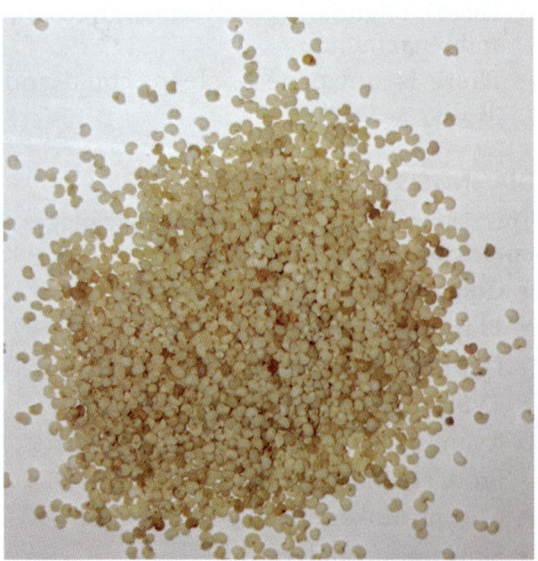 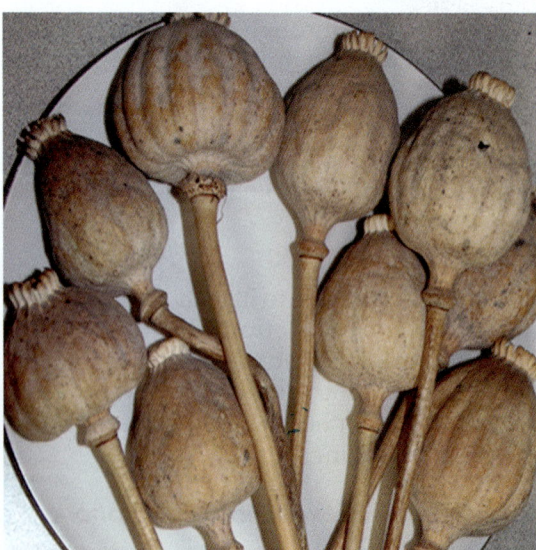

Fig. 11.4: Poppy seeds and dry poppy capsules

Internal

- **Stomach:** Contents have characteristic smell with presence of opium ingredients.
- **Respiratory tract:** Froth present.[7]
- **Lungs:** Congested, edematous [7]
- **Brain:** Congested, edematous with petechial hemorrhage on cut section.
- **Blood:** Dark and fluid.
- Visceral organs congested.

MEDICOLEGAL ASPECTS

1. Suicidal: It is a popular suicidal agents leading to painless death.
2. Homicidal: Not used due to its bitter taste, characteristic smell, and delayed death.
3. Accidental: Due to overdose in addicts and in children; and due to therapeutic misadventure.

4. Aphrodisiac: Morphine is used to increase sexual desire but it diminishes the performance.
5. Addicts can consume high dose of morphine/opium. There is moral degradation, and lack of judgment which may lead to commit any crime getting the drug out of desperation.[1]

CHEMICAL TEST

Marquis Test for Morphine

Put one drop of mixture (3 ml of conc. H_2SO_4 + 3 drops of formalin) on a blotting paper soaked with test material.

If the test material contains opium or morphine, then there is a play of color from purple to violet and finally blue.

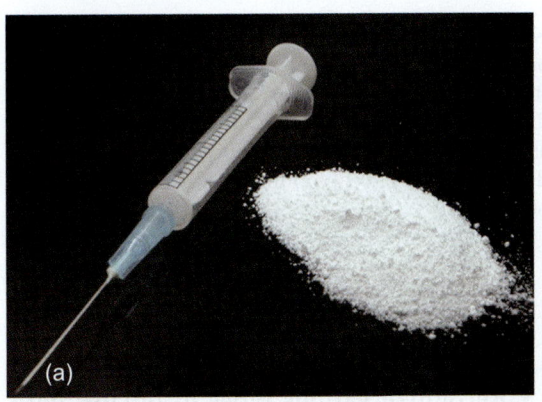
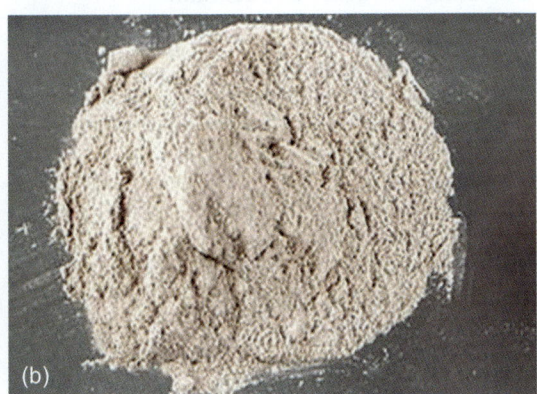

Fig. 11.5: Heroin/brown sugar

Opium/morphine addiction	Withdrawal symptoms in opium addict
Features of addiction (morphine mania)	**Features of withdrawal**
1. Irritability, fatigability, lack of interest/concentration, loss of weight and appetite, constipation, furred tongue, impotence/frigidity	1. Restlessness, anxiety, nervousness, insomnia, drug seeking behavior
2. Mental and **moral degradation**, loss of self respect and morality and a desire to procure drug by any means	2. Running nose, yawning, sweating, scratching, shivering, hot and cold flushes, goose skin appearance, dilated pupil.
3. For parentral use (skin popping in SC use and main lining in IV use): There will be **pigmentation and scar formation** at the site of injection often masked by **artificial tattooing**[1]	3. Severe twitching of muscle/muscle spasm, painful cramps in legs, tremor with vomiting, diarrhea, abdominal pain, loss of weight and appetite.
4. **Toxic dementia** may develop	4. Dangers: There may be debility, injury, intercurrent infection

Treatment of opium addiction[1]
1. Gradual withdrawal of drug
2. Substitution therapy with methadone 30–40 mg/day and then gradually tapered off
3. β-Adrenergic blocker like propranolol (80 mg) is quite effective in anxiety and craving
4. Maintenance of food, nutrition and vitamins
5. Nursing care
6. Physical restrain
7. Psychiatric counseling

Treatment of withdrawal symptoms[1]
1. Chlorpromazine 50–100 mg or pentobarbitone
2. Low dose of morphine or methadone
3. Physical restrains to protect from accident and injury
4. Maintenance of food, nutrition and vitamins
5. Nursing care
6. Antibiotic in some cases
7. Naloxone HCl: 0.4–0.8 mg IM/IV (0.01 mg/kg in children)[4]

Other opiates

Codeine (methyl morphine): (Natural)
It is popularly used as cough depressant. It is also used as an analgesic. It is less toxic than morphine and is less miotic, less constipating and more nauseating.[1] It has been used to control diarrhea[2] In toxic doses, it excites medulla and spinal cord and causes convulsion and delirium

Pethidine and methadone (synthetic opiates)
Pethidine is good analgesic, narcotic and sedative and causes mydriasis and dryness of skin. It liberates histamine from mast cells.[1–4] It has direct inhibitive action on heart muscles[4]

Brown sugar: It is crude heroin (**semisynthetic**) **Heroin (diacetyl morphine)**
It is semisynthetic opiate derived from morphine, which is 2–3 times more toxic than morphine.[1]
It is a white to dark brown colored powder.
It is more lipid soluble, therefore, enters the brain more rapidly. So, it causes more euphoria and addiction than other narcotic drugs[2]
It is 'downer' or depressant drug that affects the brain's pleasure system and interferes with the brain ability to perceive pain.

Nalorphine (N-allyl-normorphine): Semisynthetic opiate
It causes analgesic, respiratory depression, dysphoria, and hallucination.[1] It was popularly used as an antidote to morphine but because of its dysphoric and psychotomimetic effects, it is not used nowadays.[2]

IMPORTANT QUESTIONS

1. How opium is obtained? Write classification of opiates. Describe action, clinical manifestation, treatment, postmortem findings and medicolegal aspect of morphine poisoning.
2. What is afim? Write mechanism of action and management of morphine poisoning. Add a note on opium addiction and withdrawal symptoms.

SPECIFIC LEARNING OBJECTIVES

After reading this chapter, the reader should be able to:

- Define afim/opium
- Name the somniferous poisons
- Recognize various types of opiates with examples
- Enumerate different uses of opiates
- Understand the mechanism of action of opiates
- Explain clinical manifestations of poisoning due to opium/ morphine
- Recognize diagnostic features of opium poisoning
- Enumerate differential diagnosis of morphine poisoning
- Explain the management in opium/morphine poisoning
- Explain postmortem findings and medicolegal aspect of morphine poisoning
- Illustrate chemical test for morphine

References

1. Nandy A. Principles of Forensic Medicine. New Central Book Agency (P) Ltd: Calcutta, 2nd edn Reprint, 2004: 517–43.

2. Tripathi KD. Opioid Analgesic and antagonists. In: Essential of Medical Pharmacology. Jaypee Brothers Medical Publisher (P) Ltd: New Delhi, 7th edn, 2014: 469–85.

3. Shadnia S, Esmaily H, Sasanian G, Pajoumand A, Hassanian-Moghaddam H, Abdollahi M. Pattern of acute poisoning in Tehran-Iran in 2003. Human & Experimental Toxicol. 2007; 26, 753–6.

4. Dikshit PC. Textbook of Forensic Medicine and Toxicology. 2nd edn, PEEPEE Publisher and Distributors (P) Ltd. New Delhi. 2014: 547–52.

5. Bardale R. Principles of Forensic Medicine and Toxicology. 1st edn, Jaypee Brothers Medical Publishers (P) Ltd: New Delhi. 2011: 508–10.

6. Silber R, Clerkin EP. Pulmonary edema in acute heroin poisoning: Report of four cases. The American Journal of Medicine. 1959; 27(1):187–92.

7. Longo DL, Fauci AS, Kasper DL, Hauser SL, Jameson JL, Loscalzo J. (edi). Opioid drug abuse and dependence. In: **Harrison's Principles** of Internal Medicine. McGraw-Hill Companies: New York. 18th edn. (vol 2), 2012: 3552–6.

8. **Allen SC**. Problems with naloxone (letter). BMJ1975;3:434. Google Scholar.

9. Jaiswal AK, Millo T. Screening/spot/color test for different poisons. In: Handbook of Forensic Analytical Toxicology. 1st edn, Jaypee Brothers Medical Publishers (P) Ltd: New Delhi. 2014: 81–174.

Inebriant Poison: Alcohols

Inebriant means to cause drunkenness or to intoxicate. It includes alcohols and their derivatives, anesthetic drugs, and fuels like kerosene and petrol.

These are the poisons, which are characterized by two sets of manifestations:

1. Excitement
2. Narcosis—it is the combination of hypnosis + analgesia.

Definition of alcohol: It is an organic hydroxy compound obtained by replacing one or more hydrogen atoms from aliphatic hydrocarbons by hydroxyl group (–OH). Thus, alcohols are hydroxyl derivatives of aliphatic hydrocarbons. Absolute Alcohol is 99% concentrated.

Alcohol is obtained by enzymatic fermentation of: Carbohydrates (sugars and starch); Raw materials (cereals, corn, barley, etc.); Jaggery; Molasses; Potatoes; Fruits (grapes, oranges, cashew nut, etc.); and flower (mohua). The fermentation is followed by process of distillation and non-distillation method. If it is obtained by distillation method, then it is called spirit.

Spirit: Means any liquor containing alcohol and obtained by distillation after fermentation (whether denatured or not)	**Liquor:** Term used for any liquid containing alcohols obtained by any method (distillation includes spirits like brandy, gin, rum, vodka, whiskey, etc. or not distilled includes wine, beer, toddy, etc.)
Rectified spirit: It is the spirit subjected to rectification (process whereby liquor is purified or refined) for making it potable (Fig. 12.1)	**Denatured spirit:** It is the spirit subjected to a process for the purpose of rendering unfit for human consumption, e.g. French polish, varnish (Fig. 12.1)
Methylated spirit (industrial): Rectified spirit with 5–10% wood naphtha (i.e. impure methyl alcohol) so as to render it unfit for drinking. It can be applied on skin as antiseptic, cleaning and astringent purpose[1]	**Surgical spirit:** 95% ethanol + 5% methanol + oil of wintergreen (sweetish flavor for easy detection and pleasant use)
Beverages are drinks used for their flavor or stimulating effect, e.g. tea, coffee, aerated water, wines, etc. These may be alcoholic or non-alcoholic	**Toddy** is liquor not a spirit. It means fermented or unfermented juice extracted from palm tree, e.g. coconut, barb, date, etc. **Neera** is unfermented juice extracted from any palm tree

Arrack is an Eastern name for any country liquor
- Distilled from rice/sugar or jaggery, cashew nut, coco palm, and mohua flowers.

- Fortified with powerful knock out agents like potassium bromide, chloral hydrate, datura and bhang.

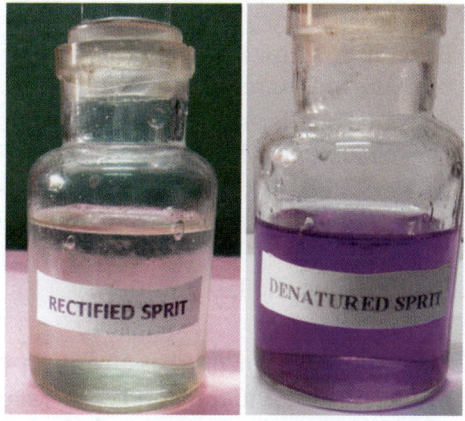

Fig. 12.1: Rectified and denatured spirit

Different names for liquor: Andhra Pradesh—Gudamba; Maharashtra—Khopri; Gujarat—Lattha; Goa—Feni; Mexico—Tequila; Japan—Sake.

Alcoholic Beverages[1]

a. Malted liquor: Obtained by fermentation of **germinating cereals**; are **un-distilled** with alcohol content of 3–6%, e.g. Beers, Stout (Fig. 12.2).

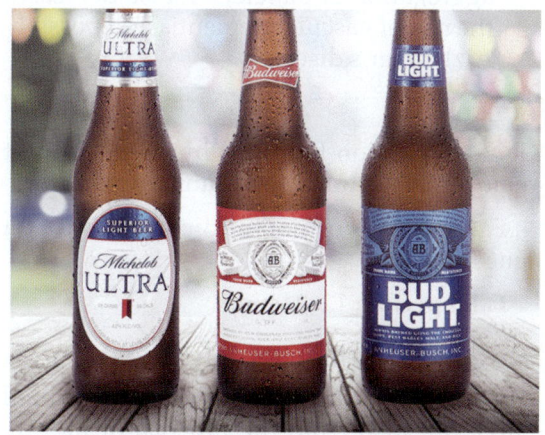

Fig. 12.2: Malted liquor—beers

b. Wines: Obtained by fermentation of natural sugars present in grapes and other **fruits**. These are also **un-distilled** containing 9–22% alcohol, e.g. claret, cider, port, sherry, champagne (Fig. 12.3).

c. Spirits: These are **distilled after fermentation**, e.g. Brandy, gin, rum,

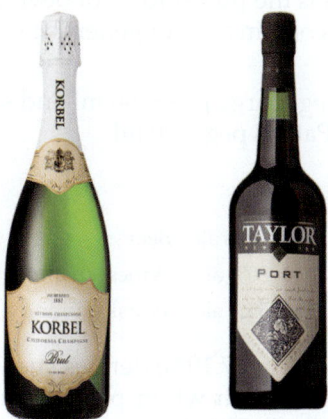

Fig. 12.3: Wines—Champagne, port

vodka, whisky, etc. It is standardized to 42.8% v/v or 37% w/w (Fig. 12.4).

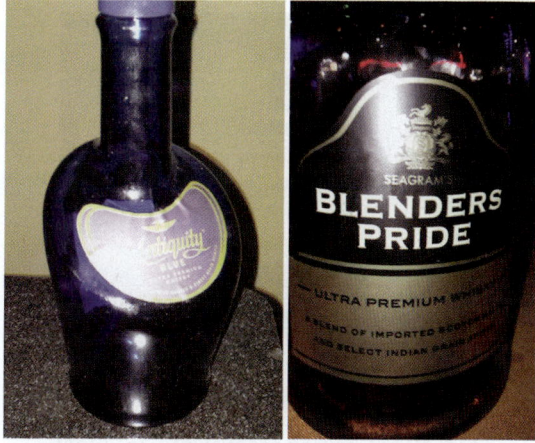

Fig. 12.4: Spirits: Whisky, vodka, gin, rum

Table 12.1: Alcohol percentage in different beverages

Beverages	Origin	Alcohol % by volume	Proof %
Rum	West Indies	42.8	75
Whisky	Scotland	42.8	75
Brandy	–	42.8	75
Gin	Holland	42.8/40.0/ 37.2	65–75
Beer	Brazil	2–10.0	3.5–17.5
Country liquor		11.4–45.7	20–80

Vodka is the purest form of beverages and does not contain any congeners. It is virtually odorless.

One peg: Large peg = 60 ml and small peg = 30 ml. Patiala peg = 90 ml

Types of drink		
Soft	04–08% alc	Beer
Moderate	10–20% alc	Wines, champagne
Hard	40–55% alc	Whisky, brandy, gin, rum

Proof spirit (57.10%) defines such strength of alcohol which when poured onto gunpowder allowed it to burn, since the remaining 42.90% of water did not prevent it. It indicates a mixture containing 57.10% by volume (or 49.28% by weight) of absolute alcohol (Fig. 12.5).

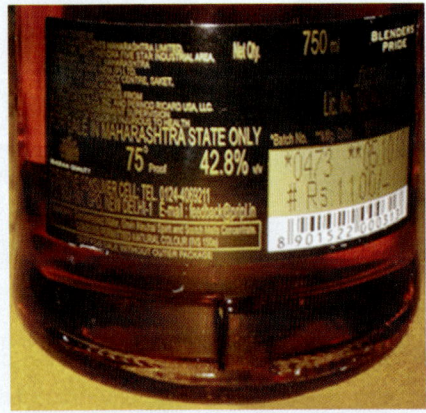

Fig. 12.5: Showing proof spirit—75° proof

Proof strength of a liquid is obtained by dividing the alcohol percent in volume by 0.571, e.g. wine—10% alcohol. Therefore, proof spirit = 10/0.571.

Similarly % of alcohol in liquid is obtained by multiplying the proof strength by 0.571, e.g. brandy 75° proof = 75 × 0.571= 42.8% by volume.

ETHYL ALCOHOL: C_2H_5OH

Properties: Colorless, sweetish/fruity (apple like) or acetone smell, sweet piercing taste, soluble in water.

Uses

1. Beverages/drink: It is used as a drink for pleasure and to reduce tension.
2. Solvent: For after-shaves, colognes, mouthwash, perfumes (15–80%).
3. Preservatives: Rectified spirit is used as preservatives of viscera for chemical analysis.
4. In industries and laboratories.
5. Medicinal uses:
   a. Surgical spirit is used as an antiseptic.
   b. Several multivitamins and cough syrups contain varying amount of alcohols—2–20%.
   c. Antidote for methanol and ethylene glycol poisoning.
   d. Ethanol sponging is an effective remedy for hyperthermia.[1]
   e. It is also used in trigeminal neuralgia.[1]
6. Decreases the risk of occlusive coronary disease and embolic strokes:[2] Relatively low doses of alcohol (1 or 2 drinks/day) have potential beneficial effects of increasing HDL cholesterol and decreasing aggregation of platelets. It also decreases the risk of vascular dementia and possibly Alzheimer's disease.

Action

CNS—excitation followed by depression. It removes the restraints on primitive behavior.

Fatal dose: For non-addicts: 150 ml at a time rapidly.

Fatal period: 12–24 hrs.

Absorption, Distribution, and Excretion

Absorbs rapidly from intestine (proximal part), but also from the mucosa of mouth, esophagus, stomach and large bowel.[2] The rate is more than glucose.

Alcohol is distributed in intracellular and extracellular fluid of the tissue. 'Walked off'— exercise sharply fall of alcohol supply to the brain.

2–10% of ethanol is excreted directly through lungs (breath), urine or sweat. But

90% is excreted/metabolised to acetaldehyde primarily in liver.[2]

Absorption of Alcohol Depends on

1. Amount of food in stomach: Empty—absorbs rapidly.
2. Quality of food: Fat and protein—delays absorption.
3. Concentration of alcohol:
   a. Higher concentration is absorbed rapidly due to irritation and inflammation of gastric mucosa.
   b. But in chronic user, it is not rapidly absorbed as higher concentration destroys the mucosa.
   c. The absorption is maximum at 20% v/v dilution of ethanol.[2]
4. Presence of CO_2: Increases absorption by increasing the absorption surface and induce rapid gastric emptying.[2]
5. Condition of stomach wall: Gastrectomy, chronic gastritis—increases the absorption.
6. Quantity and rate of drinking.
7. Weight of person.
8. Development of tolerance.

Metabolism

Ethyl alcohol → acetaldehyde → acetic acid → CO_2+H_2O

80% of the ethanol is oxidized by alcohol dehyrogenase and then aldehyde dehydrogenase in the cell cytosol and mitochondria (Fig. 12.6). But 20% metabolized in the microsomes of the smooth endoplasmic reticulum called microsomal ethanol oxidizing system (MEOS).[2]

Oxidation yields 7 cal of energy/gm and causes reduction of intake of other food by alcoholic (vitamin and nutrients), leading to degenerative changes in liver.[3]

Blood Alcohol Concentration (BAC)

Blood levels of ethanol are expressed as milligrams or grams of ethanol/decilitre (e.g. 100 mg/dL = 0.10 g/dL) or milligram/ml of blood (e.g. 100 mg/100 ml = 0.1% = 0.1 g/dL) with values of ~0.02g/dL resulting from ingestion of one typical drink.[2]

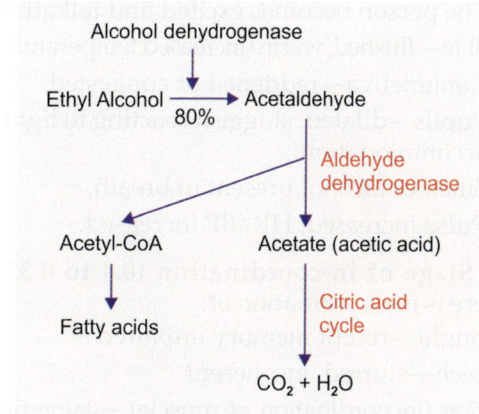

Fig. 12.6: Alcohol metabolism

Blood alcohol level reduces by about 10 mg% per hours and about 7 ml is washed out per hour in this way.

BAC reaches a maximum (peak) in about 1 to 1½ hours after ingestion. However, it is present in the blood within 30 min and urine within 60 min.

Level of alcohol in mg/100 ml of blood (BAC)	Minimum consumed volume of 75° proof spirit in ml
50 (0.05%)	69.5 ml
100 (0.1%)	139.0
200 (0.2%)	278.0
300 (0.3%)	417.0
400 (0.4%)	556.0
500 (0.5%)	695.0

Acute poisoning: Result from consumption of any preparation containing alcohol either in small doses at short interval or one big dose.

Clinical Features and Stages

I. Stage of excitement: 0.05% to 0.1% blood alcohol (>0.1% not fit to drive a vehicle)
- Inhibits the higher centers, which controls judgment and behaviour leading to unrestrained and unabstained character of a person.
- There is loss of restraints of code of conduct (habit, duty, behavior).

- The person becomes excited and talkative.
- Skin—flushed, warm (increased temperature).
- Conjunctiva—reddened or congested.
- Pupils—dilated, sluggish reacting to light/accommodation.
- Smell of alcohol present in breath.
- Pulse increased, HR/BP increased.

II. Stage of in-coordination (0.1 to 0.3%)
There is in-coordination of:

Thought—recent memory impaired

Speech—slurred, incoherent

Action (incoordination of muscle)—staggering gait, and skill movement impaired and reaction time increased.

- Impaired judgement
- Eyes—suffused,
- Vision—blurred, double,
- Pupil—dilated, sluggishly reacting to light,
- Mouth—dry, and
- Tongue—furred.

III. Stage of narcosis (0.3 to 0.5%)
- Deep sleep responds to strong stimuli
- Pulse—rapid, temperature—subnormal,
- **Pupil—constricted,**

- **Macewen's sign** present (pinching of skin of neck/face leads to dilation of pupil).
- A fine lateral **nystagmus**—oscillatory movement of eyeball (alcoholic gaze nystagmus—AGN). Alcohol causes nystagmus by two mechanisms.
  1. Firstly by acting on vestibular system, it causes positional alcoholic nystagmus (PAN), when the person is lying supine with head turned either left or right.
  2. Secondly by inhibiting smooth pursuit system due to alcohol effect on ocular movement via neural mechanism results in horizontal gaze nystagmus (HGN).

IV. Stage of medullary paralysis (>0.5%):
- Slow, stertorous respiration,
- Cold calmly cyanotic skin,
- Dilated pupil, abolished reflexes, very weak pulse,
- Dilated pupil,
- Abolished reflexes, very weak pulse.

Chronic poisoning: Result from continued use of alcohol and is characterized by **physical, moral and mental deterioration.**

Physical: Lack of personal hygiene, loss of appetite, gastroenteritis, wasting, peripheral

Treatment—acute alcoholic	Treatment—chronic alcoholic
1. 25% dextrose drip	1. Gradual withdrawal of alcohol
2. Inj B[1] (thiamine) 100 mg IM stat followed by 100 mg thiamine in 500 ml glucose IV infusion[1] daily till the patient becomes conscious. Then, switch to oral B-complex	2. **Antabuse: Disulfiram**—It is alcohol dehydrogenase inhibitor; and produces vomiting and autonomic nervous system instability due to accumulation of acetaldehyde in the blood.[2] **Dose:**[1] 500 mg × 7 days followed by 250 mg daily. It should be given only when the patient has not consumed alcohol within 12 hours and who sincerely desire to leave the habit.
3. **Proton pump inhibitor:** Inj pantoprazole/rabeprazole/ranitidine	3. **Citrated calcium carbimide (CCC):**[3] Temposil—50 mg—OD (similar to antabuse)
4. Sucralfate—if GIT bleeding	4. Chlorpromazine— 50 mg
5. IV fluids maintenance	5. Diet
6. Respiration is safeguarded by artificial respiration and O[2] inhalation, if needed	6. Supportive
7. Stomach wash, if required	

neuropathy, fatty changes in liver and heart, impotence and sterility.

Moral: Wide sociological abnormalities.

Mental: Loss of memory, impaired judgement.

Thus, there is GIT disturbance, liver damage with jaundice, ascitis, peripheral neuritis, tremor, insomnia, intermittent infection.[3] Approximately 35% of drinkers experienced temporary anterograde amnesia and disturbed sleep.[2]

Complication resulting from chronic alcoholism (alcohol withdrawal syndrome)

1. **Delirium tremens:** It is a psychotic condition in chronic alcoholic and its withdrawal. It is characterized by tremor, convulsions, insomnia, amnesia, confusion, disorientation, and failure to recognize known things, hallucination and agitated behavior

   Causes
   i Sudden increase in quantity
   ii. Sudden withdrawal of alcohol
   iii. Injury/infection
   iv. Shock from injury
   v. Exposure to cold

   Treatment[3]
   i. Largactil—100 mg orally
   ii. Meprobamate—2.4 gm daily
   iii. Sedation—phenobarbitone, paraldehyde or chlorpromazine injection is given
   iv. 5% dextrose IV drip, vitamins
   v. Symptomatic

2. **Korsakoff's psychosis:** It is a psychological and neurogenic deranged condition occurring in some alcoholics.[3] It is characterized by hallucinogens, disorientation, multiple neuritis and muscular degeneration, i.e. weakness, wasting and unsteady gait, retrograde amnesia—loss of recent memory.

3. **Acute hallucinosis:** Auditory hallucinogens, delusion of persecution.

4. **Alcoholic confusional insanity:** It is one of the withdrawal problems in chronic alcoholic with disorientation of time and place, hallucinations, delusions and mania/attack.

PM Findings

- Clothes are dirty, torn, soiled with vomitus and earth particle.
- There may be minor and major external injuries.

- Visceral organs are congested.
- Stomach contents—smell of alcohol with mucosa congested, hemorrhagic at places.
- Lungs and brain are congested and edematous.
- Liver may be cirrhotic, fatty.
- Other signs of hazards of alcohol may be present.

Material Preserved

1. Routine viscera—in saturated solution of common salt. (Rectified spirit—not to be used.)
2. Blood—in sodium fluoride/oxalate.
3. Urine—without any preservatives.

Medicolegal Aspects

1. Alcohol causes death mostly due to its associated hazards.
2. Accidental death—due to inhalation of vomitus or due to adulterated drinks or due to consumption of synergistic drug along with alcohol.
3. Suicide—alcohol is commonly used with other poison to commit suicide. Poisons were also taken under the influence of alcohol.
4. Homicide—for this the poison is mixed with alcohol to mask taste and smell. The person was killed by inflicting fatal injury or by pushing from height or by drowning after intoxicate by giving alcohol.
5. Aphrodisiac agent—it is used to increase sexual desire but it decreases the performance.
6. It is used to accomplish a criminal act or to give strength before committing crime.

Hazards Associated with Alcohols

1. Vehicular accidents.
2. Fall from height.
3. Electrocution/drowning/burns
4. Choking-café coronary
5. Cooking gas poisoning
6. Death

7. **Saturday night paralysis**—by compression of circumflex nerve. In intoxicated condition, the person rests his armpit on the back of his chair causing sustained pressure on circumflex nerve leading to temporary paralysis of his arm.

CHEMICAL TEST: DICHROMATE TEST

Filter paper soaked with potassium dichromate is placed at the mouth of test tube containing test material (urine).

Heat the test tube for 1 min.

If alcohol is present, color of filter paper changes from orange to green.

DETERMINATION OF BLOOD/ URINE ALCOHOL

1. **Kozelka-Hine/Cavett method**—aeration/distillation method:

Alcohol $\dfrac{\text{Potassium dichromate or } H_2SO_4}{\text{Oxidized}}$ acetic acid

Each ml of 0.05 N dichromate solution that is reduced in the process is equivalent to 0.575 mg of alcohol.

2. **Gas chromatography**

3. **Alcohol dehydrogenase method**

4. **Breathalyzer**—it is a device for estimating blood alcohol concentration (BAC) from a breath sample (Fig. 12.10). The driver/ rider is asked to blow through the plastic tube, the level of alcohol is displayed on the screen. It is legally admissible as per the section of MV Act, 1988. The false positives are[4]: Mouthwash containing alcohol used within 20–30 min, hyperventilation, physical exercise, emesis, regurgitation of stomach content.

WIDMARK FORMULA

It is used to estimate alcohol absorbed in the body by

- $a = CPR$, therefore $C = a/PR$
- R is the constant, for male = 0.68, for female = 0.54,
- C is the blood alcohol concentration (gm/kg); 'a' is the total amount of alcohol in gm absorbed in the body.
  P = Weight of person
- For urine, a = 3/4 qpr, where q is the concentration of alcohol in urine (gm/L)
- **Example:** 70 kg male has consumed 120 ml of 25° proof liquor. What will be the blood alcohol level?
- a = CPR, but proof spirit and density of alcohol (ml/kg) consumed should be considered for calculation.

Therefore,
C = a × proof spirit × density of alcohol/PR
  = 120 × 0.428 × 0.8/70 × 0.68 = 86 mg%

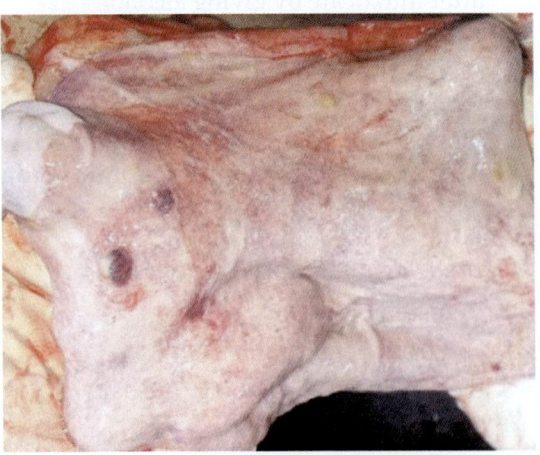

Fig. 12.7: Submucosal hemorrhage of stomach in acute alcoholic intoxication

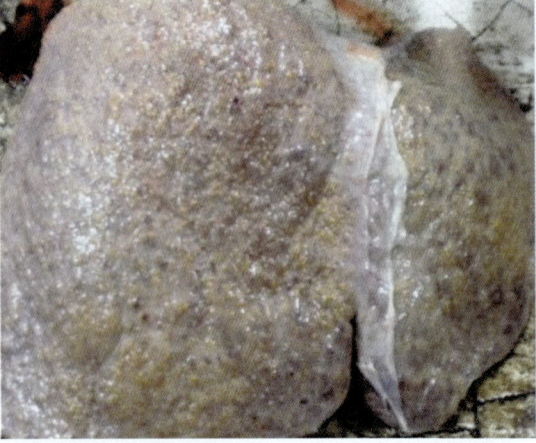

Fig. 12.8: Cirrhosis of liver in chronic alcoholic

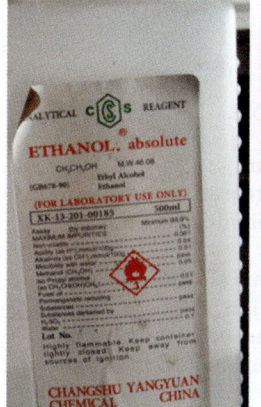 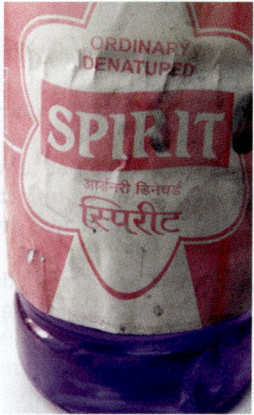

Fig. 12.9: Ethanol and denatured spirit

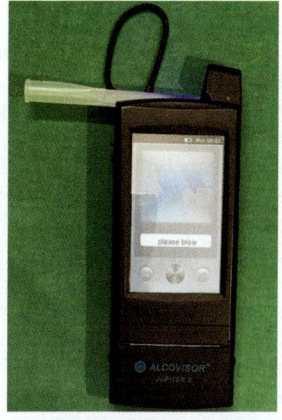

Fig. 12.10: Breathalyzer

METHYL ALCOHOL: CH_3OH (METHANOL)	ISOPROPYL ALCOHOL: C_3H_7OH
It is a volatile, colorless, flammable liquid with distinct odor similar to ethanol, but highly toxic and unfit for human consumption (Wood naphtha/spirit)	It is a colorless flammable liquid with a strong odor, used in disinfecting pads/hand sanitizers It is 3 times more toxic than methyl alcohol, which is more toxic than ethyl alcohol
Uses 1. Used as industrial solvents 2. With ethanol, used as antiseptic spirit 3. Methylated spirit = Mixture of ethanol + methanol 4. Embalming fluid, leather dyes, paint remover, varnish	**Uses** 1. Used as industrial solvents 2. Used as gasoline additive 3. Alternative to formaldehyde as tissue preservatives 4. Antiseptic spirit/hand sanitizer.
Fatal dose: 60–120 ml	**Fatal dose:** >100 mg% in blood
Fatal period: 24–36 hours	**Fatal period:** A few hours
Action: CNS depression.	**Action:** Cerebral depressant and renal damage as it oxidizes to acetone.[3]
Absorption, distribution, excretion Same as ethanol. However, methanol is metabolized to formaldehyde and formic acid by alcohol dehydrogenase and aldehyde dehydrogenase respectively, but the rate is 1/7th that of ethanol.[1] Methyl alcohol → formaldehyde → formic acid	**Absorption, metabolism, excretion** Absorption through mucosa of GIT/RT. It is metabolised (oxidized) to acetone by alcohol dehydrogenase in liver.[5] Excreted through urine as such or acetone, and small amount through breath.
Clinical features • Nausea, vomiting, abdominal pain, epigastric pain, dehydration, smell present. • Tachypnea, dyspnea, bradycardia, low BP, collapse • Headache, dizziness, vertigo, muscular pain/ weakness, cramp, restlessness, disorientation, convulsion, coma. • Acidosis due to formic acid which leads to **retinal changes leading to blurring of vision and blindness.**[1] • Death due to respiratory failure.	**Clinical features**[5] • Nausea, vomiting, abdominal pain, dehydration, smell present • Low BP, hypothermia • Headache, dizziness • Diminish reflexes • Constriction of pupils • Renal damage • Shock, respiratory depression and coma

Treatment
1. Patient must be hospitalized and kept in quiet dark room.
2. Eyes—covered and protected from light
3. Stomach wash with $NaHCO_3$[1]
4. Combat acidosis by IV $NaHCO_3$ infusion (2 gm in 250 ml water every 2 hrs) prevents retinal damage and other symptoms (dehydration).[1,4,6] Potassium chloride infusion for hypokalemia due to alkali therapy.[1]
5. Hemodialysis: It clears methanol/ formic acid[6]
6. Antidote: Oral ethyl alcohol[7] and Fomepizole
7. *Folate therapy:*[1] Calcium Leucovorin 50 mg injected 6 hourly to reduce formic acid level.

Treatment
1. Stomach wash
2. Symptomatic
3. Protection of the kidneys:
   • Hemodialysis
   • Dialysis if renal failure
4. Oxygen therapy to excrete acetone from lungs
5. Fluid replacement if dehydration

Clinical diagnosis of methyl alcohol poisoning is made in the presence of high index of suspicion of toxic alcohol ingestion, early visual symptoms, unexplained anion gap metabolic acidosis and significant osmolar gap.[7]

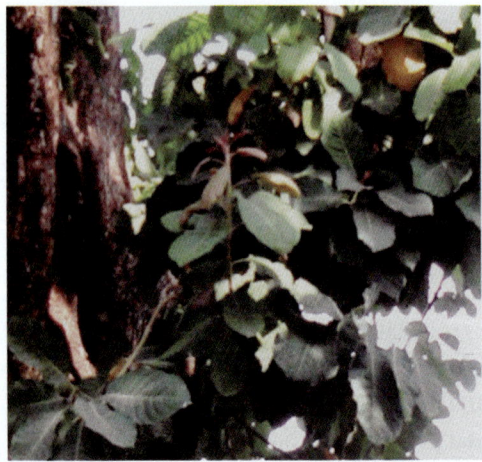

Fig. 12.11: Mohua plant and seeds

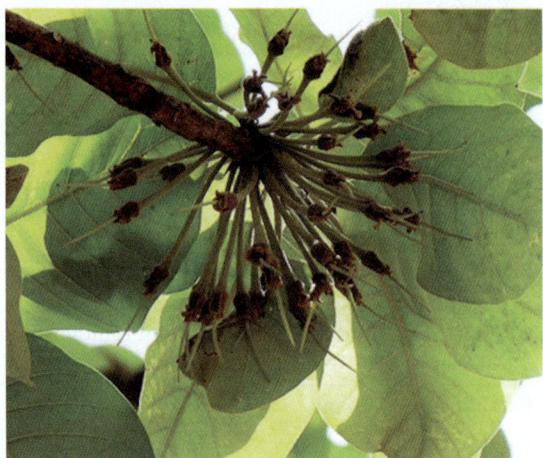

Fig. 12.12: Mohua flower

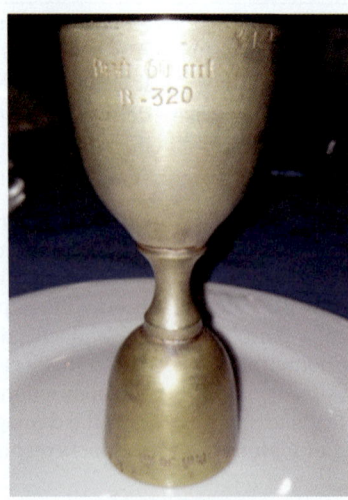

Fig. 12.13: Large and small pegs—measurement

Specific antidote of methanol poisoning[1]

1. Ethanol 100 mg/dl in blood saturates alcohol dehydrogenase and retards methanol metabolism and thereby reduces the rate of generation of toxic metabolite. No IV formulation of ethanol is available. Ethanol 10% in water is given through nasogastric tube in a loading dose of 0.7 ml/kg followed by 0.15 ml/kg/hr
2. **Fomepizol** is a specific alcohol dehydrogenase inhibitor, is given in 15 mg/kg IV followed by 10 mg/kg 12 hrly till serum methanol falls below 20 mg/dl

Methyl alcohol	Isopropyl alcohol
PM findings • S/o asphyxia with cyanosis and marked PM staining. • Frothing from mouth with presence of smell. • Stomach/intestine—mucosa congested, alcoholic smell present • Lungs/brain—congested and edematous • Liver—fatty changes • Kidney—tubular degeneration	**PM findings** • Nothing specific • Visceral organs—congested • Liver/kidneys—congested, edematous • Renal degeneration
ML aspects 1. Accidental: Most of cases are accidental due to adulteration of alcoholic drink with methylated spirit 2. Suicidal and homicidal uses may occur but are not common	**ML aspects** 1. Accidental—mostly by way of external medicinal use 2. Suicidal—due to easy availability as it is the main ingredient in many cleaning products

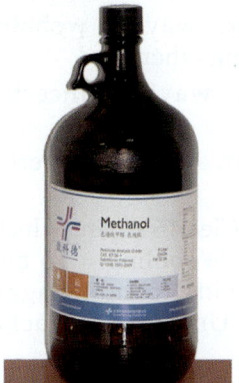 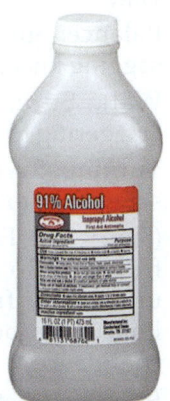

Fig. 12.14: Methanol and isopropyl alcohol

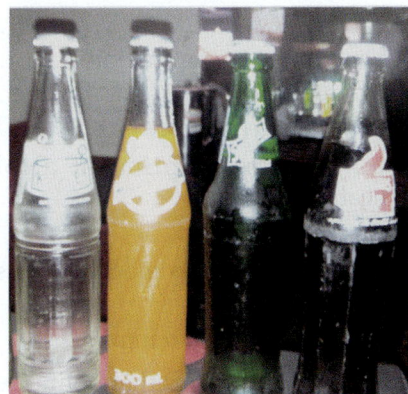

Fig. 12.15: Non-alcoholic beverages

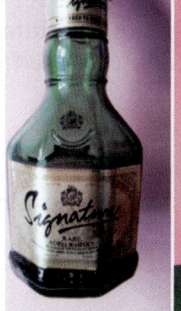 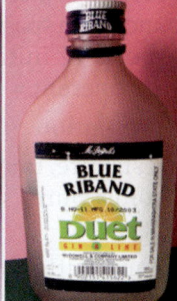 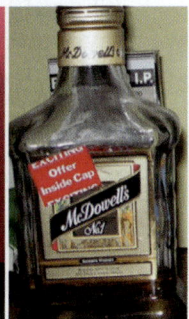 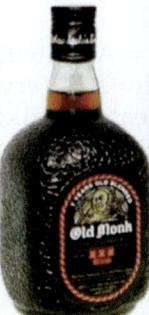 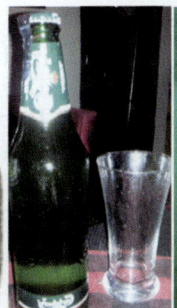 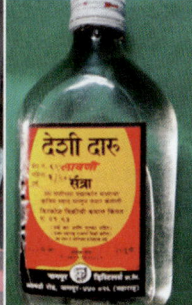

Fig. 12.16: Different types of alcoholic beverages

EXAMINATION OF ALCOHOLIC PERSON

Medical man is often required to examine a person and certify whether the person is under the influence of alcohol or not. So it is examined as per the following proforma:

Examination of Alcoholic

To

The Investigating Officer

PS ....

Ref: Your letter No. ...., dated ....

1. Name: .... Age: ..... Sex: ......
   Address: ....
   ....

2. **Identification marks** (two)

3. **Consent**
   Under Section 53(1) of CrPC: Examination of accused can be carried out by a medical practitioner at the request of police even without his consent and by use of force, if necessary.
   Brought by PC: .... No.: .... PS ....
   Date and time of examination: ....
   Place of examination: ....
   Examination in presence of: ....

4. **History** of consumption of alcohol/medication:
   - Type, duration
   - Consumption of any mouthwashes
   - History of diabetes
   - Past history of: Head injury

5. **General behavior:** Whether polite, excited, hilarious, talkative, carefree, sleepy, cooperative, indifferent, antagonistic, combating, insulting, etc.
   (Polite = Polished; Excited = Agitated, roused emotionally; Hilarious = Very funny; Talkative = Repeated talk; Indifferent = Not very good, uninteresting; Antagonistic = One who straggles with other; Combating = Opposing)

6. **Memory:** Recent event
   - Whether having orientation of time/place/person.

- Ask a few personal questions and then ask the same at the end of examination.
- Ask about some article/object in the examination room like number of tube light/tables, etc. and then ask the same in the last.

7. **Mental alertness:** Ask simple sums of addition or subtraction and see how much time person will take.
   How quickly the person responds to you and your question during examination.

8. Temp

9. Pulse

10. Resp

11. BP

12. **Skin:** Dry, moist, flushed, pale

13. **Smell of alcohol in breath**

14. **Eye:** Normal, watery, congested, suffused.
    Pupils: Normal, dilated, constricted.
    Reaction to light: Normal, poor.

15. **Gait**
    Balance: Sure, fair, swaying, wobbling, sagging knee, falling other.
    Walk: Sure, fair, swaying, uncertain, staggering to reel.
    Turning: Sure, fair, swaying, uncertain, staggering to reel.
    (Sure = Safe; Fair = Clear; Swaying = Incline from side to side; Wobbling = To move unsteadily from side to side; Sagging knee = To bend; Uncertain = Lacking confidence)

16. **Speech:** Whether fair, slurred, stuttering, confused, incoherent, other.
    (Slurred = Blurred; Stuttering = To speak, say or pronounce with spasmodic repetition of words, especially initial; Confused = Disordered; Incoherent = Loose)

17. **Muscular coordination**
    Finger nose test: Sure, uncertain.
    Picking up coins: Sure, slow, uncertain, unable.
    Unbuttoning and buttoning of shirt.

18. **Handwriting and copying of sentence:** Missing of letters; not in straight line

19. **Reflexes:** Knee and ankle: Delayed and sluggish.

20. **Systemic examination**

    RS

    CVS

    P/A

21. **Investigation**

    Blood: Spirit must not be used

    Preservatives: 10 mg sodium fluoride + 30 mg Potassium oxalate per 10 ml of blood

    Urine: 100 ml

    Preservatives: 30 mg phenyl mercuric nitrate for 10 ml urine or 5 ml conc. HCl for 200–500 ml urine.

    Note: The samples are preserved, sealed and handed over to police on duty at the earliest for chemical analysis.

Opinion

1. The above person has not consumed alcohol.

2. The above person has consumed alcohol but is not under its influence.

3. The above person has consumed alcohol and is under its influence.

    Place .... Signature ....

    Date ....

    Name of doctor ....

    Time ....

    Designation ....

    Seal ....

But, the opinion whether the person is under or not under the influence of alcohol is purely based on the clinical examination. The signs and symptoms of alcoholism are based on the personal tolerance to alcohol and various other factors. The same amount of alcohol consumed or same BAC (blood alcohol concentration) in two individuals give different clinical manifestation; one may be under influence and other may not be under influence of alcohol. Chemical analysis of the blood in this examination reveals only the amount or concentration of alcohol.

Alcoholic anonymous: It is an association (without having a formed body and place) of people who have given up alcohol. The addicts, who desire to give up alcohol, narrate their bad experiences to other alcoholics through meetings, symposiums, letters, press, etc.

Alcoholic intoxication: It is a state occurring in a person due to consumption of alcohol in a quantity sufficient to loose control of his faculty to such an extent that he is unable to perform his activities.

Drunkenness: It is a condition which results from excessive intake of alcohol and the person concerned is so much under its influence that:

1. He loses control over his mental faculties.

2. He is unable to perform his duties in which he is engaged at a particular time.

3. He may be a source of danger to himself or others.

Features at Different States of Alcohol Consumption

Slight: Flushed face, dilated pupils, euphoric, loss of restraints.

Under the influence: Flushed face, dilated and sluggish pupils, loss of restraints, increase in reaction time, stagger in sudden turning.

Drunk: In addition to the above symptoms, there is staggering gait with reeling and lurching while making sudden turn.

Bombay Prohibition Act

It is the Act (operated in Maharashtra/Gujarat) in relation to drinking, drunkenness, pleas in relation to drinking of nonprohibited preparation and possession of intoxicant. Some important sections of BP Act are as follows:

Sec. 65 and 66(1): Provide penalty for illegal import, export, manufacture, sale, and purchase of an intoxicant without proper license, permit or authorization.

Sec. 62(2): If blood alcohol concentration is not less than 0.05% (50 mg%), then accused person is supposed to prove the cause.

Sec. 84: Provides penalty for being found drunk or drinking in a common drinking place/house or being present for the purpose of drinking. Punishment of ₹500.

Sec. 85: Provides punishment for being drunk and disorderly in any public place, street, thoroughfare. Punishment for imprisonment of 1–3 months with or without fine of ₹500.

Sec. 129(A): A prohibition officer who has reasonable ground for believing that the person has consumed an intoxicant, is authorised to get such a person medically examined and his blood test for quantitative estimation of alcohol.

Rule 3 of BP Act: Deals with clinical examination and certification of a person by RMP in alleged consumption case.

Rule 4: Provides for the manner of collection of blood and forwarding to CA.

Rule 5: Deals with certificate of test in relation to blood sample examined by the chemical examiner.

Rule 117: Prohibition officer authorized to search any person, article or premises believed to provide evidence of possession of intoxication.

Rule 121(1): Opens any package and examines any goods and stop and search any vehicle.

Rule 123(1): Seize and detain any articles likely to contain intoxicant.

Rule 123(2): Forward the article to nearest police station for CA.

Section 117 of Motor Vehicle Act: Offence to drive/attempt to drive a motor vehicle with any quarter of alcohol in blood. In India, the statutory limit of alcohol in blood is 30 mg% u/s 185b of MVA, 1988[8]. The punishment for 1st offence is up to ₹2000/– or 6 months imprisonment; and for subsequent offence is ₹3000/- or 2 years imprisonment or both.

Table 12.2: BAC in relation to different stages of alcohols intoxication

BAC	Different stages
0.05% (0.05 g/dL)	Changes in special test
0.10%	Stimulation
0.2% (0.2 g/dL)	Incoordination
0.3% (0.3 g/dL)	Confusion
0.4%	Stupor
0.5%	Coma
0.6% (0.6 g/dL)	Death

If the BAC is 0.1% and above, then person is usually considered to be under the influence.

FORMALDEHYDE	KEROSENE	NAPHTHALENE (MOTH BALLS)
40% formaldehyde is formalin. It is colorless, pungent irritating odor	It is a clear liquid formed from hydrocarbons obtained from the fractional distillation of petroleum between 150 and 275°C	**Properties:** White scaly powder which volatiles at room temperature[9]
Uses 1. Preservation of tissue for histopathology 2. Embalming fluid	**Uses** 1. Used as fuels/and solvent in paints, pesticides 2. For preserving yellow phosphorus	**Uses** 1. Moth repellent—as mothballs 2. Deodorant cakes
Action Locally—GIT irritation, and precipitation of protein After absorption it causes systemic acidosis[3]	**Action** Locally—irritation of GIT Systemic—nephrotoxic, neurotoxic, respiratory depression	**Action** The metabolites alpha and beta naphthol and naphthaquinone are powerful hemolytic agents,[4] especially in individual with G6PD deficiency[9]

Absorption, fate, and excretion	Absorption, fate, and excretion	Absorption, fate, and excretion
Absorption through mucosa of GIT/RT After absorption it is changed to formic acid (like in methyl alcohol)[3]	Kerosene is poorly absorbed from GIT but there is often aspiration into respiratory tract especially, if child vomits	Absorbed through mucosa of GIT. It is metabolized in liver and distributed to visceral organs and excreted in urine
Fatal dose: 30–90 ml **Fatal period:** Within 24 hrs	**Fatal dose:** 30 ml **Fatal period:** Not fixed	**Fatal dose:**[8] 2–5 gm **Fatal period:** Uncertain
Clinical features • Nausea, vomiting, diarrhea, abdominal pain confusion, • After absorption it produces systemic acidosis and other features similar to methyl alcohol poisoning.[3] • When vapor is inhaled—it causes bronchitis, pneumonitis.[3]	**Clinical features** • Vomiting, diarrhea, abdominal pain, smell of kerosene in breath • Headache, giddiness, drowsiness, confusion, convulsion, coma • Cough, cyanosis, labored breathing, with respiratory failure, pneumonitis, pulmonary edema due to aspiration • Fever[10] • Glycosuria, proteinuria[10] • The features of kerosene intoxication are due to aspiration after swallowing.[11]	**Clinical features** • General—nausea, vomiting, abdominal pain, fever, convulsion • Hemolytic manifestation—pallor, weakness, jaundice, cyanosis, and dark urine (hemoglobinuria) with increase WBC count, fragmented RBC, anisopoikilocytosis, Heinz bodies[9] • Chronic exposure leads to aplastic anemia, hepatic neurosis and jaundice[8]
Treatment 1. Stomach wash: 0.1% ammonia solution and sodium bicarbonate solution[3] 2. Demulcent 3. Antidote: Sodium bicarbonate IV infusion[3]	**Treatment** 1. Stomach wash: Sodium bicarbonate. Although relatively CI, if done with good care to avoid aspiration, it is beneficial.[10] 2. Artificial respiration and O₂ inhalation 3. Liquid paraffin—250 mg oral 4. Symptomatic: Steroids, pantoprazole, IV fluids, antibiotics	**Treatment** 1. Stomach wash and emesis 2. Avoid demulcent 3. Treat hemolysis with blood transfusion, packed/red cell transfusion or exchange transfusion[9]
PM findings Stomach: Mucosa—inflamed; Wall—hard and leathery; Content—formalin smell present Adjacent organs: Also becomes hard and inflamed due to the transudation of formalin through stomach Lungs/brain: Congested, edematous Liver/kidneys: Shows fatty degeneration	**PM findings** On opening the body cavities—smell of kerosene present. Stomach: Mucosa—inflamed; Wall—soft; Content—kerosene smell present Organs: Congested Kidneys: Degenerative changes Lungs: Congested, edematous, pneumonitis	**PM findings** Not specific Stomach: Mucosa—inflamed; Wall—soft; Content—naphthalene particle with peculiar smell present Organs: Congested Kidneys: Hemorrhagic on cut section Lungs: Congested, edematous
ML aspects 1. Suicidal: Rarely 2. Homicidal: Not occur 3. Accidental: Mostly	**ML aspects** 1. Suicidal: Rarely 2. Homicidal: Not occur 3. Accidental: Mostly in children	**ML aspects** 1. Suicidal: Rarely 2. Homicidal: Not occur 3. Accidental: Mostly in children

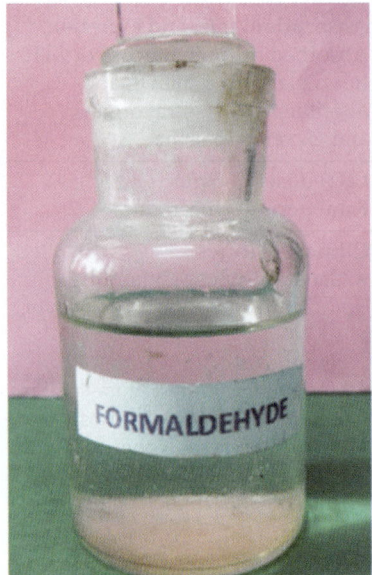

Fig. 12.17: Formaldehyde

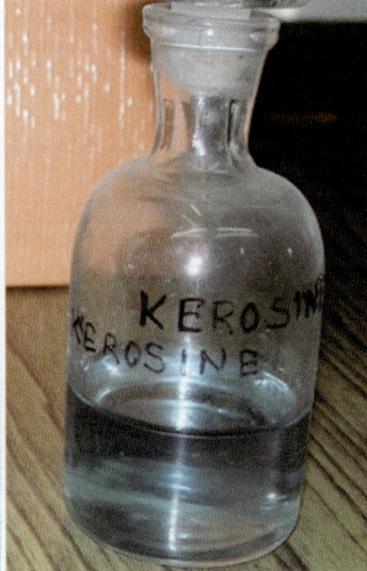

Fig. 12.18: Kerosene

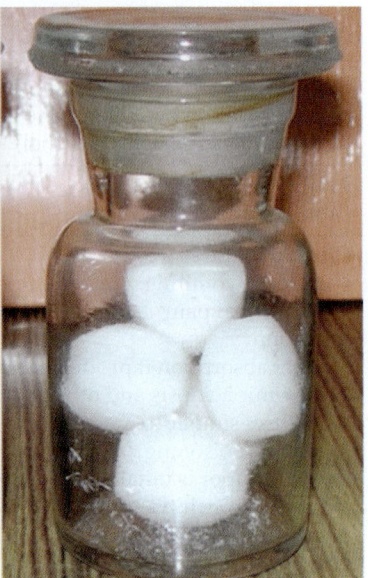

Fig. 12.19: Naphthalene balls

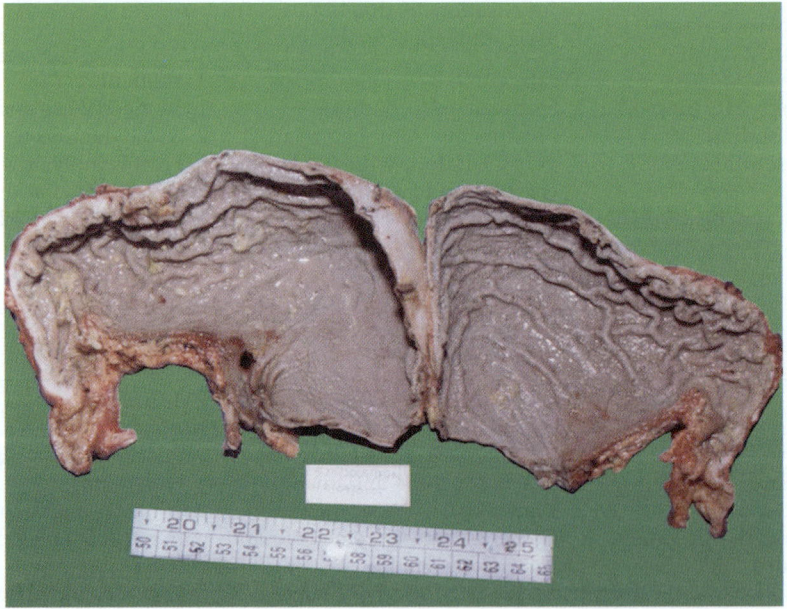

Fig. 12.20: Stomach in formalin poisoning

Table 12.3: Types and examples of different hydrocarbons[8]

Types	Examples
Aliphatic hydrocarbons	Gasoline, naphtha, mineral spirits, kerosene, turpentine
Halogenated (chlorinated) HC	Organochlorines, CCl_4, TCE (trichloroethylene)
Aromatic hydrocarbons	Benzene, toluene, xylene

IMPORTANT QUESTIONS

1. Explain the term 'spirit' and 'liquor' with examples. Describe metabolism, clinical features and management of ethyl alcohol intoxication.

2. Write different types of beverages with examples. Describe metabolism, clinical manifestation, treatment and medicolegal aspect of methyl alcohol intoxication.

3. What is rectified and denatured spirit? Add a note on Breathalyzer and Widmark formula. Write different hazards and medicolegal aspect of alcohol.

4. What is inebriant poison? Describe clinical features, management and medicolegal aspect of formaldehyde or kerosene poisoning.

5. What are distilled and un-distilled products of alcohols? Describe different factors affecting rate of absorption of alcohol. Describe management of ethyl and methyl alcohol intoxication. Add a note on Bombay Prohibition Act.

SPECIFIC LEARNING OBJECTIVES

After reading this chapter, the reader should be able to:

- Define inebriants and related terms like alcohols, spirit, liquor, beverages, arrack, proof spirit, etc
- Name different inebriant poisons
- Classify alcoholic beverages with examples
- Enumerate the uses of ethyl/methyl alcohol
- Recognize the metabolism of alcohol with fatal dose and fatal period
- Explain clinical manifestations, treatment, postmortem findings and medicolegal aspect of ethyl/methyl alcohol intoxication
- Enumerate different tests for alcohol
- Define drunkenness and BP Act and recognize the basics of breathalyzer

- Examine alcoholic person and to certify the opinion
- Explain clinical features, treatment, postmortem findings and medicolegal aspect of isopropyl alcohol/ kerosene poisoning

References

1. Tripathi KD. Ethyl and methyl alcohols. In: Essential of Medical Pharmacology. Jaypee Brothers Medical Publishers (P) Ltd: New Delhi, 7th edn, 2014: 388–96.

2. Longo DL, Fauci AS, Kasper DL, Hauser SL, Jameson JL, Loscalzo J. (edi). Alcohol and alcoholism. In: **Harrison's Principles** of Internal Medicine. McGraw-Hill Companies: New York. 18th edn. (vol 2), 2012: 3546–52.

3. Nandy A. Principles of Forensic Medicine. New Central Book Agency (P) Ltd: Calcutta, 2nd edn Reprint, 2004: 517–43.

4. Dikshit PC. Textbook of Forensic Medicine and Toxicology. 2nd edn, PEEPEE Publisher and Distributors (P) Ltd. New Delhi. 2014: 536–47.

5. Slaughter RJ, Mason RW, Beasley DM, Vale JA, Schep LJ. "Isopropanol poisoning". Clinical Toxicology. 2014; 52 (5): 470–8. doi:10.3109/15563650.2014.914527. PMID 24815348.

6. Kruse JA, Methanol poisoning. Intensive Care Med. 1992; 18: 391. https://doi.org/10.1007/BF01694340.

7. Nand L, Chander S, Kashyap R, Gupta D, Jhobta A. Methyl alcohol poisoning: a manifestation of typical toxicity and outcome. J Assoc Physicians India. 2014 Aug;62(8):756–9.

8. Reddy KSN, Murthy OP. The Essential of Forensic Medicine and Toxicology. 32nd edn, Om Sai Graphics: Hyderabad. 2013: 537–53.

9. Pillay VV. Textbook of Forensic Medicine and Toxicology. Paras Medical Publisher: Hyderabad, 17th edn, 2016: 581–601.

10. Nouri L, Al-Rahim K. Kerosene poisoning in children. Postgraduate Med J. 1970; 46: 71–5.

11. Maheswari A, Gulati S. Kerosene poisoning. Indian Journal of Medical Specialities. 2018; 9(3): 163–6. https://doi.org/10.1016/j.injms. 2018.06. 009

Deliriant Poisons: Datura, Cannabis and Cocaine

Deliriants are the substance, which causes delirium, means great excitement and ecstasy. Delirium is an acutely disordered state of mind characterized by altered consciousness, agitation, confusion, delusion, hallucination[1] with incoherent speech, and frenzied excitement, occurring in intoxication, fever, metabolic states, etc. Important examples are Datura, cannabis, and cocaine. However, cocaine is potent CNS stimulant, but is described in this chapter.

DATURA

Common Name

Thorn apple, Jimson weed, stinkweed.

Family: Solanaceae.

Plant: Characteristics

Datura stramonium—grows in Himalayan altitudes.

Datura fustuosa—grows on plains all over India.

There are two varieties of *Datura fustuosa*—niger (with purple flowers), and alba (with white flowers) (Figs 13.1 and 13.2).

Toxic part: All parts of the plant are poisonous but maximum concentration is in the seeds present in the fruit commonly called 'Thorn Apple', which is spherical in shaped having multiple spikes on the surface and containing about 400–500 seeds. The white or purple color flowers are tubular in shape.

Datura seeds: Odorless, bitter taste, yellowish brown, larger and thicker than chilli, kidney-shaped, rough surface, have two ridges on their convex surface, on dissection embryos are curved outward near hilum (Fig. 13.3). Datura seeds are similar to chilli (Capsicum) seeds. Points of differences are shown in Table 13.1.

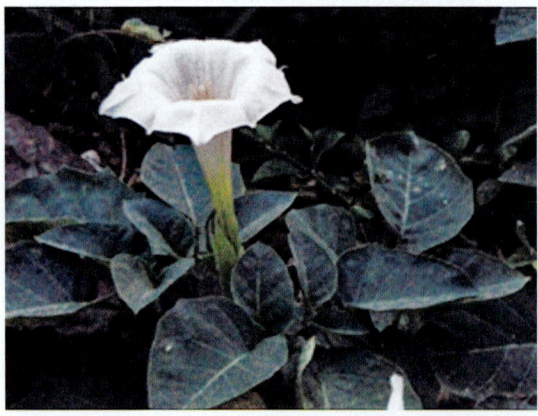

Fig. 13.1: *Datura fustuosa*—Alba variety

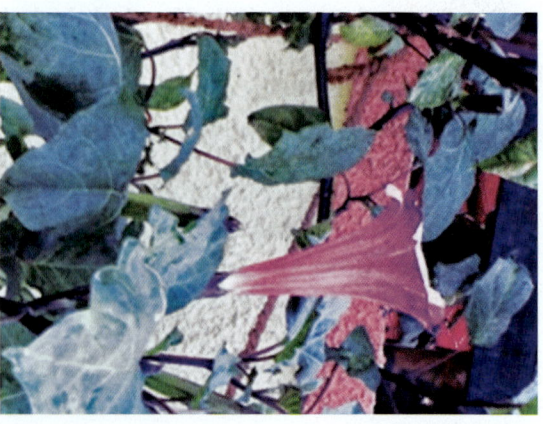

Fig. 13.2: *Datura fustuosa*—Niger variety

Table 13.1: Difference between seeds of Datura and Capsicum (chilli)

Points	Datura	Chilli
1. Odor	Odorless	Pungent
2. Taste	Bitter	Burning Irritating
3. Color	Yellowish brown	Pale yellow
4. Size	Larger	Smaller
5. Thickness	Thick	Thin
6. Shape	Kidney	Round
7. Surface	Rough	Smooth
8. Ridge on convex surface	Two ridges	No ridge
9. On cut section[2]	Embryo curved outward	Embryo curved inward

Capsicum seeds: Pungent irritating smell, burning irritating taste, pale yellow, smaller and thinner, roundish, smooth surface, no double ridges on the margins, on dissection embryos are curved inward near hilum (Fig. 13.4).

Active Principles (Belladonna alkaloids)[1]

- Hyoscine (scopolamine)
- Hyoscyamine
- Atropine.

Uses

1. Atropine as one of the active principles is used as medicine in:[3]
   a. Antidote for organophosphates and carbamates poisoning and mushroom poisoning.
   b. Anti-secretory in pre-anesthetic medication.
   c. Mydriatic.
   d. Antispasmodic.
   e. Bronchial asthma.
2. Datura seeds powder is used as kicking agent in the alcohol.
3. The seeds are also used in preparing *sui* (needle) from *Abrus precatorius* seeds.

Fatal Dose

Atropine—50–60 mg, hyoscine—10 mg.
  Seeds—75–100 seeds, for stupefying uses—40–50 seeds.

Fatal Period

24 hours.

Absorption, Metabolism, and Excretion

- It is absorbed through mucosa of GIT/RT.
- Metabolized in liver (atropine is destroyed by enzyme atropinase).
- Excreted through urine.

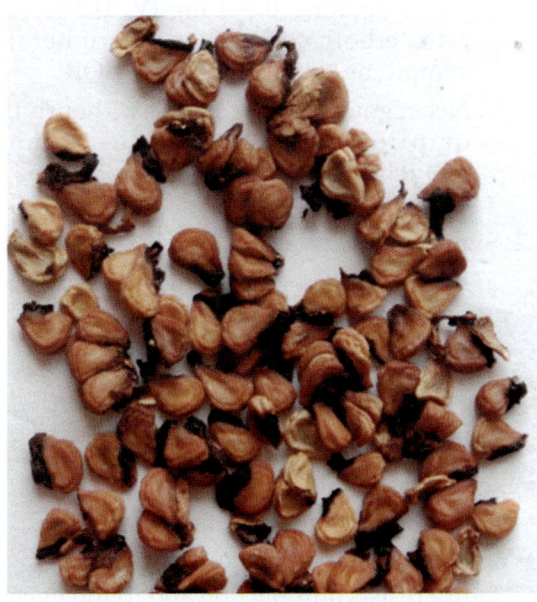

Fig. 13.3: Datura seeds

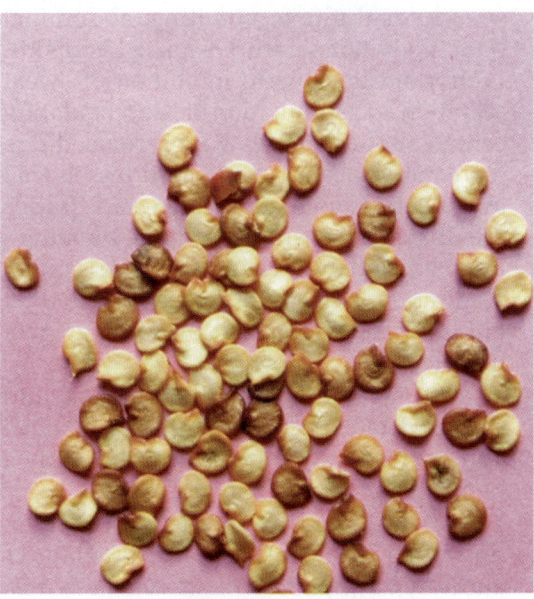

Fig. 13.4: Capsicum seeds

- Atropine is retained for long periods in dead bodies.

Action

- It blocks the ACh receptor and thus produces sympathomimetic or parasympatholytic action.
- CNS—it first stimulates and then depresses.

Clinical Manifestation

The alkaloids of datura stimulate the higher centers of the brain and then the motor centers. Thus, they inhibit secretion, dilate the cutaneous blood vessels, dilate the pupils and stimulate the heat regulating center. The initial stimulation (stage of delirium) is followed by depression and paralysis of the vital centers in the medulla (stage of coma).

Central effects of alkaloids are usually *psychotic-like symptoms* with photophobia, blurred vision, seizure and even coma,[4,5] whereas it causes *peripheral symptoms* like mydriasis, dry mouth, flushing, tachycardia, fever and urinary retention.[4,5]

The symptoms are classically described as classic phrase—**dry as a bone, red as a beet, blind as a bat, hot as a hare, and mad as a wet hen.**

- There is bitter taste in mouth, difficulty in speech/deglutition, vomiting, abdominal pain. Body temperature is raised and **skin is dry** and hot due to inhibition of sweat secretion and stimulation of heat regulating centers **(hot as a hare)**. Face is flushed due to dilatation of cutaneous blood vessels **(red as a beet)**. Conjunctiva congested, pupils are dilated, insensitivity to light, blurring/double vision **(blind as a bat)**. Pulse is rapid, respiration is hurried. This is followed by giddiness, staggering gait, incoordination of muscle.
- The mind is affected, first restless and confused, later becomes delirious, talkative and mutters indistinct words **(mad as a hen)**.
- This is followed by mania, convulsion, delirium and hallucination (visual/auditory). *The person tries to run away from the place, grasp imaginary object, and put imaginary threads in the imaginary needles with fingers.*[6]
- This excitation phase is followed by depressive phase, where the person is in deep sleep/coma, respiratory depression and death.

Thus, the main features can better be summarized under 9 Ds[1] mistaken for drunkenness and anticholinergic poisoning:

1. Dryness of mouth/throat, nausea, vomiting.
2. Difficulty in talking.
3. Dysphagia.
4. Dilated pupils, diplopia.
5. Dry, hot skin.
6. Drunken gait (ataxia).
7. Delirium, with disorientation, confusion, agitation, and hallucinations.
8. Drowsiness leading to coma.
9. Dysuria (urinary retention).

Death is due to respiratory failure or cardiac arrhythmias.

Treatment

1. Stomach wash with $KMnO_4$ or Tannic acid
2. Purgatives
3. Antidotes:
   a. Physostigmine[7] 0.5–2 mg IV, 1–2 hrly, relieve both cerebral and peripheral symptoms (usually preferred). OR
   b. Neostigmine (2.5 mg IV every 3 hourly), or pilocarpine nitrate (6–15 mg SC) relieves only peripheral symptoms. OR
4. Symptomatic:
   a. Inj chlorpromazine (50–100 mg) or inj diazepam, if patient is violent.
   b. Cold sponging.

Postmortem Findings

- Not specific.
- Signs of asphyxia.
- **Stomach:** Broken seeds of datura.
- Visceral organs are congested.
- Datura resists putrefaction and found even in decomposed bodies.

Medicolegal Aspect

1. **Accidental:** While using for other purposes, mistaken with capsicum seeds usually by children, adulterated country liquor/toddy (mixed with datura seeds powder, chloral hydrate for kicking effect).
2. **Suicidal:** Mostly reported from rural areas.
3. **Homicidal:** Extremely rare.
4. **Stupefying agents:** Prior to robbery, kidnapping or rape, the seeds are crushed and mixed with food, tea, drink, paan, prasad and given to unwary travellers by co-passengers to produce confusion, disorientation, and loss of consciousness.

Children may be easily kidnapped by giving them candy or sweet mixed with datura. They follow all the instructions of the person (who gave these sweet) to follow him. Likewise, women have been abducted, robbed or raped.

5. **Aphrodisiac agent:** To increase sexual desire.
6. **Datura abuse** due to its hypnotic and hallucinogenic properties.[1]

Chemical Test: Mydriatic Test[2]

If a drop of stomach content (having Datura) is poured in rabbit's eye, then there is dilatation of pupil.

Laboratory Investigation

Raised liver enzymes like LDH, CPK, etc. without myoglobinuria and normal kidney function test.[8]

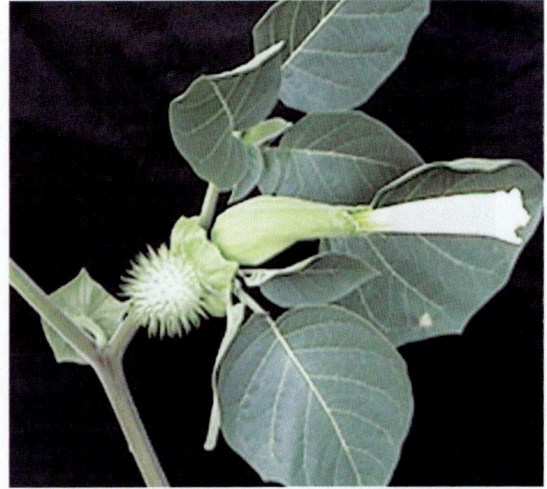

Fig. 13.6: *Datura fustuosa*—alba variety

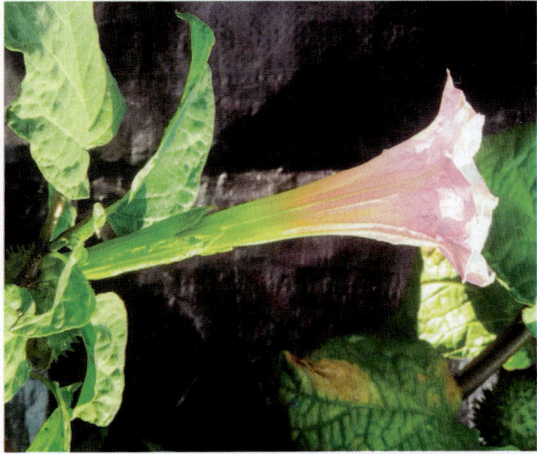

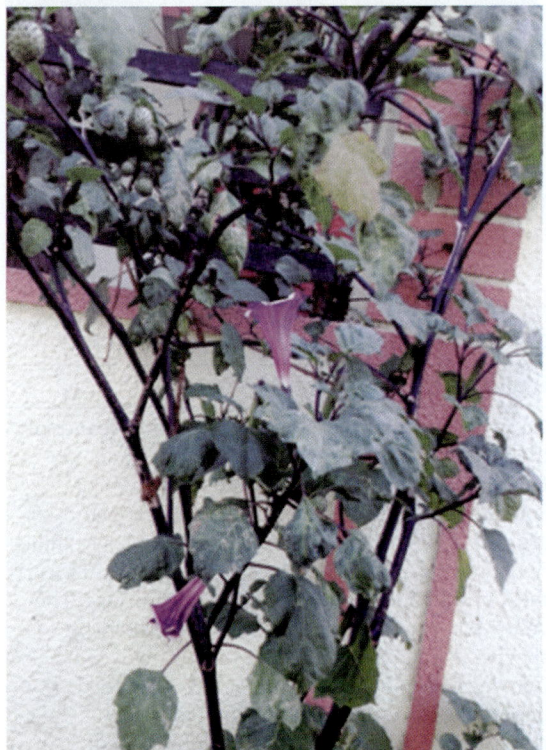

Fig. 13.5: *Datura fustuosa*—niger variety (*Courtesy:* Dr. Manish Shrigiriwar)

Fig. 13.7: *Datura fustuosa*—niger variety with purple flower

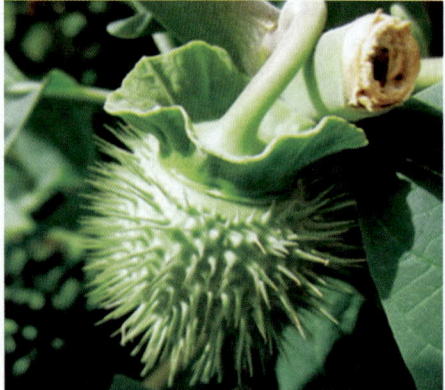

Fig. 13.8a: Thorn apple—Datura fruit (alba)

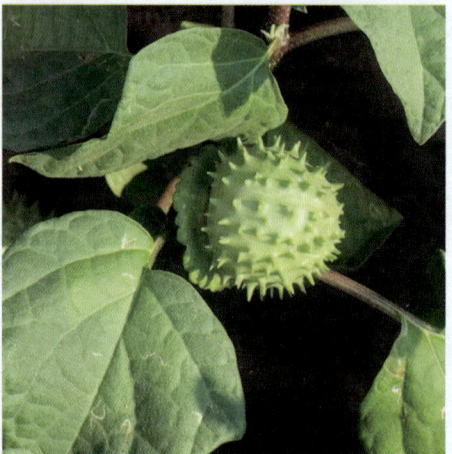

Fig. 13.8b: Thorn apple—Datura fruit (niger)

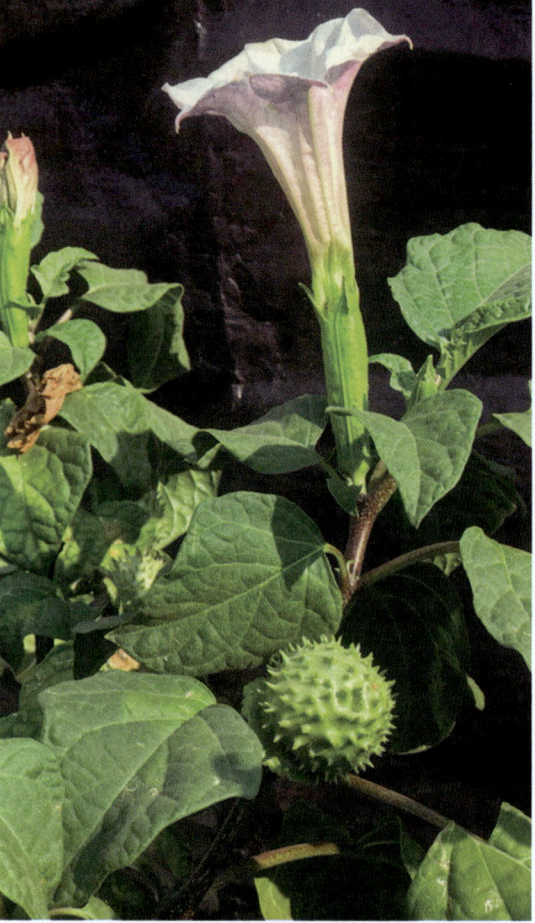

Fig. 13.9: *Datura fustuosa*—purple flower

CANNABIS	COCAINE (*Erythroxylum Coca*)
Common name: Indian hemp	**Common names:** Coke, snow, cadillac, white lady, etc.
Family: Cannabaceae	**Family[1]:** Erythroxylaceae
Cannabis sativa is having two varieties: *Cannabis indica*—grows all over India. *Cannabis mexicana*—grows in Mexico. The term cannabis refers to the flowering and fruiting tops of Cannabis plant. Cannabis is a tall weed growing up to 15 feet in height and it is a dioecious plant, i.e. the sexes are separated. All part of the plant is toxic. But its cultivation and marketing is under strict legislation and control under government. It is a drug of dependence and consumed in different preparations containing different concentrations of **active principle,** namely **Tetra-hydrocannabinol (THC).**	**Cocaine is an alkaloid,** extracted from the leaves of the coca tree, namely *Erythroxylum coca* and *E. novogranatense*. They grow in mountains of South America, Indonesia, and India. The plant grows to a height of 7–10 feet. The green leaves have two longitudinal curved lines on either side of the thick midrib, clearly seen on the undersurface. The yellowish-white flowers are small in clusters on short stalk, which mature into red berries. Cocaine is the strongest **drug of psychological** dependence but also causes strong **physical dependence** that makes it a notorious drug of addiction.

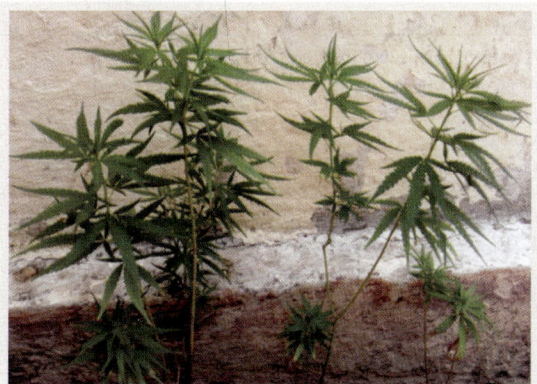

Fig. 13.10: Cannabis plant

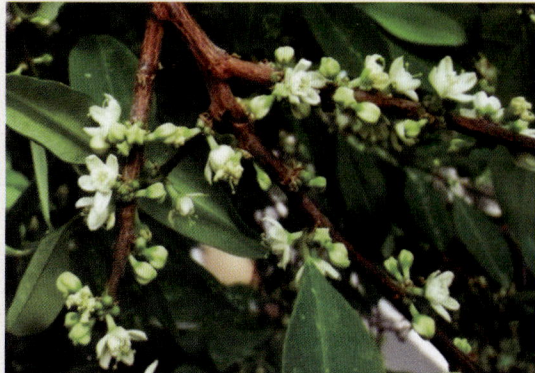

Fig. 13.11: *Erythroxylum coca* (cocaine plant)

Cannabis is usually abused among sadhus-sanyasis, college students and western musicians/painters, however, physical dependence is not common.[1]

Cocaine is usually abused by the upper classes of society to enhance self-image or improve professional performance[1]

Common preparations/forms of cannabis[2,9] and concentration of THC in brackets
1. **Bhang:** (Siddi/patti) prepared from dried leaves and stem (2–5% THC), and consumed orally.
2. **Majun:** Sweet preparation of bhang after treating with sugar, flour, milk
3. **Ganja:** Prepared from flowering tops of female plant (5–10%). It is rusty brown and is smoked
4. **Charas/hashish:** It is resinous extract from flowering tops and leaves. It is dark green or brown-colored powder[2] (25–40%) is usually smoked along with tobacco.

Cocaine is available in various forms:[2]
1. **Cocaine hydrochloride:** It is white, shiny crystalline odorless substance with a bitter, numbing taste. Typically used for injection/snorting, but can also be ingested.
2. **Cocaine sulphate (Cocoa paste):** It is a crude product contaminated with solvents, used for smoking.
3. **Crack:** It is prepared by heating cocaine with baking soda and water. It is used for smoking, gives off cracking sound, hence named.
4. **Speedball:** Cocaine is taken with heroine by IV route for higher euphoria.

Ganja is smoked either as it is or mixed with tobacco in a pipe/hookah/chilam or in the form of cigarette. The cigarette preparation of ganja is called '**Reefer**'.[2] When ganja is smoked in a pipe, then it is called **Marijuana**.[1] Bhang is mixed with fruit juice or milk and consumed during Holi and Navaratri in North India.[1]

There is a characteristic **odor** like that of a **burnt rope** in all cannabis preparations when smoked.

Uses:[9]
At present, cannabis is a banned drug in India and most parts of the world. Cannabis has been the most popular recreational and ritualistic intoxicant used for millennia
1. **Antiemetic** against vomiting induced by anticancer drugs
2. Treatment of convulsions/anxiety[1] and migraine
3. As bronchodilator in asthma.
4. To reduce IOT in glaucoma.

Uses:
1. Medicinally used as local **anesthetic agent** in minor surgery/procedures
2. **Brompton's cocktail:** It contains cocaine, morphine, chlorpromazine, and alcohol. It was previously popular as a pain reliever in terminal cancer[1]
3. Used as a snuff to reduce appetite and feeling of fatigue[10]
4. Used as aphrodisiac and as a pleasant intoxicant[10]

Fatal dose:[2] Very high, fatality is uncommon
   Charas—2 gm; Ganja—8 gm
   Bhang—10 gm/kg body weight
Fatal period: 12 hours to a few days

Fatal dose
   Oral—1.5 gm
   Injection—1 gm (hypodermic injection 40 mg)
Fatal period: A few min to 2 hours

Cannabis	Cocaine
Absorption, fate, and excretion	**Absorption, fate, and excretion**
Absorbed through mucosa of GIT and also through RT when smoked Metabolized in liver Excreted through urine, feces, bile	Absorbed through mucosa of GIT/RT/nose (when used as snuff) Metabolized in liver Excreted through urine
Action	**Action**
1. It is a **hallucinogen** causes excitement followed by sleep 2. CNS—stimulant	1. It is a strong **amino-oxidase inhibitor** and potentiates the effects of adrenaline or noradrenaline 2. CNS—stimulant and local anesthetic[11]

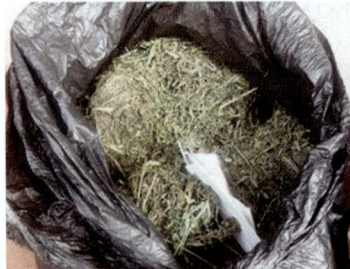

Fig. 13.12: Ganja   **Fig. 13.13:** Chilam   **Fig. 13.14:** Cocaine powder

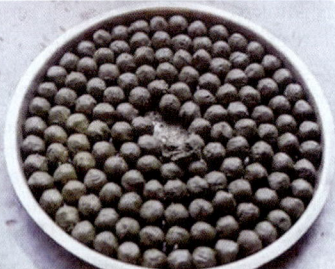

Fig. 13.15: Bhang   **Fig. 13.16:** Majun   **Fig. 13.17:** Charas

Clinical features

Acute cannabis poisoning:

Generally considered, cannabis is not very toxic and fatal. It is a hallucinogen. In acute poisoning, it causes excitement followed by sleep.

The manifestations depend on individual tolerance and routes of administration and are grouped into two stages.

a. Stage of excitement/euphoria and release of inhibition

• Sense of well-being, excitement, euphoria, talkativeness, **uncontrollable laugh,** marked

Clinical features

Acute cocaine poisoning

Cocaine toxicity produces a hyper-adrenergic state characterised by hypertension, tachycardia, tonic-clonic seizures, dyspnea, and ventricular arrhythmias.[12]

It is a powerful CNS stimulant causing in sequence euphoria—excitement—confusion—restlessness—tremor and twitching of muscle—convulsion—unconsciousness—respiratory depression—death, in a dose dependant manner.[11] It also stimulates vagal centre—bradycardia; vasomotor centre—rise in BP;

increase in appetite specially sweet, craving for sleep, purposeless muscular movement and **visual hallucination and ideas** (sees nude beautiful women dancing before him, playing music, and singing romantic songs)

- **Motor incoordination,** tachycardia, conjunctival congestion, miosis
- There may be **disorientation** of time, place and person and gradually patient passes to next stage

b. **Stage of narcosis**

- It is characterized by giddiness, confusion and ataxia. The person is in **dreamy state,** with frightful hallucination and delirium. Sometimes there is development of homicidal tendency or thanatophobia
- There is **tingling and numbness** of skin or generalized anesthesia and becomes deeply narcotized
- Intravenous use can cause headache, vertigo, dyspnea, diplopia, hypotension, and renal failure[1]
- Usually recovery occurs after a deep sleep.
- Death is due to respiratory failure

Vomiting centre—nausea, vomiting; temperature regulating centre—pyrexia (fever).[11]

The manifestations are grouped in two stages.

a. **Stage of stimulation:**

- Initially there is a sense of well-being, euphoria with excitement, confusion, restlessness, increases reflexes **with increase in the BP, heart rate, and respiratory rate, and ventricular arrhythmia.**
- There may be sudden rise of temperature with rigor **(cocaine fever),** dryness of mouth, dysphagia, tingling and numbness of tongue/mouth.
- Pupils—dilated
- There may be hallucination, muscle twitching, tremor, and convulsion and gradually passed to next stage.

b. **Stage of depression:**

- There may be paralysis of muscle, loss of reflexes, collapse, coma and death.
- Cocaine washed out syndrome[1]: Sometimes, there may be lethargy and decreased level of consciousness persisting up to 24 hours followed by recovery.

Chronic cannabis poisoning: Seen in person who consumed for long period with the development of strong psychological dependence

- There is **general loss of weight/appetite,** weakness, emaciation, tremor, impotence
- There is **mental and moral deterioration/degradation,** insanity and sometimes person turns violent and may **'run amok',** who go on killing person who comes in his way to either surrender or killing himself ultimately. The person suffers from some **hallucination or delusion** of persecution/infidelity, due to which the patient is overpowered by an irresistible impulse to destroy life and property
- **Amotivational syndrome:**[1,9] Chronic young abusers gradually become lethargic, apathetic with lack of interest and concentration in work
- **Toxic psychosis:** Decreased concentration, memory and learning abilities[2]
- **Hashish insanity:**[1] Heavy abuse causes paranoid psychosis with violent behavior, culminating in homicide or suicide (run amok)
- **Increased susceptibility to** pharyngitis, bronchitis, asthma, and gynecomastia (in males)

Chronic cocaine poisoning: Cocainism/cocainomania—Immediately upon intake, there is euphoria (rush), for an hour or more followed by rebound depression (crash). To get rid of the unpleasant effects of the later, the individual feels compelled to take the drug again, and the vicious cycle continues until physical, financial, or drug resources are exhausted.

- There is **loss of weight/ appetite,** weakness, tremors, impotence, insomnia, and emaciation
- There is **mental and moral degradation.** There is degeneration of CNS with development of dementia and may get involved in crimes
- **Psychosis:**[1] There is **tactile hallucination** with feeling of insects crawling on the skin, or of sand lying under the skin **(cocaine bugs, Magnan's syndrome).** The person may suffer from dreadful hallucination and delusion of persecution and melancholia
- **Sexual perversion** in males and erotic tension/nymphomania in females are characteristic feature of chronic cocaine takers
- There is **blackish pigmentation of tongue and teeth,** perhaps due to the action of saliva and lime on cocaine when **taken orally,** and ulceration/**perforation of nasal septum when cocaine is sniffed**

Treatment of acute poisoning—cannabis

1. Stomach wash with warm water, in case the drug has been ingested, and purgatives
2. Artificial respiration
3. Antidotes—no specific antidotes
4. Supportive:
   - Benzodiazepines (0.5 mg/kg IV) for agitation and convulsion[12]
   - Haloperidol or other antipsychotic for psychosis
   - Maintenance of nutrition and
   - Strong tea/coffee by oral or per rectum

DEATH occurs due to hazards like:
a. Inhalation of vomitus
b. Accidents—injury, electrocution, drowning, etc. when the person takes cannabis

Treatment of acute poisoning—cocaine

1. Stomach wash with activated charcoal[1] when ingested
2. Antidote: Amyl nitrite inhalation
3. Artificial respiration and O_2 inhalation
4. Symptomatic/supportive:
   - Benzodiazepines (0.5 mg/kg IV over an 8 hours period[13]) for restlessness and convulsions
   - Haloperidol or other antipsychotic for psychosis, and
   - Ice bath for hyperthermia
5. For cardiac irritability:[6]
   a. Vagal stimulant—acetylcholine HCl 1 mg IV or carbachol 0.25 mg IV
   b. Inhibit cholinesterase enzyme—100 mg procainamide IV
   c. Slow injection of dilute phenoxybenzamine 10 mg has antiadrenaline action
   d. Propranolol (0.5–1 mg IV)[13] for hypertension and ventricular arrhythmia

DEATH due to respiratory failure or cardiac arrest.

Treatment of chronic poisoning:[1]

1. Gradual withdrawal of the drug
2. Diazepam for anxiety
3. Antipsychotics for psychosis; Psychotherapy

Treatment of chronic poisoning

1. Gradual withdrawal of the drug
2. Psychotherapy

PM findings
- Not specific
- Suggestive of asphyxia

PM findings
Acute poisoning: Nothing specific
- Suggestive of asphyxia and cardiac failure
- Cerebral and pulmonary edema
- Generalized visceral congestion

Chronic poisoning:[1]
- Evidence of nasal erosions, ulceration, or perforation (in "snorters"). Nasal swabs must be taken for chemical analysis

Medicolegal aspects

1. Accidental: Mostly due to over indulgence. Death has been reported in young adult male (who had undergone open heart surgery) after consuming bhang during Hindu festival[14]
2. Suicidal: Rare
3. Homicidal: Rare
4. Stupefying: Used prior to robbery, kidnapping or rape
5. The person committing a crime under this condition will not be held responsible for the Act under Section 84 of IPC
6. Abrupt stoppage after habitual use can result in a mild withdrawal reaction characterized by restlessness, insomnia, anorexia, and nausea

Medicolegal aspects

1. Suicidal: Not used
2. Homicidal: Not popular
3. Accidental: Due to overdose from its intradermal/urethral or other uses as a drug of abuse/addiction (causes both **psychological** and **physical dependence**)
4. Aphrodisiac: Increases the duration of sex performance when used locally by causing desensitization of the glans penis
5. To improve professional performance

Body packer:[15] The smuggler smuggled contraband drugs (mostly cocaine/heroine and amphetamines, hashish and marijuana), across international border in specially devised packages in the carrier's rectum, vagina or alimentary canal. Typically the drug is wrapped in several layers of latex by using condoms, gloves or even toy balloons. Up to 214 packages have been found in a single "mule" means 'potli or sack containing packages'. The packages, which are round or oval of 1–2 cm in diameter, usually contain 3–7 gm of narcotics.

The smugglers are termed "packer", "swallowers" or "stuffers". All these packages are removed from GIT by taking cathartics or rectal suppositories or disposable enemas. Sometimes the packing may burst, leading to overdose, collapse and acute poisoning (c/s body packers syndrome/ Minipacker syndrome).

Diagnosis of an asymptomatic body packer: It can be diagnosed by abdominal X-ray or ultrasound/ CT scan (if X-ray is unclear).[15] Water-soluble iodinated contrast material has been given orally to confirm or exclude body packages.

Treatment of body packer syndrome:[1]
1. Asymptomatic patients:
   a. Whole bowel irrigation with polythylene glycol solution. However, it can dissolve the heroin from a package, rupturing it and increasing absorption of heroin.
   b. Hence, low volume phosphosoda enemas or high volume saline enemas are given when all packages pass into the colon from the stomach.
   c. Metoclopramide 10 mg, 8 hourly, may be administered to encourage gastric emptying.
   d. It may be advisable to empty the rectum first by a bisacodyl suppository.

2. Symptomatic patients: It must be managed with specific drugs, activated charcoal, and whole bowel irrigation. Intestinal perforation or obstruction by packets requires surgical intervention.

IMPORTANT QUESTIONS

1. Enumerate deliriant poisons. Describe clinical manifestation, treatment, post-mortem features and medicolegal aspect of Datura poisoning.

2. Write differences between Datura seeds and capsicum seeds. Describe clinical features and treatment of Datura poisoning. Add a note on uses of Datura.

3. Write different preparations of Cannabis. Describe clinical features, treatment and medicolegal aspects of Cannabis poisoning.

4. Describe clinical features and treatment of cocaine poisoning. Add a note on body packer syndrome.

SPECIFIC LEARNING OBJECTIVES

After reading this chapter, the reader should be able to:

- Name the different deliriant poisons
- Differentiate Datura and Capsicum seeds
- Enumerate active principles, uses and fatal dose/period of Datura
- Explain clinical manifestations, treatment, postmortem findings and medicolegal aspects of Datura intoxication
- Enumerate 9 Ds of Datura poisoning
- Enlist active principle, uses and different preparations of Cannabis
- Define run amok and explain clinical manifestations of acute and chronic Cannabis poisoning
- Explain the management and medicolegal aspect of Cannabis poisoning
- Enlist various uses and different forms of cocaine
- Define cocaine fever/Magnan's syndrome and explain clinical manifestations of acute and chronic cocaine poisoning
- Explain the treatment and medicolegal aspect of cocaine poisoning
- Understand the significance of body packer syndrome with its diagnosis and treatment

References

1. Pillay VV. Textbook of Forensic Medicine and Toxicology. 17th edn, Paras Medical Publisher: Hyderabad. 2016: 618–33.

2. Dikshit PC. Textbook of Forensic Medicine and Toxicology. 2nd edn, PEEPEE Publisher and Distributors (P) Ltd. New Delhi. 2014: 528–35.

3. Tripathi KD. Anticholinergic drugs and drugs acting on autonomic ganglia. In: Essential of Medical Pharmacology. 7th edn, Jaypee Brothers Medical Publishers (P) Ltd: New Delhi. 2014: 113–23.

4. Krenzelok EP. Aspects of Datura poisoning and treatment. Clinical Toxicology 2010;48(2):104–10.

5. Forrester MB. Jimsonweed (Datura stramonium) Exposures in Texas, 1998–2004. Journal of Toxicology and Environmental Health. 2006;69 (19):1757–62.

6. Nandy A. Principles of Forensic Medicine. 2nd edn, Reprint. New Central Book Agency (P) Ltd: Calcutta. 2004: 517–43.

7. Tripathi KD. Cholinergic system and drugs. In: Essential of Medical Pharmacology. 7th edn, Jaypee Brothers Medical Publishers (P) Ltd: New Delhi. 2014: 99–112.

8. Mohammad Arefi, Nasrin Barzegari, Mahboubeh Asgari, Siamak Soltani, Naeimeh Farhidnia, Fardin Fallah. Datura poisoning, clinical and laboratory findings. Report of five cases. Rom J Leg Med. 2016;24:30–11. DOI: 10.4323/rjlm.

2016.308. © 2016 Romanian Society of Legal Medicine

9. Tripathi KD. Antipsychotic and antimanic drugs. In: Essential of Medical Pharmacology. 7th edn, Jaypee Brothers Medical Publishers (P) Ltd: New Delhi. 2014: 435–53.

10. Singhal SK. Singhal's Toxicology at a glance. 9th edn, National book depot: Mumbai.2016: 81–6.

11. Tripathi KD. Local anaesthetics. In: Essential of Medical Pharmacology. 7th edn, Jaypee Brothers Medical Publishers (P) Ltd: New Delhi. 2014: 360–71.

12. Bui QM, Simpson S, Nordstrom K. Psychiatric and Medical Management of Marijuana Intoxication in the Emergency Department. West J Emerg Med. 2015 May; 16(3): 414–7. doi: 10.5811/westjem.2015.3.25284.

13. Longo DL, Fauci AS, Kasper DL, Hauser SL, Jameson JL, Loscalzo J. (edi). Cocaine and other commonly abused drugs. In: **Harrison's Principles** of Internal Medicine. 18th edn. (vol 2), McGraw-Hill Companies: New York. 2012: 3556–60.

14. Gupta BD, Jani CB, Shah PH. Fatal Bhang poisoning. Med Sci Law. 2001; 41: 349–52.

15. Brogdon BG. Forensic Radiology. 1st edn, CRC Press: Boca Raton (USA).1998: 251–5.

Cerebral Depressant

Cerebral depressants are the drugs which cause CNS depression. These drugs are sedative (that subduces excitement without sleep) and hypnotic (that induces sleep). It includes barbiturates and benzodiazepines. Bromide, chloral hydrate, and paraldehyde are no longer used as sedative–hypnotic.

BARBITURATES	BENZODIAZEPINES
It is the derivative of barbituric acid (malonylurea).[1,2] Barbiturates have been popular hypnotic and sedatives up to 1960s.	Initially BDZs introduce as anti-anxiety drug, but replaced barbiturates as hypnotics and sedatives after 1960s.
Uses: Medicinal uses in:[1] 1. Psychiatric disorder 2. Epilepsy/seizure disorder (grand mal) 3. For induction and maintenance of general anesthesia (when given IV) 4. IV thiopentone—used as truth serum in narcoanalysis	**Uses:** Medicinal uses in:[1] 1. Insomnia 2. Epilepsy/seizure disorder and strychnine poisoning 3. Anxiety disorders 4. As sedatives and hypnotics displacing the barbiturates 5. As muscle relaxant—centrally acting
Classification: According to duration of action a. Long acting barbiturates (6–12 hours): Mephobarbitone, phenobarbitone b. Intermediate acting (3–6 hours): Amobarbitone, aprobarbitone, butobarbitone c. Short acting (<3 hours): Hexobarbitone, pentobarbitone d. Ultrashort acting (<15–20 m): Thiopentone sodium Except for phenobarbitone in epilepsy and thiopentone in anesthesia, no other barbiturates are used now[1]	**Classification of BZDs:**[1] a. Hypnotic: Diazepam, flurazepam, alprazolam, nitrazepam, triazolam b. Antianxiety: Diazepam, oxazepam, lorazepam, alprazolam c. Anticonvulsant: Diazepam, lorazepam, clonazepam, clobazam Benzodiazepines are the example of minor tranquilizers. Whereas, phenothiazine derivatives (chlorpromazine, thioridazine) and butophenone derivatives (haloperidol, carbamazepine, tegritol) are major tranquilizers.

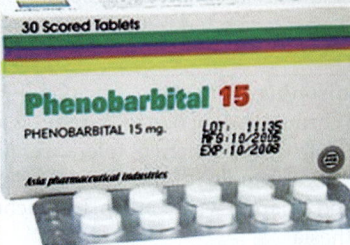

Fig. 14.1: Phenobarbitone

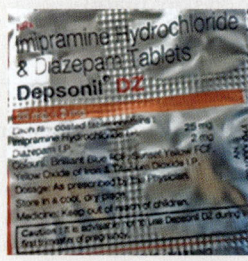 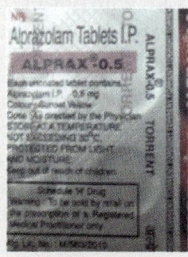

Fig. 14.2: Diazepam and alprazolam tablets

Barbiturates	*Benzodiazepines*
Fatal dose: 4–5 gm **Fatal period:** 1–2 days	**Fatal dose:** 5–10 gm/variable **Fatal period:** 1–2 days
Absorption, fate, and excretion Absorption: Through GIT Distribution: Equally in all tissues as also in red cells and plasma Metabolism: Detoxified in liver by oxidation and dealkylation Excreted: Slowly in urine up to a week. The rate of excretion reduces in liver and renal disease	**Absorption, fate, and excretion** Absorption: Through GIT Distributed: In all tissues Metabolism: Metabolised extensively in liver by oxidation and conjugation with only 20% excreted unchanged through urine.[3]
Action 1. CNS depressant (act on midbrain): It acts at GABA: BZD receptor—chloride channel complex without binding to BZD receptor. It potentiates GABAergic inhibition by increasing the lifetime of chloride channel opening (in contrast to BZDs which increase the frequency of chloride channel opening).[1] 2. Sedative, hypnotic, anticonvulsant and anesthetic action 3. Synergistic action of barbiturates[4] with • Sedatives/hypnotics/tranquilizers • Anticonvulsants • Antipyretic, analgesics, antihistaminic • Alcohol Alcohol + barbiturates: Causes dangerous coma Chlorpromazine + barbiturates: Potentiates the effect	**Action** 1. CNS depressant: It acts by enhancing pre-/post-synaptic inhibition through BZD receptors in GABA: BZD receptor—chloride channel complex, thereby opening the chloride ion channel resulting in the increased conduction of chloride ion across the nerve cell membrane.[1] This lowers the potential difference between the interior and exterior of the cell, blocking the ability of the cell to conduct nerve impulses. 2. It acts on midbrain, ascending reticular formation (maintain wakefulness), limbic system (thought and mental function), medulla (muscle relaxation) and cerebellum (ataxia).[1] 3. Synergistic action with alcohol and other CNS depressant.
Clinical features With therapeutic doses, it results in drowsiness with repeated self-administration of a drug without memory for taking it leading to **barbiturate automatism**.[5] **Acute poisoning: It is due to excessive CNS depression**[1] • Headache, confusion, giddiness • Flaccid limbs, areflexia, comatose • Diplopia and pupils show **alternate constriction and dilatation**, nystagmus. • Respiration is slow, BP fall, and skin is cold, with blister/bullae on skin[1] **(barbiturate blister)** seen in 6% cases[7] • There is oliguria and albuminuria.	**Clinical features** With therapeutic doses, it results in sleep and feels relaxed. **Acute poisoning:** • Nausea, headache, giddiness, dizziness • Disorientation, ataxia, weakness • Diplopia, nystagmus, blurring of vision and constriction of pupil[3] • Followed by amnesia, vertigo, slurred speech, lethargy • Sometimes there may be restlessness, agitation and hallucination. • Deep coma with fall of BP and respiration, diminished reflexes and retention of urine[3]
Chronic poisoning Lack of interest and concentration, vertigo, tremor, ataxia, hallucination and barbiturate blisters. Abrupt stoppage is associated with withdrawal symptoms characterized by anorexia, insomnia, headache, tremor, cramps, seizures, and delerium	**Chronic poisoning** It is due to chronic user of benzodiazepines and is associated with development of tolerance. Abrupt stoppage is associated with withdrawal symptoms characterised by anxiety, insomnia, headache, tremor, and paresthesia

Barbiturates	*Benzodiazepines*
Diagnosis:	**Diagnosis:**
1. Gas chromatography (GC) can be used to analyse urine level of barbiturate	1. Gas chromatography—mass spectrometry can be used to analyze urine level of BD
2. Thin layer chromatography (TLC)—of urine, gastric aspirate or other residue	2. Thin layer chromatography (TLC)—of urine, gastric aspirate or other residue
3. High pressure liquid chromatography is also useful	3. Estimation of plasma level of BD is usually not necessary
Treatment[1]	**Treatment**
1. Maintain respiration by: Foot end raised, suction of airway, artificial respiration and O_2 inhalation, tracheostomy or endotracheal intubation	1. Maintain respiration by: Suction of airway, artificial respiration and O_2 inhalation, tracheostomy or endotracheal intubation
2. Maintain circulation: IV fluid and electrolyte, vasopressor—dopamine is preferred[1]	2. Correction of hypotension with dopamine or levarterenol with IV fluids
3. Antidote: Not specific	3. **Antidote:**[8] **Flumazenil**—0.2 mg/min IV till the patient regains consciousness[1] OR 0.3–1 mg IV, resedation occurs within 1 hour
4. **Forced alkaline diuresis** (with soda bicarb—50 cc IV 6 hourly with or without mannitol/frusemide in 1 litre of Ringer lactate solution.[1,6]	4. Stomach wash with activated charcoal (if <6–12 hrs)
5. Stomach wash with activated charcoal[1] (if patient is not in coma)—500 mg.[6]	**In chronic poisoning:** Phenobarbitone is used. However, replacement of short half-life BD (alprazolam) with long half-life BD (clonazepam) is recommended before tapering and final discontinuation of BD.
6. Hemodialysis and hemoperfusion through column of activated charcoal or other adsorbent.[1,6]	(For acute somatic symptoms in withdrawal of BD, propranolol is used)
7. Cerebral stimulant or analeptic like *bemigrid (50 mg IV)*, daptazol (15 mg IV), metrazol have been used in the past, but dangerous.[1]	
PM findings	**PM findings**
• Suggestive of asphyxia, cyanosis	• Suggestive of asphyxia
• Froth at mouth/nostril	• Froth at mouth/nostril
• Visceral organs—congested	• Visceral organs—congested
• Lungs and brain are congested and edematous with punctate hemorrhages	• Lungs and brain are congested and edematous
• Bronchopneumonia	
• Stomach—parts of tablet may be present, mucosa may be congested, erosion present	• Stomach—parts of tablet may be present, mucosa may be congested
• **Barbiturate blisters**—on the buttocks, inner and posterior aspect of thigh and forearms	
ML aspects	**ML aspects**
1. Suicidal—ideal, mostly used	1. Suicide/homicide—it is used to commit suicide[3] peacefully, usually by hospital staff.
2. Homicidal—rare	2. It is used deliberately to induce amnesia in order to accomplish an illegal or immoral act **(Date rape).** Gamma-hydroxybutyric acid (GHB); Rohypnol-flunitrazepam, a strong benzodiazepine; Ketamine and alcohol are commonly used for date rape
3. Accidental—due to overdose or automatism, abuse, due to drug addiction. (Marilyn Monroe was addicted to alcohol and barbiturate and was found dead at home following an overdose of barbiturate.)	3. Accidental—due to overdose or abuse. In spite of having wide safety margin, death has been reported even in unexpectedly low dose of BD.

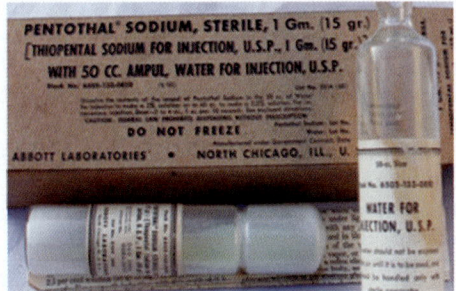

Fig. 14.3: Thiopentone sodium injection

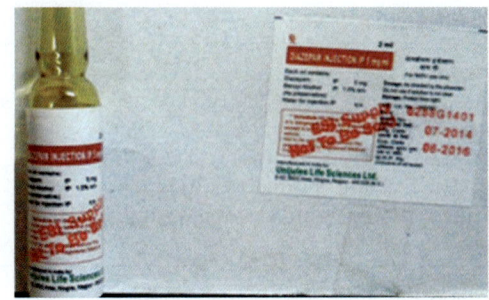

Fig. 14.4: Diazepam injection

BROMIDES	CHLORAL HYDRATE—DRY WINE	PARALDEHYDE
Salts of Na/K or calcium/ lithium: Sodium bromide is a high melting, white crystalline solid resembling NaCl	It is a white, crystalline powder, freely soluble in water, bitter to taste, and has pungent odor. It is a synthetic product	Synthetic drug It is a colorless, volatile liquid with an ethereal odor
Uses 1. For insomnia, epilepsy nervous breakdown[2] 2. Disinfectant for swimming pool in conjunction with chlorine	**Use[7]** For kicking effect in alcohol Alcohol + CH → Mickey Finn	**Use** As an effective anticonvulsant
Absorption, fate, and excretion Absorbed through S/L intestine. Metabolized in liver and distributed in tissue Excreted mostly through urine, sweat and other body secretions	**Absorption, fate, and excretion** Absorbed through mucosa of GIT, usually stomach Metabolized in liver mainly to trichloroethanol and then to trichloroacetaldehyde and trichloroacetic acid. Excreted mostly through urine, either alone or combined with glucuronic acid.[2,7]	**Absorption, fate, and excretion** Absorbed through mucosa of stomach/intestine **Metabolism:** Oxidized in liver to acetaldehyde and acetic acid. Excreted mostly through kidneys and lungs without alteration
Action **Cerebral depressant:** It replaces chlorides from plasma and cells and causes fatal depression of nervous systems both sensory and motor function[7]	**Action** **Cerebral depressant:** It enhances the GABA receptor complex	**Action** Cerebral depressant and basal anesthetics[2]
Fatal dose: 30–45 gm **Fatal period:** 6–8 hrs	**Fatal dose:** 5–10 gm **Fatal period:** 8–12 hrs	**Fatal dose:** 100 ml **Fatal period:** Within a few hours
Clinical features • Nausea, vomiting, abdominal pain. Headache, confusion. • Fall of BP/temperature/ respiration/pulse • Vertigo, weakness, skin rash, paralysis, coma	**Clinical features** (resembles like barbiturates[7]): • Nausea, vomiting, headache, confusion, giddiness, drowsiness. • BP—low, and temperature is low, respiration—depressed, pulse— slow, weak, irregular.	**Clinical features** • Nausea, vomiting, headache, confusion, giddiness, drowsiness • BP—low, temperature is low, respiration—depressed, pulse—weak • Etheral smell in breath • Coma

- Bromide rash[7]—seen in 30% of chronic exposure poisoning (Bromism). The rashes (acneiform eruption) start over face followed by all over body.

- Cardiac arrhythmia, muscle relaxed, albuminuria, deep sleep, coma
- Urticarial rash may be present on skin[7]

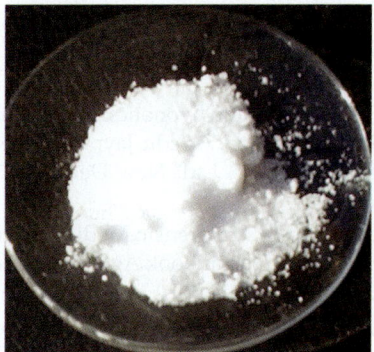

Fig. 14.5: Sodium bromide powder

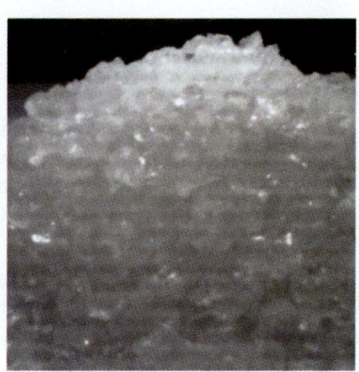

Fig. 14.6: Chloral hydrate crystal

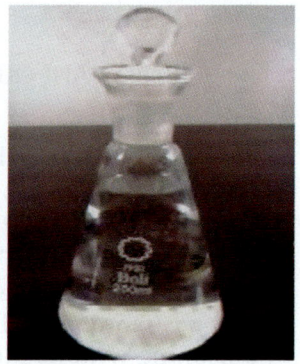

Fig. 14.7: Paraldehyde liquid

Treatment
1. Stomach wash
2. Antidotes[7]: NaCl orally or in drip as it increases the elimination of bromides
3. Hemodialysis[7]
4. Symptomatic

Treatment
1. Stomach wash—alk sol.
2. Antidotes[7]: Naloxone or flumazenil produce dramatic improvement
3. Caffeine etsodibenzoate IV repeated after 15 mins and 1 hr
4. Artificial respiration
5. For liver protection—glucose
6. To protect heart—strophanthine[2] 0.3 mg
7. Forced diuresis/dialysis[7]

Treatment
1. Stomach/colonic wash[7] with NaHCO$_3$
2. Antidotes: Not specific
3. Artificial respiration
4. Respiratory stimulant
5. Calcium gluconate IV.[7]

PM finding
Nothing specific

PM findings
- Suggestive of asphyxia
- Liver damage in chronic cases
- Renal damage

PM findings
- Suggestive of asphyxia
- Organs—congested
- Lungs—congested, edematous.
- Smell of paraldehyde on opening the body cavities[2,7]

ML aspects
1. Suicidal: Rare
2. Homicidal: Rare
3. Accidental: Mostly, chronic Medication due to cumulative poisoning[2]

ML aspects
1. Suicidal: Rare
2. Homicidal: Not possible due to smell/taste
3. Accidental: Due to overdose, chronic use as 'knockout drop' due to addiction and gradual accumulation

ML aspect
1. Suicide: Rare
2. Homicidal: Not used due to smell
3. Accidental: Overdose due to addiction

4. For the purpose of rape/
robbery by mixing it in food
or drink to render a person
suddenly helpless.[7]

Chemical test:[7]
Br + AgNO$_3$ —**whitish/**
yellowish ppt which is soluble
in potassium cyanide

IMPORTANT QUESTIONS

1. Classification, action and uses of benzo-diazepines. Describe clinical mani-festation, treatment, autopsy findings and medicolegal aspect of intoxication with benzodiazepines.

2. Describe clinical features, treatment and postmortem findings in barbiturate poisoning with its mechanism of action and uses.

SPECIFIC LEARNING OBJECTIVES

After reading this chapter, the reader should be able to:

- Name the different cerebral depressant
- Classify barbiturates/benzodiazepines (BDZ) and delineate its mechanism of action
- Enumerate different uses of barbiturates/BDZ
- Explain clinical manifestations, treatment and medicolegal aspects of barbiturate/BDZ poisoning
- Explain clinical features, treatment and medicolegal aspects of chloral hydrate

References

1. Tripathi KD. Sedatives and hypnotics. In: Essential of Medical Pharmacology. 7th edn, Jaypee Brothers Medical Publishers (P) Ltd: New Delhi. 2014: 397–410.

2. Nandy A. Principles of Forensic Medicine. 2nd edn, Reprint. New Central Book Agency (P) Ltd: Calcutta. 2004: 528–30.

3. Kakkar A, Sushil Kumar. Alprazolam Poisoning. J Indian Acad Forensic Med. 2014; 36 (4): 432–3.

4. Dikshit PC. Textbook of Forensic Medicine and Toxicology. 2nd edn, PEEPEE Publisher and Distributors (P) Ltd. New Delhi. 2014: 552–6.

5. Gokhale S, Ciro Ramos-Estebanez. An Interesting Case of Barbiturate Automatism and Review of Literature. Case Reports in Neurological Medicine. Volume 2013, Article ID 713065, 2 pages. http://dx.doi.org/10.1155/2013/713065

6. Kiran Shashi, Chhabra B, Nandini. Management of barbiturate poisoning—a case report. Indian J. Anaesth. 2002;46 (6):480–2.

7. Reddy KSN, Murthy OP. The Essential of Forensic Medicine and Toxicology. 32nd edn, Om Sai Graphics: Hyderabad. 2013: 557–9.

8. Votey SR, Bosse GM, Bayer MJ, Hoffman JR. Flumazenil: a new benzodiazepine antagonist. Ann Emerg Med. 1991; 20(2):181–8.

Cerebral Stimulant

Cerebral stimulants are the drugs which cause CNS stimulation. It includes cocaine, camphor, caffeine, theophylline and theobromine.

CEREBRAL STIMULANTS

Examples

1. Cocaine and its synthetic derivatives like procaine, butacaine, lidocaine, tetracaine and dibucaine. They are used as local and spinal anesthetic agents. The synthetic substitutes of cocaine like Nuvacaine, Nupercaine and Xylocaine are used as local anesthetics.

2. Camphor, amphetamine

3. Caffeine, theophylline, theobromine.

COCAINE

It is already discussed in the previous chapter. It should never be injected. It is a protoplasmic poison and causes tissue necrosis.[1]

PROCAINE

It is a synthetic product almost one-third as toxic as cocaine, i.e. less potent.

Uses: It is used as local infiltration anesthesia or spinal anesthesia.

Absorption, fate, and excretion: Same as Cocaine

It is partly hydrolyzed by esterase while in circulation and partly by liver to PABA (which is excreted through urine) and diethylamino-ethanol.[2]

Properties and action: Same as cocaine

Clinical features: Same as cocaine.

The intoxication occurs only when it is injected wrongly into a vein or when giving intrathecally.[2]

In case of spinal use, there may be post-anesthetic myelitis with cord degeneration[2] pulmonary edema and pneumonitis.

Treatment

- Prophylactic premedication with barbiturate and ephedrine is necessary before using as spinal anesthesia.[2]
- For circulatory collapse—noradrenaline drip.
- For respiration—oxygen inhalation and artificial respiration.

PM findings: Same as cocaine.

ML aspect

Accidental: Due to its overdose.

BUTACAINE, LIDOCAINE, TETRACAINE, AND DIBUCAINE

These are the synthetic derivative of cocaine. Butacaine and lidocaine are almost two times as toxic as cocaine. Tetracaine and dibucaine are four times as toxic as cocaine.[2]

Action, clinical features, treatment, PM findings and medicolegal aspect: same as cocaine.

CAMPHOR	**AMPHETAMINE**
1. Camphor is naturally obtained from stem/bark of *Cinnamomum camphora* 2. Synthetically, it is produced from turpentine oil	Chemically, amphetamine is phenylpropanolamine. Amphetamine was first synthesized in 1887, but used therapeutically only after 1930s.[3] Because of potential, abuse of amphetamine, its therapeutic administration is greatly restricted today.[4]
Uses 1. Pain reliever in various ayurvedic medicines. Also used in nasal congestion and cold 2. Deodorant 3. Mosquito/cockroaches repellents 4. In worshipping (*pooja*)	**Uses** 1. Abuse—to enhance the performance or to stay awake 2. Narcolepsy and obesity 3. Attention deficit disorder 4. Hypotension (mephentermine as IV solution)
Absorption, fate, and excretion • Absorbed from GIT • It is partly oxidized and partly conjugated with glycuronic acid.[2] • Excreted mostly through the kidneys (urine)[2] and small amount through lungs	**Absorption, fate, and excretion** • Absorbed from GIT • Excreted mostly through the kidneys and small amount through lungs
Fatal dose: 15 gm **Fatal period:** 24 hours	**Fatal dose:** 250 mg (addicts can tolerate larger doses) **Fatal period:** Uncertain
Action 1. CNS—stimulant 2. GIT—irritant	**Action** 1. CNS: They are powerful CNS stimulants, add weaker peripheral cardiovascular actions[5] 2. Increases synaptic concentration of norepinephrine[4] and inhibits neuronal reuptake of dopamine[5]

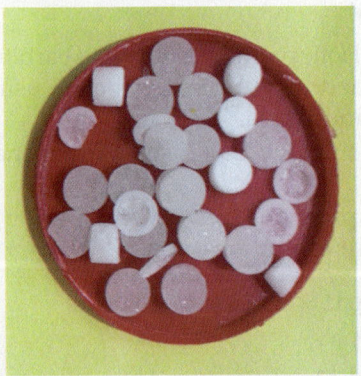

Fig. 15.1: Camphor cakes

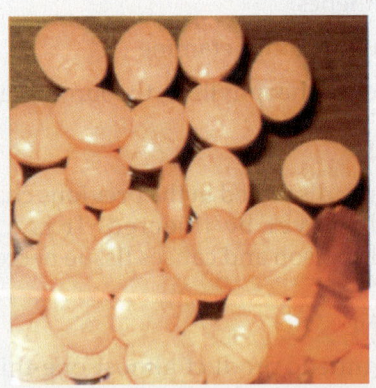

Fig. 15.2: Amphetamine 30 mg tablet

Clinical features *Acute poisoning occurs in two phases:* **1. Convulsive phase** **2. Depressive phase** • Abdominal pain, vomiting, diarrhea, circulatory collapse, *excitement, anxiety, epileptiform, convulsion, delirium, hypertension, cyanosis*[2] • There may be hallucination and delusion followed by depression, collapse and coma	**Clinical features** **Acute poisoning:** It is not common in India. • It causes increase concentration—attention span and alertness with euphoria, talkativeness, **increased work capacity and postponement of sleep,** but for shorter duration.[5] This is followed by restlessness, anxiety, tremor, dysphoria and agitation (hyperactivity).[5]

• Higher/toxic doses produce insomnia, aggression, confusion, delirium, hallucination, hypertension, palpitation, sweating, arrhythmias, hyperpyrexia vomiting, abdominal cramps and vascular collapse, convulsion, coma, death.

Chronic poisoning	**Chronic poisoning**
There are neurological symptoms with convulsion	1. **Amphetamine psychosis**
	2. **Gilles de la Tourette's syndrome**

Treatment	**Treatment**
In acute poisoning	*In acute poisoning*
1. Benzodiazepam or inhalation of ether vapor (for convulsion)	1. Benzodiazepines or antipsychotics for agitation and convulsions.
2. Stomach wash	2. Stomach wash and emesis
During depressive phase:[2]	3. Acidic diuresis[3,4] (controversial)
1. Caffeine	4. IV Na-nitroprusside for hypertension[4]
2. Maintenance of circulation and IV fluids	5. Cold sponging for hypertension[4]
3. Hemodialysis	6. Supportive measures
4. Supportive	**In chronic poisoning:** Chlorpromazine
In chronic poisoning—precaution against exposure.	for amphetamine psychosis/toxicity[5] and haloperidol for Gilles de la Tourette's syndrome
Death is due to respiratory or cardiac failure	

PM findings	**PM findings**
• S/o asphyxia	• Not specific
• Organs—congested	• S/o asphyxia
• Stomach—congested, smell present	• Organs—congested with SAH present

ML aspects	**ML significance**
1. Suicide—rare	1. Suicide: Due to bizarre behaviour
2. Homicidal—not occur	2. Homicide: Due to bizarre behaviour
3. Accidental—mostly, in children due to	3. Accidental deaths may occur in **abuser** when
i. Mistaken with other medicine/castor oil	combined with alcohol and other CNS
ii. Chronic exposure in workers and users	depressant or due to overdose
	4. Aphrodisiac

Amphetamine abuse

1. Formerly, it was used (abused) by truck driver, guard or night shift workers who were compelled **to stay awake at nights.**

2. Abused by **athletes to excel their performance** like increases stamina/strength and alertness.[6] But its use is prohibited at sporting events regulated by national and international anti-doping agencies,[7] so 'DOPE TEST' is carried out for athletes[3]

3. Today "designer drugs" are abused in **rave parties, for dancing all night long** by youngsters

Chronic amphetamine poisoning

1. Amphetamine psychosis:[4,8]

Stereotype—obsessed with repetitive activities involving grooming, rearranging, cleaning, etc.
Paranoid behaviour—characterized by suspicion, hostility, and anxiety
Delusions of persecution
Hallucinations—usually visual

2. Gilles de la Tourette's syndrome:[4] Characterized by tic, eye blinking, jaw jerks, humming, etc.

CAFFEINE (TRIMETHYL XANTHINE)	THEOPHYLLINE	THEOBROMINE
Caffeine is extracted from the leaves of tea and coffee beans	It is 1, 3-dimethyl xanthine. It is extracted from tea leaves	It is 3, 7-dimethyl xanthine. It is extracted from the seeds of Theobroma cacao
Absorption, fate, and excretion 1. Absorbed through GIT 2. It is demethylated and further metabolized in liver[2] 3. Excreted through kidneys, partly as methylated xanthine and partly as xanthine[2]	**Absorption, fate, and excretion** Same as caffeine	**Absorption, fate, and excretion** Same as caffeine
Action[2] Cerebral and spinal stimulation	**Action** Same as caffeine	**Action** Same as caffeine
Fatal dose/period: Not certain	**Fatal dose/period:** Not certain	**Fatal dose/period:** Not certain
Clinical features 1. Headache, anxiety, insomnia, vertigo, tremor, convulsion, delirium 2. Due to adrenocortical stimulation, there is a rise in serum catecholamines and increase excretion of 11-hydroxycorticosteriod[2]	**Clinical features** • Same as caffeine • Theophylline causes hematuria	**Clinical features** • Same as caffeine • It is irritant to stomach and also causes palpitation
Treatment 1. Sedatives/tranquilizers: Barbiturates, or diazepam to counter cerebral/spinal stimulation 2. Artificial respiration and O_2 inhalation 3. Symptomatic	**Treatment** Same as caffeine	**Treatment** Same as caffeine
PM findings Nothing specific S/o asphyxia	**PM findings** Same as caffeine	**PM finding** Same as caffeine
ML aspects 1. Accidental: Mostly mistaken with other drugs or overdose 2. Suicidal/homicidal: Not reported	**ML aspect** Same as caffeine	**ML aspect** Same as caffeine

IMPORTANT QUESTION

1. Enumerate cerebral stimulant drugs. Describe clinical manifestation in acute and chronic amphetamine poisoning with its treatment and medicolegal aspect.

SPECIFIC LEARNING OBJECTIVES

After reading this chapter, the reader should be able to:

- Enlist different cerebral stimulants
- Enumerate the uses of camphor and amphetamine

- Explain clinical manifestation, treatment and medicolegal aspect of camphor/amphetamine poisoning
- Appreciate amphetamine abuse

References

1. Tripathi KD. Local Anaesthetics. In: Essential of Medical Pharmacology. 7th edn, Jaypee Brothers Medical Publishers (P) Ltd: New Delhi. 2014: 360–71.

2. Nandy A. Principles of Forensic Medicine. 2nd edn, Reprint. New Central Book Agency (P) Ltd: Calcutta. 2004: 517–43.

3. Dikshit PC. Textbook of Forensic Medicine and Toxicology. 2nd edn, PEEPEE Publisher and Distributors (P) Ltd. New Delhi. 2014: 577–8.

4. Pillay VV. Textbook of Forensic Medicine and Toxicology. 17th edn, Paras Medical Publisher: Hyderabad. 2016: 629–30.

5. Tripathi KD. Adrenergic system and drugs. In: Essential of Medical Pharmacology. 7th edn, Jaypee Brothers Medical Publishers (P) Ltd: New Delhi. 2014: 124–39.

6. Westfall DP, Westfall TC. "Miscellaneous Sympathomimetic Agonists". In Brunton LL, Chabner BA, Knollmann BC. Goodman & Gilman's Pharmacological Basis of Therapeutics (12th ed.). New York, USA: McGraw-Hill. ISBN 9780071624428.. 2010: 297–9.

7. Docherty JR. "Pharmacology of stimulants prohibited by the World Anti-Doping Agency (WADA)". Br. J. Pharmacol. 2008; 154 (3): 606–22. doi:10.1038/bjp.2008.124. PMC 2439527. PMID 18500382.

8. Reddy KSN, Murthy OP. The Essential of Forensic Medicine and Toxicology. 32nd edn, Om Sai Graphics: Hyderabad. 2013: 503–9.

Hallucinogens

Hallucinogens (psychedelics) are the drugs which cause hallucinations. Hallucination is a false sense of perception. It includes Lysergic acid diethylamide, Phencyclidine, Mescaline. These are the drugs which alter mood, behavior, thought and perception similar to psychosis.[1]

LYSERGIC ACID DIETHYLAMIDE (LSD)	PHENCYCLIDINE
It is an Indole Amines derivatives LSD is the most powerful hallucinogen known to man, synthesized by Hoffman in 1938. It was popular among the hippies in the West in the 1960s. It is usually impregnated in stamp sized paper **(LSD blotter)** which is licked or consumed	**It is an Arylcyclohexyl Amines derivatives** Phencyclidine is a popular drug of abuse in the West. A common mode of intake involves sprinkling the drug on parsley or marijuana leaves, and then smoking it. It is sometimes used as an adulterant in expensive drugs of abuse such as cocaine
Common name[2] Acid, microdot, purple haze, white lightning, etc.	**Common name[2]** Angel dust, PCP, peace pill, hog, rocket fuel, etc.
Physical appearance It is colorless, odorless, tasteless and water-soluble crystalline substance. It is effective in extremely small doses (micrograms)[2]	**Physical appearance** White granular powder which is usually smoked sniffed or injected (IV/SC) or ingested.[3]
Clinical features • Tachycardia, hypertension, hyperpyrexia, mydriasis, and tremor.[3] • Panic attacks, flashback phenomena, mania with visual illusion, delusion, hallucination and disturbed behavior.[2,4] • Convulsion, coma and bleeding disorder. • Post-hallucinogenic perception disorder.[2]	**Clinical features** • Low dose (5 mg) produce agitation, excitement, impaired motor coordination, dysarthria and analgesia with nystagmus, flushing and diaphoresis.[3] • Higher dose (5–10 mg may produce excessive salivation, vomiting, fever, stupor or coma).[3] • Dose >10 mg may produce convulsion, tremor, opisthotonus, coma.[3] • Tachycardia, hypertension, acute psychosis, with violent tendency, bizarre behavior, delusions and hallucinations.
Treatment 1. Stomach wash should be avoided as it is rapidly absorbed and ingested in very less amount.[3] 2. Quiet, secluded environment 3. Antipsychotics 4. Benzodiazepines	**Treatment** 1. Stomach wash is needed only when taken orally. 2. Acid diuresis—increases renal excretion[4] 3. Diazepam for convulsion 4. Haloperidol (5 mg IM) to reduce psychotic behavior.[3]

5. Supportive measures—reassurance 6. Psychiatric follow-up	5. Supportive care 6. Psychiatric follow-up
ML significance Suicidal and accidental deaths arising out of bizarre behavior induced by the drug have been reported.[2] Repeated use by an addict can lead to permanent psychosis	**ML significance** Addiction leads to violent tendency, psychosis, and suicidal as well as homicidal behavior[2,4]

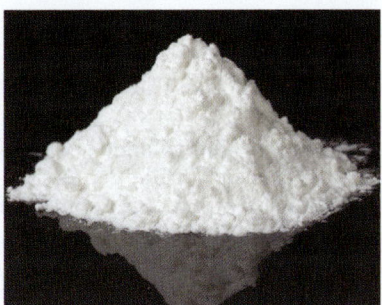

Fig. 16.1: LSD powder

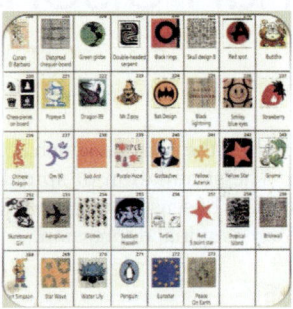

Fig. 16.2: LSD blotter

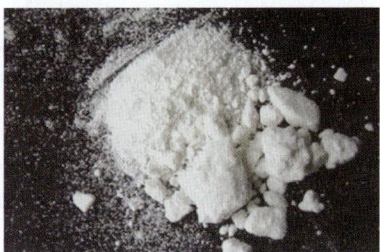

Fig. 16.3: Phencyclidine

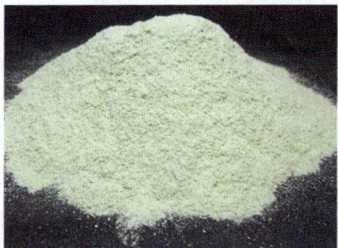

Fig. 16.4: Mescaline

MESCALINE

It is a phenyl alkyl amines derivative from Mexican 'Peyote Cactus' Lophophora Williamsi.[1] It is less potent hallucinogens used by natives during rituals.

IMPORTANT QUESTIONS

1. LSD blotters.
2. Enumerate different hallucinogens. Describe clinical manifestation, treatment and medicolegal aspect of intoxication with LSD.

SPECIFIC LEARNING OBJECTIVES

After reading this chapter, the reader should be able to:

• **Define hallucinogens and enlist different hallucinogens**
• **Identify LSD blotter**

References

1. Tripathi KD. Antipsychotic and antimanic drugs. In: Essential of Medical Pharmacology. 7th edn, Jaypee Brothers Medical Publishers (P) Ltd: New Delhi. 2014: 435–53.

2. Pillay VV. Textbook of Forensic Medicine and Toxicology. 17th edn, Paras Medical Publisher: Hyderabad. 2016: 631–3.

3. Longo DL, Fauci AS, Kasper DL, Hauser SL, Jameson JL, Loscalzo J. (edi). Opioid drug abuse and dependence. In: Harrison's Principles of Internal Medicine. 18th edn. (vol 2), McGraw- Hill Companies: New York. 2012: 3552–64.

4. Dikshit PC. Textbook of Forensic Medicine and Toxicology. 2nd edn, PEEPEE Publisher and Distributors (P) Ltd. New Delhi. 2014: 574–6.

Spinal Poisons

Spinal poisons are the poisons which act on the spinal cord. It may either cause stimulation or depression of spinal cord. The stimulation of spinal cord results in spasm and convulsion while depression causes paralysis and loss of sensation.[1] It includes Nux vomica and Gelsemium. Nux vomica is a spinal stimulant and Gelsemium is spinal depression.

STRYCHNINE

Common Name: Kuchila

Plant: Strychnos nux vomica

Three varieties: Colubrina, Ignati, Tiute.

The tree is a native of South East Asia and grows in most part of India, belong to a family Loganiaceae. The fruit is globular yellowish brown to orange colour with hard covering containing seeds, which contains highly poisonous alkaloid—strychnine and brucine.

Toxic part: All part of the plant (maximum concentration in seeds)

Seeds: Biconvex button-shaped seeds, 2–2.5 cm in diameter and 0.5 cm thick, bitter to taste, yellowish brown, shiny, hard pericarp with fine hairs over surface (Fig. 17.1).

Active principle: Strychnine, brucine, loganine. Strychnine is odorless, colorless crystals having very bitter taste.

Uses

1. Medicinal: As CNS stimulant.
2. Used in popular homeopathic remedy 'Nux Vomica'.
3. Also used in herbal medicine to elevate BP.
4. Used as vermin paste.
5. Rodenticidal agent.
6. For killing stray dogs[2]

Route of administration: Usually oral

Action

It is a spinal poison acts particularly on the anterior horn cell of spinal cord. It acts by blocking post-synaptic inhibition produced by inhibitory transmitter glycine.[3]

It is a CNS stimulant—produces excitation of all portion of nervous system by increasing the ongoing neuronal activity causing convulsion.

Fatal dose: 1–2 seeds, 30–60 mg strychnine.

Fatal period: 30 mins to 2 hrs.

Clinical Features

1. When swallowed/crushed: Bitter taste with choking sensation in throat. The patient is restless, sensitive, and apprehensive and has anxious look. Froth at mouth and nostrils.
2. Twitching/tremor of muscle: First clonic followed by tonic type.[1]
3. Due to extreme degree of contraction of muscle, the **body may assume one of the following positions** (Fig. 17.2) along with the contraction of the muscle of the face leading to widening of angle of mouth with creases appearing in and around the eyelids (a state known as **'risus sardonicus'**—monkey-like face):[4,5]

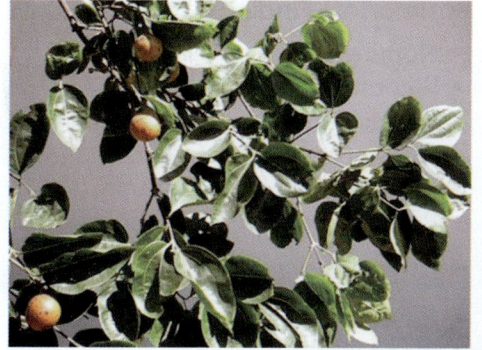 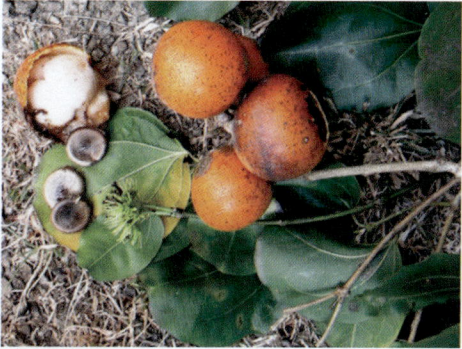

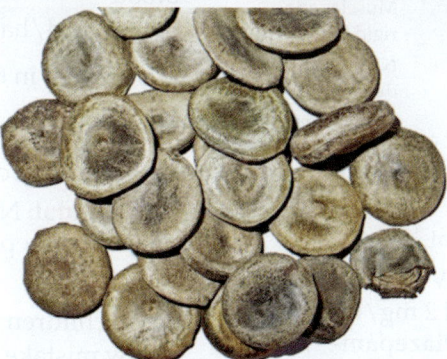

Fig. 17.1: Nux vomica plant, fruit, and seeds

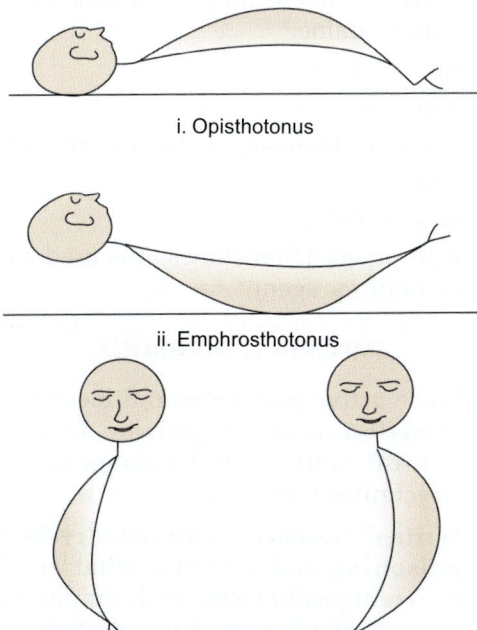

i. Opisthotonus

ii. Emphrosthotonus

iii. Pleurosthotonus

Fig. 17.2: Different body positions

i. Opisthotonus: Bend backward with convexity facing forward with head—heel touches the ground surface.

ii. Emphrosthotonus: Bend forward

iii. Pleurosthotonus: Bend sidewise

4. In between the contraction: Muscles are relaxed. The intercostal muscles fixed leading to difficulty in breathing and cyanosis.

5. The mind is not affected nor is the consciousness.

The clinical features are similar to tetanus and have to be differentiated (Table 17.1).

Death Due to

1. Respiratory failure due to asphyxia.
2. Medullary paralysis.

Treatment

1. Keep the patient in a dark, noiseless room (because they are easily stimulated).

Table 17.1: Differences between strychnine poisoning and tetanus

Differences	Strychnine poisoning	Tetanus
1. Onset:	Sudden	Gradual
2. History of:	Ingestion of some bitter white powder followed by convulsion	Injury
3. Muscle involvement:	All muscles are involved at a time	Muscles are gradually involved
4. Muscle during interval:	Muscles are relaxed	Muscles are rigid throughout
5. Chemical analysis:	Strychnine is detected	No poison detected
6. Microbiological exam:	Nil	*Clostridium tetani* present

2. Antidote: Anticonvulsant [3]

   i. Lorazepam—4 mg IV (0.1 mg/kg in children) at the rate of 2 mg/min, is the drug of choice. OR **Diazepam**—10 mg IV (0.2–0.3 mg/kg) at 2 mg/min. The dose is repeated after 10 min if required.

   ii. Fosphenytoin 100–150 mg/min IV infusion (max 1 gm) under ECG monitoring, if seizures fail to respond to above drugs. OR **Phenobarbitone sodium** 50–100 mg/min IV is alternative to Fosphenytoin to maintain seizure free state before oral therapy is started.

3. Stomach wash with mixture of 0.1% $KMnO_4$, 2% tannic acid or activated charcoal—50 gm[6], after controlling the convulsion.

4. Muscle relaxant:[7]

   i. Succinylcholine (0.5–0.8 mg/kg IV) OR **Pancuronium** (0.04–0.1 mg/kg IV) is used as d-tubocurarine is not used nowadays.

   ii. Mephenesin (30 mg/kg slow IV drip) OR Methocarbamol is used as alternative muscle relaxant.

5. Artificial respiration[3] (by tracheostomy) and O_2 supply.

6. Supportive.

Postmortem Findings

- Nothing specific.
- Rigor mortis—stays longer.
- Detected even in decomposed bodies.[8]
- Signs of asphyxia present.
- Rupture of stretched muscle.
- Postmortem caloricity present.[2]

Preservation of Viscera

- Routine viscera
- Blood
- Spinal cord/half of brain and entire heart.[2]

It is present in the tissue for days to years.

ML Aspects

1. **Suicidal:** Not common due to painful death.

2. **Homicidal:** Not common, but a few cases have been reported.

3. **Accidental**
   i. In children
   ii. By mistake
   iii. Overdose
   iv. It is found to be adulterant in street drugs such as amphetamines, heroin and cocaine.[9]

4. **Abortifacient**

5. **Arrow poison**

6. **Cattle poison**—it is also useful to kill dogs.[2]

7. **Rodenticidal**[6]

8. **Aphrodisiac:** Sometimes, it is used as an aphrodisiac agent.[4]

IMPORTANT QUESTIONS

1. **Write active principles and mechanism of action of spinal poison. Describe clinical features and management of strychnine poisoning.**

2. **Write differences between strychnine poisoning and tetanus. What are the different positions the body may assume in case of consumption of strychnos nux vomica seeds. Write its postmortem findings and medicolegal aspects.**

SPECIFIC LEARNING OBJECTIVES

After reading this chapter, the reader should be able to:

- **Enumerate active principles and uses of strychnos nux vomica**
- **Understand the mechanism of action of strychnine**
- **Explain clinical manifestation, treatment, postmortem findings and medicolegal aspect of strychnine poisoning**
- **Enlist different positions of body in strychnine poisoning**
- **Distinguish between strychnine poisoning and tetanus**

References

1. Dikshit PC. Textbook of Forensic Medicine and Toxicology. 2nd edn, PEEPEE Publisher and Distributors (P) Ltd. New Delhi. 2014: 557–9.

2. Pillay VV. Textbook of Forensic Medicine and Toxicology. 17th edn, Paras Medical Publisher: Hyderabad. 2016: 611–3.

3. Tripathi KD. CNS stimulants and cognition enhancers. In: Essential of Medical Pharmacology. 7th edn, Jaypee Brothers Medical Publishers (P) Ltd: New Delhi. 2014: 486–91.

4. Reddy KSN, Murthy OP. The Essential of Forensic Medicine and Toxicology. 32nd edn, Om Sai Graphics: Hyderabad. 2013: 580–3.

5. Bardale R. Principles of Forensic Medicine and Toxicology. 1st edn, Jaypee Brothers Medical Publishers (P) Ltd: New Delhi. 2011: 535–7.

6. Wood DM, Webster E, Martinez D, Dargan PI, Jones AL. Case report: Survival after deliberate strychnine self-poisoning, with toxicokinetic data. Crit Care. 2002; 6(5): 456–9. Published online 2002 Jul 10. doi: 10.1186/cc1549.

7. Tripathi KD. Skeletal muscle relaxants. In: Essential of Medical Pharmacology. 7th edn, Jaypee Brothers Medical Publishers (P) Ltd: New Delhi. 2014: 347–59.

8. Benomran FA, Henry JD. Homicide by strychnine poisoning. Med Sci Law. 1996 Jul; 36(3):271–3.

9. O'Callaghan WG, Joyce N, Counihan HE, Ward M, Lavelle P, O'Brien E. Unusual strychnine poisoning and its treatment: report of eight cases. Br Med J (Clin Res Ed). 1982; 285(6340): 478.

Peripheral Nerve Poisons

Peripheral nerve poisons are the poisons which block the action of acetylcholine at nerve ends causing skeletal muscle relaxation. These are basically the skeletal muscle relaxants that act peripherally at neuromuscular junction/muscle fibre to reduce muscle tone and/or cause paralysis.[1] Pancuronium, d-tubocurarine, vecuronium, mivacurium, succinylcholine are examples of neuromuscular blocking agents. Peripheral nerve poisons include Curare and Conium.

CONIUM	CURARE
Common name Poison hemlock, Socrates poison	**Common name** Vine
Plant: *Conium maculatum* **Toxic part:** All parts of plant. It belongs to carrot family, grows between 5 and 8 feet tall with smooth green hollow stem. Flowers are small white, clustered in umbels up to 4–6 inch across. When crushed, leaves and root emit a rank, unpleasant mousy[2] odor	**Plant:** *Chondrodendron tomentosum* **Toxic part:** All parts of plant (maximum concentration in bark and stem) It is a long poisonous vine that can stretch up to the canopy. Leaves are large, heart shaped, covered with tiny hairs. Flowers are small and greenish white. Fruits are fleshy but very tiny

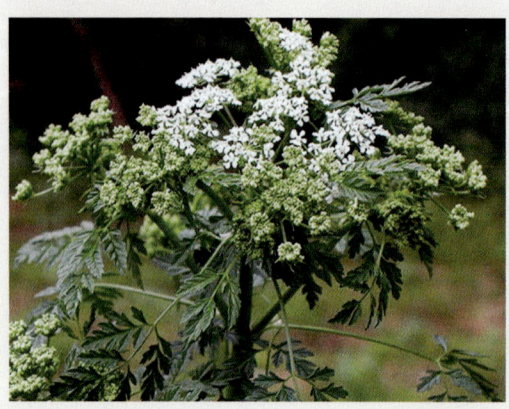 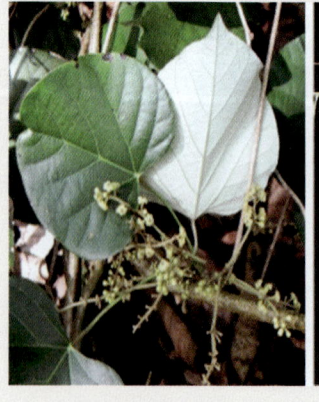 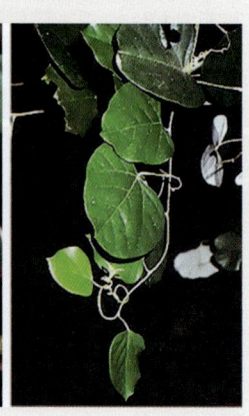

Active principle Coniine, Gamma—Coniceine	**Active principle** Curare, Curariform, Curarine, d-Tubocurarine, Syncurine, Succinylcholine chloride

Conium	*Curare*
Uses 1. Medicinal: As muscle relaxant 2. Execution of capital punishment	**Uses** 1. Medicinal: As muscle relaxant during anesthesia/surgery[1,3] 2. As anticonvulsant 3. Used to treat bruise and kidney stones
Route of administration: Usually oral	**Route of administration:** Injectables only
Action 1. It acts at neuromuscular junction as non-depolarizing blockers and causes flaccid paralysis (similar to curare) 2. It also acts on autonomic ganglia producing nicotinic effects	**Action** 1. It acts at neuromuscular junction as both depolarising and non-depolarising blockers and causes muscle paralysis[1] 2. It is a skeletal muscle relaxant
Fatal dose:[2] 1 cm of any part of plant or 60 mg Coniine **Fatal period:** A few hours	**Fatal dose:**[2] 30–60 mg curarine **Fatal period:** 1–2 hours
Clinical features 1. Nausea, vomiting, abdominal pain 2. Sweating, salivation 3. Mydriasis, tachycardia followed by bradycardia, hypotension with confusion and blurring of vision 4. Muscle weakness and paralysis extending upward followed by coma and respiratory failure	**Clinical features** 1. When swallowed: No poisonous[2] 2. When injected: Inability to move due to flaccidity of muscle which gets paralyzed leading to respiratory failure (due to involvement of muscles of diaphragm and intercostal muscles) 3. Muscle relaxed/flaccid all the time 4. There may be altered consciousness 5. There is also headache, confusion, vertigo, mydriasis, blurring of vision, hyperthermia, hypotension
Death due to Respiratory failure: Due to asphyxia	**Death due to** Respiratory failure: Due to asphyxia without convulsion and without pain[4]
Treatment 1. Artificial respiration and O_2 supply 2. Antidote: Not specific 3. Stomach wash: With activated charcoal/KMnO$_4$ 4. Stimulant 5. Supportive	**Treatment** 1. Artificial respiration and O_2 supply 2. Antidote:[5] Administration of Cholinesterase inhibitor like Neostigmine (0.5–1 mg SC) and Physostigmine (1–2 mg SC) after pre-treat with atropine (0.6 mg IV) [2] 3. 100 mg of Congo Red in 10 ml of 5% glucose by slow IV drip[6] 4. Stimulant 5. Supportive
PM findings • Nothing specific • Stomach—peculiar (mousy) odor • Suggestive of asphyxia • Organs—congested	**PM findings** • Nothing specific • Evidence of injection mark • Suggestive asphyxia
Preservation of viscera Routine viscera Blood	**Preservation of viscera** Routine viscera Blood Skin and underlying muscle at the site of injection

ML aspects

1. Suicidal: Rare
2. Homicidal: In ancient period, it was used for execution of punishments. Socrates was executed by poison hemlock
3. Accidental: Rarely occur

ML aspects

1. Suicidal: Administered usually by person in medical profession—to impart painless death
2. Homicidal: Administered usually by person in medical profession—in dyadic death
3. Accidental:
   i. By mistake
   ii. Overdose during anesthesia
4. Abortifacient
5. Arrow poison—by natives of South America[4]

IMPORTANT QUESTION

1. **Enumerate different peripheral nerve poisons with its mechanism of action and active principles. Write clinical features, treatment and medicolegal aspect of poisoning due to any one of them.**

SPECIFIC LEARNING OBJECTIVES

After reading this chapter, the reader should be able to:

- **Name different peripheral nerve poisons and skeletal muscle relaxant**

- **Delineate the mechanism of action of curare/conium**

- **Enumerate active principles of curare/ conium**

- **Explain clinical features, treatment, post-mortem findings and medicolegal aspect of conium/curare poisoning**

References

1. Tripathi KD. Skeletal muscle relaxant. In: Essential of Medical Pharmacology. 7th edn, Jaypee Brothers Medical Publishers (P) Ltd: New Delhi. 2014: 347–59.

2. Reddy KSN, Murthy OP. The Essential of Forensic Medicine and Toxicology. 32nd edn, Om Sai Graphics: Hyderabad. 2013: 580–3.

3. Carl J, Schwarzer M, Klingelhoefer D, Ohlendorf D, Groneberg DA. Curare—A Curative Poison: A Scientometric Analysis. PLoS One. 2014; 9(11): e112026. Published online 2014 Nov 19. doi: 10.1371/journal.pone.0112026.

4. Lee MR. Curare: The South American Arrow Poison. J R Coll Physicians Edinb. 2005;35:83–92.

5. Thomas Morgan III, Bernadette Kalman (2007). Neuroimmunology in Clinical Practice. Wiley-Blackwell. ISBN 978-1-4051-5840-4: Page 153. https://books.google.co.in/books?isbn= 1405158409

6. Nandy A. Principles of Forensic Medicine. 2nd edn, Reprint. New Central Book Agency (P) Ltd: Calcutta. 2004: 546–7.

Cardiac Poisons

Cardiac poisons are the systemic poison which acts on the heart. Aconite, *Cerbera thevetia*, *Nerium odorum*, Tobacco, Quinine, and Digitalis are the examples of cardiac poisons.

Aconitum ferox/napellus

Synonyms: Aconite, *Mitha Zaher* (sweet poison), monkshood

Properties

Grows in Himalayan altitude

Toxic part: All parts of plant are toxic (maximum concentration in dried root). The root is brownish yellow, conical and long shrivelled, sweet taste

When fresh root is cut—white surface turns red

When fresh horseradish root is cut, it remains white

Active principles: Aconitine, pseudo-aconitine, aconine, picraconitine

Uses

1. Aconite is a pharmacological product marketed as tincture aconitum, has **anodyne properties** (able to relieve pain/mentally soothing)
2. Used in ayurvedic/homoepathic medicines

Action[1,2]

Stimulates and then depresses heart, smooth/skeletal muscle, CNS and peripheral nerves.

Absorption, Fate, and Excretion

- Aconite is absorbed through MM of GIT
- It is metabolized in liver
- Excreted through urine

Fatal dose: Root—1 gm, aconitine: 2–6 mg

Fatal period: 1–6 hours

Clinical Manifestation

- Tingling/numbness/burning sensation in mouth/tongue/throat with bitter sweet taste and feeling of constriction in chest, increase salivation, nausea, vomiting, and abdominal pain.
- Tingling/numbness/weakness of muscle and limbs, ringing in ear, impairment of hearing/vision/speech.
- There may be low BP, pulse, and respiration with cardiac irregularities, like extrasystole, ventricular fibrillation and bundle brunch block.
- This is followed by headache, confusion, vertigo, dizziness, dyspnea, delirium, convulsion, collapse, and coma.
- Pupils show **hippus reaction**[1,3] (alternate constriction and dilatation).

Treatment

1. Emesis
2. Stomach wash:[1,3] $KMnO_4$/tannic acid/charcoal
3. Demulcent
4. Artificial respiration and O_2 inhalation

5. Symptomatic: Atropine 1 mg SC to avoid vagal inhibition[3]

Lignocaine—0.1% of 50 ml slow IV drip—to relieve

PM Findings

- Nothing specific
- Froth in respiratory tract.
- Pallor of mucous membrane of mouth
- Stomach: Root remains present

Viscera Preservation

- Routine viscera
- Heart
- Preserved in saturated solution of NaCl or rectified spirit acidified with acetic acid

Medicolegal Aspects

1. Suicidal: Not common, as it is painful
2. Homicidal: Ideal homicidal poison given by oral route, mixed with *paan* and drinks
3. Accidental: Mostly due to:
   i. Mistaken with horseradish root
   ii. Mixed with country liquor for kicking effect[1,3]
   iii. Quackery medicine
4. Abortifacient—by root
5. Arrow poison: By parenteral route by tribal people/hilly areas
6. Cattle poison: By parenteral route by tribal people/hilly areas

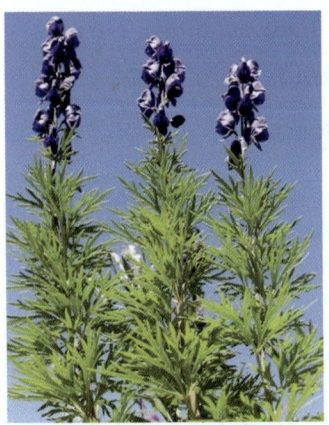

Fig. 19.1: *Aconitum napellus*

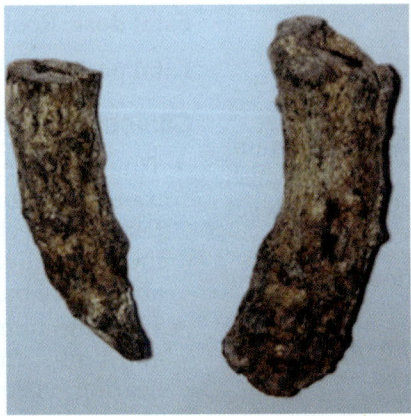

Fig. 19.2: Root of aconite

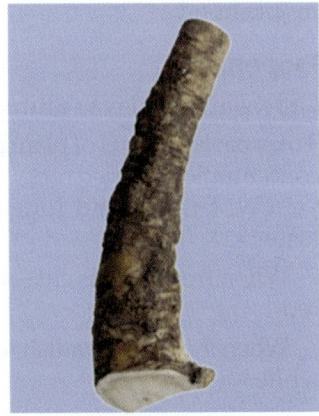

Fig. 19.3: Root of horseradish

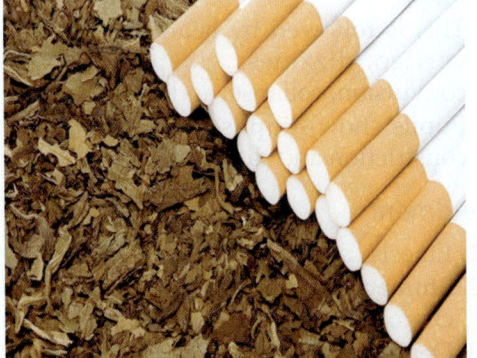

Fig. 19.4: Nicotine dry leaves (tobacco) and cigarette

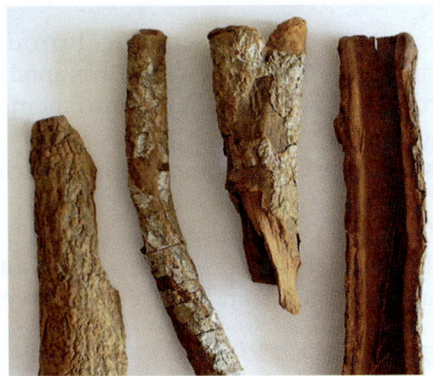

Fig. 19.5: Cinchona bark

Digitalis purpurea/lanata	Nicotiana tabacum	Cinchona pubescens
Synonyms: Digitalis/fox glove	**Synonyms:** Tobacco (*tambakhu*)	**Synonyms:** Quinine, quina
Grows in: All over world	**Grows in:** All over world	**Grows in:** All over world
Toxic part: All parts of plant (max concentration leaves)	**Toxic part:** All parts of plant (max concentration leaves)	**Toxic part:** All parts of plant (max concentration bark)
Toxic principles: Digitalin, digitoxin, digitonin, digoxin	**Toxic principles:** Nicotine, nicotianine, lobeline	**Toxic principles** Quinine, quinidine, cinchonine, cinchonidine
Uses T/t of congestive heart failure and atrial fibrillation/flutter	**Uses** 1. Dried leaves—smoking, chewing 2. In agriculture—for fumigation and spraying as insecticide and fumigants[2]	**Uses**[4] 1. Malaria/cerebral malaria 2. Nocturnal muscle cramps 3. Antiarrhythmias
Action: It increases excitability/force of cardiac contraction and prolong diastolic period.[5]	**Action:** It is a selective (nicotinic cholinergic receptors) ganglionic stimulants.[6] Stimulates and depresses heart.	**Action:**[4] Quinidine blocks myocardial Na^+ channel—reduces automaticity/contractility
Fatal dose: Dried leaves: 1–2 gm Digitoxin: 2–3 mg **Fatal period:** 1–24 hours	**Fatal dose:** Dried leaves: 20–40 gm, nicotine: 1–2 drops **Fatal period:** 1–5 hours	**Fatal dose:** Bark: 2–8 gm **Fatal period:** 1–5 hours
Clinical features • Slow pulse/heart/respiration rate, with extrasystole, ventricular fibrillation, pericardial distress • Nausea, vomiting, abdominal pain, and diarrhea with fatigue, malaise • Headache, confusion, dyspnea, dizziness, delirium, dilated pupil, convulsion, collapse, coma • Visual disturbance, psychosis and disorientation[5] • Skin rashes and gynecomastia are rare.[5]	**Clinical features** • Cardiovascular collapse, cardiac irregularities, increased heart rate, extrasystole, ventricular fibrillation, pericardial distress. • Nausea, vomiting, abdominal pain. • Headache, confusion, dyspnea, dizziness, delirium, dilated pupil, convulsion, collapse, coma • **Chronic:** Cough, bronchitis, tingling, numbness, tremor, weakness, loss of memory, cardiac systole, anorexia	**Clinical features**[3, 4] (Cinchonism—due to large single dose or higher dose for few days) • Ringing in ears, dimness of vision, loss of vision/hearing. • Nausea, vomiting, abdominal pain. • Headache, confusion, dyspnea, dizziness, delirium, dilated pupil, convulsion, collapse, coma • Fever, marked weakness, hypotension, cardiac arrhythmias with hemolysis, hemoglobinuria, renal damage. • Hypersensitivity to quinine: Rashes, itching, edema, bronchoconstriction
Treatment[1,3,5] 1. Emesis/stomach wash (with $KMnO_4$)/demulcent.[1] 2. For ventricular arrhythmia:[5] Lidocaine (100 mg Lignocaine) IV–suppresses excessive automaticity	**Treatment** 1. Emesis/stomach wash (with $KMnO_4$)/demulcent.[1] 2. Artificial respiration and O_2 inhalation. 3. Specific antidote:[1,6] Mecamylamine tablets	**Treatment** 1. Emesis/stomach wash (with $KMnO_4$ or $MgSO_4$)/demulcent.[1,3] 2. Artificial respiration and O_2 inhalation. 3. Forced acid diuresis[3]

Digitalis purpurea/lanata	*Nicotiana tabacum*	*Cinchona pubescens*
3. For supraventricular arrhythmia: Propranolol may be given IV or orally. 4. For AV block and bradycardia:[5] Atropine 0.6–1.2 mg IM 5. Digoxin specific antibody: (Fab fragment—marketed as Digibind in Europe—38 mg vial).[5] It combines to form digoxin—Fab complex and excreted in urine. Given 1 vial IV in 30 min[3] 6. Artificial respiration and O_2 inhalation.	4. Supportive:[1,7] Atropine/ adrenaline. **Treatment of smoking cessation:**[6] 1. Nicotine transdermal: This patch formulation is applied once daily on the hip/abdomen/arm as an aid to smoking cessation. 2. Nicotine chewing gum (Nulife:1, 2, 4 mg) for those smoking >20 cigarettes/day. Start with 4 mg chewed gum and retained in mouth for 30 min when urge to smoke is felt. 3. Mecamylamine (ganglion blocking agent) alone or in combination with nicotine patch has been tried for smoking cessation.	4. Bilateral stellate ganglion block causes immediate return of vision.[3] 5. Supportive:[7] Procainamide Protect kidney/vision by giving nitrate
PM findings • Nothing specific • Stomach: Fragment of leaves or tablet	**PM findings** • Nothing specific • Suggestive of asphyxia • Stomach: Inflammation, smell present with leaves ingredient	**PM findings** • Nothing specific • Hemolysis of RBC[3] • Renal tubules blocked by hemoglobin[3]
ML aspects • Suicidal: Not known • Homicidal: Occasionally used • Accidental: Overdose	**ML aspects** • Suicidal: Unusual • Homicidal: Unusual • Accidental: In chronic case • Malingering purpose: The leaves are soaked in water and placed in axilla[3]	**ML aspects** • Suicidal: Rare • Homicidal: Rare • Accidental: Overdose • Abortifacient

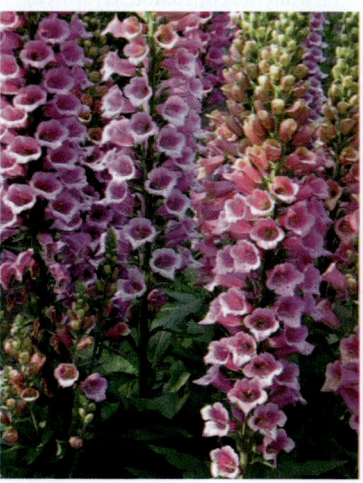 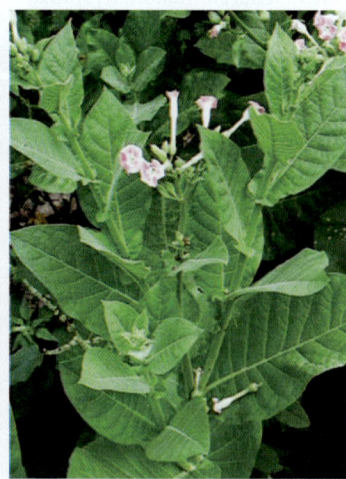 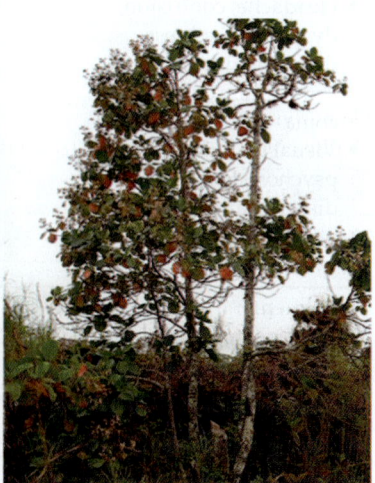

Fig. 19.6: *Digitalis purpurae* plant   **Fig. 19.7:** *Nicotiana tabacum* plant   **Fig. 19.8:** *Cinchona pubescens* plant

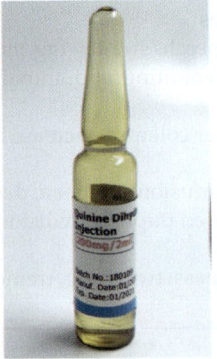

Fig. 19.9: Quinine

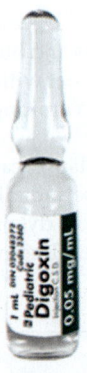

Fig. 19.10: Digoxin

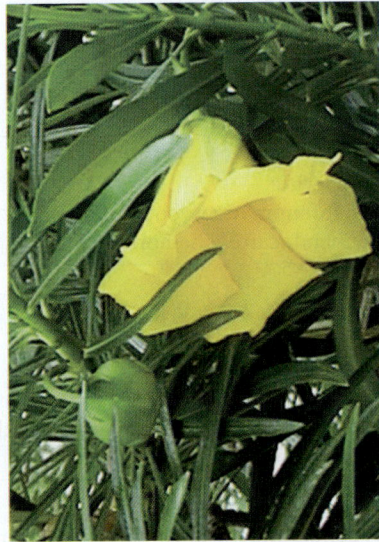

Fig. 19.11: *Cerbera thevetia* with yellow flower and fruit

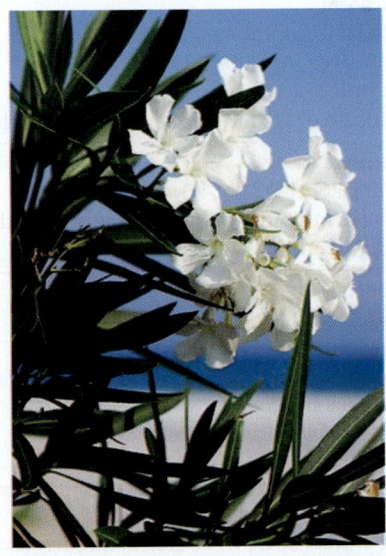

Fig. 19.12: *Nerium odorum* with white flower

Cerbera thevetia	*Nerium odorum*
Synonyms: Pila Kanher Yellow oleander, bitta-green globular fruit	**Synonyms:** Safed Kanher, White oleander
Grows in: All over India	All over India
Toxic parts: All parts of plant (maximum concentration—roots, seeds)	**Toxic parts:** All parts of plant (maximum concentration—roots)
Toxic principles: Cerberin, Thevetin, Thevotoxin	**Toxic principles:** Nerin
Use: Seeds used for playing in rural areas	**Use:** Medicinal use on ulcer/cancer/venereal disease[3]
Action: Cardiac depressant	**Action:** Cardiac depressant
Fatal dose **Roots:** 15 gm; **Seeds:** 8–10 seeds **Fatal period:** 2–3 hours	**Fatal dose** **Roots:** 15 gm **Fatal period:** 24–36 hours

Clinical features
- Tingling, numbness and burning sensation in mouth/tongue/throat with bitter taste, increase salivation, nausea, vomiting, abdominal pain, and diarrhea
- Cardiovascular collapse, cardiac irregularities, slow irregular pulse and fall of BP[1]
- Headache, confusion, dyspnea, dizziness, delirium, dilated pupil, convulsion, collapse, and coma

Clinical features
- Difficulty in speech/swallowing, increase salivation with nausea, vomiting, abdominal pain, and diarrhea.
- Cardiovascular collapse, increase in pulse and fall of BP.
- Headache, confusion, dyspnea, dizziness, delirium, dilated pupil, convulsion, collapse, coma
- Muscle weakness, twitching, tremor, tetany, lock jaw

Treatment
- Emesis
- Stomach wash: $KMnO_4$
- Demulcent
- Artificial respiration and O_2 inhalation
- Supportive:[7]
  - Atropine
  - Infusion of sodium molar lactate with glucose

Treatment
- Emesis
- Stomach wash
- Demulcent/purgatives
- Artificial respiration and O_2 inhalation
- Supportive

PM findings
- Nothing specific
- Stomach: Inflammation, seeds/root ingredient
- Heart: Subendocardial hemorrhage[1]

PM findings
- Nothing specific
- Stomach: Inflammation, root ingredient
- Heart: Subendocardial hemorrhage

ML aspects
- Suicidal: Usually in rural areas
- Homicidal: Rare
- Accidental: Usually to children (by seeds/flower)
- Abortifacient: Root
- Cattle poison: Leaves/fruit

ML aspects
- Suicidal: Rare
- Homicidal: Rare
- Accidental: Quack medicine
- Abortifacient: Root
- Cattle poison: Juice applied on piece of cloth and inserted into anus[3]

Keller's Test: for *Cerbera thevetia*:[8]

1. Ether extract of CT in viscera is dissolved in 1 ml of Glacial AA containing 5% ferric sulphate. It is then put over the mixture containing 100 part of conc H_2SO_4 + 1 part of Ferric sulphate → blue color appears on AA layer and mauve color on H_2SO_4 layer.
2. TM+ dil HCl → Blue color if yellow oleander

Test for cardiac glycosides of digitalis:[8]

TM+ conc H_2SO_4 → green color—if digitoxin and no change with bromine. Yellow to brick red—if digitalin and violet red with bromine. Red color—if digitonin and color deepens with bromine

IMPORTANT QUESTIONS

1. Enumerate different cardiac poisons. Describe action, clinical manifestation, management and medicolegal aspect of digitalis or quinine intoxication.

2. Enumerate cardiac poisons of vegetable source with its different active principles. Describe clinical features, treatment and medicolegal aspect of aconite poisoning.

3. Enumerate roadside cardiac poisons. Describe clinical features, treatment and medicolegal significance of any one.

4. Enumerate cardiac poisons which are of medicinal utility. Describe action, clinical manifestation, treatment and medicolegal aspect of nicotine poisoning. Add a note on treatment of smoking cessation.

SPECIFIC LEARNING OBJECTIVES

After reading this chapter, the reader should be able to:

- Name different cardiac poisons
- Enumerate active principles and uses of different cardiac poisons and their fatal dose and fatal period
- Explain clinical manifestation, treatment, postmortem findings and medicolegal aspect of aconite poisoning
- Differentiate root of aconite and horse radish
- Explain clinical features, treatment and medicolegal aspect of nicotine and quinine intoxication
- Explain clinical features, treatment and medicolegal aspect of *Cerbera thevetia/ Nerium odorum* poisoning

References

1. Dikshit PC. Textbook of Forensic Medicine and Toxicology. 2nd edn, PEEPEE Publisher and Distributors (P) Ltd. New Delhi. 2014: 560–9.

2. Singhal SK. Singhal's Toxicology at a glance. 9th edn, National book depot: Mumbai.2016: 88–93.

3. Reddy KSN, Murthy OP. The Essential of Forensic Medicine and Toxicology. 32nd edn, Om Sai graphics: Hyderabad. 2013: 583–7.

4. Tripathi KD. Antimalarials drugs. In: Essential of Medical Pharmacology. 7th edn, Jaypee Brothers Medical Publishers (P) Ltd: New Delhi. 2014: 816–35.

5. Tripathi KD. Cardiac glycosides and drugs for heart failure. In: Essential of Medical Pharmacology. 7th edn, Jaypee Brothers Medical Publishers (P) Ltd: New Delhi. 2014: 512–25.

6. Tripathi KD. Cholinergic drugs and drugs acting on autonomic ganglion. In: Essential of Medical Pharmacology. 7th edn, Jaypee Brothers Medical Publishers (P) Ltd: New Delhi. 2014: 113–23.

7. Nandy A. Principles of Forensic Medicine. 2nd edn, Reprint. New Central Book Agency (P) Ltd: Calcutta. 2004: 551–8.

8. Jaiswal AK, Millo T. Screening/spot/color test for different poisons. In: Handbook of Forensic Analytical Toxicology. 1st edn, Jaypee Brothers Medical Publishers (P) Ltd: New Delhi. 2014: 81–174.

Asphyxiant and Irrespirable Poisons

Asphyxiant poisons are the gases which cause asphyxia due to one of the following causes.

Causes of asphyxia due to poisons

1. Lack of sufficient oxygen in inspired air: Vitiated air
2. Spasm of RT/larynx: SO_2, mineral acid fumes.
3. Agent which prevents diffusion of gases at alveolar membrane: Phosgene (choking gas)
4. Failure of RBC to pick up oxygen in the lungs: CO
5. Poisons which interfere with the transport of oxygenated blood to tissue: Circulatory depressant.
6. Poisons which prevent the use of oxygen at tissue level: Cyanides, HCN
7. Agent which causes paralysis of respiratory muscle used for respiration: Curare
8. Agents which cause failure of respiratory center: CO_2, H_2S.

Classification of asphyxiant agents:

1. Simple asphyxiants: These are inert gases act mechanically by displacing oxygen—CO_2, NO_2
2. Irritants: These agents cause destruction of respiratory tract—smoke, formaline, chlorine
3. Chemical: These combine with hemoglobin or prevent oxygen from reaching the tissue—HCN, CO
4. Systemic asphyxiants: These agents causes systemic toxicity when inhaled—Arsine, insecticidal spray
5. Volatile: These agents act as anesthetic agents—Aliphatic/aromatic/halogenated hydrocarbons.

CARBON DIOXIDE (CO₂)	CARBON MONOXIDE (CO)
Properties Colorless, odorless, tasteless, heavier than air	**Properties** Colorless, odorless, tasteless, lighter than air
Source: Product of complete combustion • Present in expiration • Decomposition gases • Fermentation, in manholes and wells • Explosion of mines	**Source:**[1,2] Product of incomplete combustion of fuel (Automobiles –5%CO, Coal gas— 5–15%, Fuel gas—30%) • Explosion gas—60% CO • Decomposition of organic matter
Uses 1. As respiratory stimulant 2. Fire extinguisher 3. Refrigerant 4. Carbonation of beverages[3]	**Uses** 1. Cheap source of fuel and burns with blue flame[4] 2. It is used as safety measure where it is mixed with other gas to detect the leakage easily

Action: Respiratory depressant

Action:[5,6] Greater affinity (210 times) for Hb than O_2 and produce carboxy-Hb. It affects carrying capacity of O_2 leading to anemic anoxia. It is diagnosed by measuring the CO-Hb level in heparinized blood sample[7]

Fatal dose: 2000 ppm
Fatal period: Min to hrs

Fatal dose: 1500 ppm
Fatal period: Min to hrs

Clinical features
Depends on percentage (%) of CO_2 in air:
- 0.04% : Normal in air
- 2%   : Respiratory stimulants with tachypnea[3]
- 5%   : Difficulty in breathing
- 10%   : Vasoconstriction → increase HR, pulse, BP
- 20–30%: Respiratory discomfort with sudden fall of respiration
- 40%   : Headache, dyspnea, dizziness, confusion, giddiness, tightness in chest, ringing in ears, dimness of vision
- 50%   : Paralysis of respiratory centers
- 50–60%: Convulsion, cardiac irregularities, collapse
- >60% : Unconsciousness, rapid death

Clinical features
Depends on saturation% of CO in blood:
- Normally, CO is not found in blood
- 0–10% : No signs
- 10–20% : Headache, dyspnea
- 20–30% : Throbbing headache, dyspnea, weakness
- 30–40% : Headache, dyspnea, dizziness, confusion, giddiness, tightness in chest, ringing in ears, dimness of vision, with increase pulse and BP
- 40–50% : In addition to above features, there is pinkish discoloration of skin. Bullous eruption on skin[5]
- 50–60% : Convulsion, collapse, coma, paralysis of respiratory centers
- >60%   : Respiratory arrest

Treatment[3]
- Quick removal from source
- Artificial respiration and oxygen inhalation
- Supportive

Treatment
- Quick removal from source
- Artificial respiration and 100% O_2 inhalation[2]
- Carbogen inhalation (95% O_2 + 5% CO_2)[1]
- Supportive: 5% dextrose, antibiotic cover, mannitol.
- Blood transfusion

PM findings
- PM staining: Prominent bluish color (Fig. 20.1)
- Organs: Congested, bluish, petechial hemorrhages
- Blood: Dark red fluid blood
- Marked cyanosis of nails (Fig. 20.3)
- Thoracic musculature congested (Fig. 20.5)

PM findings
- PM staining: Cherry red color (Fig. 20.2) to be differentiated from cold exposure and cyanide poisoning. Froth present at mouth and nostrils
- Organs: Congested, bright red, petechial hemorrhages (Figs 20.4, 20.6 and 20.7)
- Blood: Bright red fluid blood/skin blisters

ML aspects
- Suicidal: Rare
- Homicidal: Rare
- Accidental:[1,4] In vulnerable circumstances like inside mines, wells, leakage of fire extinguisher and outbreak of fire, and overcrowding in ill-ventilated room

ML aspects
- Suicidal: Common in male, Western countries[4]
- Homicidal: Rare by placing a gas tube inside the room of victim when he is sleeping at night
- Accidental: In vulnerable circumstances like outbreak of fire and by cooking gas. Also due to inhalation of exhaust fumes[8] of vehicles, generator, and air conditioner.

Bedside test for carbon monoxide poisoning: 1 ml of blood + 10 ml of water. Add 1ml of 5% NaOH solution. If >20% saturation of CO → turns pink. Normal blood turns brown.[9]

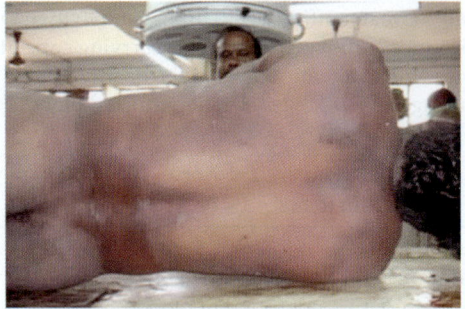

Fig. 20.1: Marked purple PML lividity

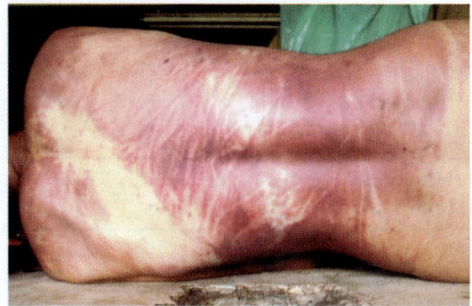

Fig. 20.2: Cherry red PM lividity in CO poisoning

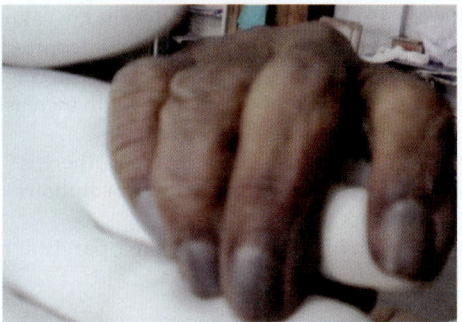

Fig. 20.3: Cyanosis of nails

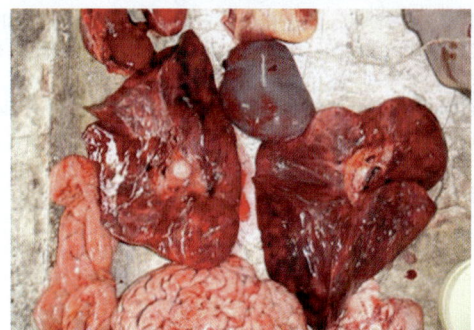

Fig. 20.4: Organs—bright red in CO poisoning

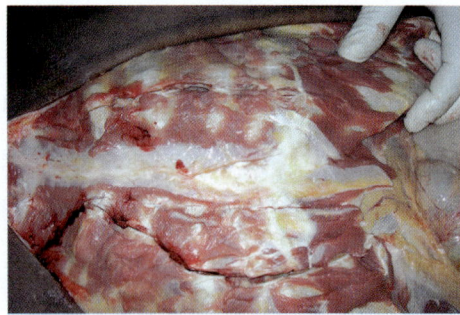

Fig. 20.5: Purplish colored congestion of muscles

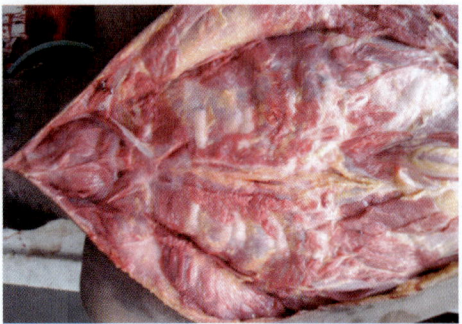

Fig. 20.6: Bright red discoloration of muscles in CO poisoning

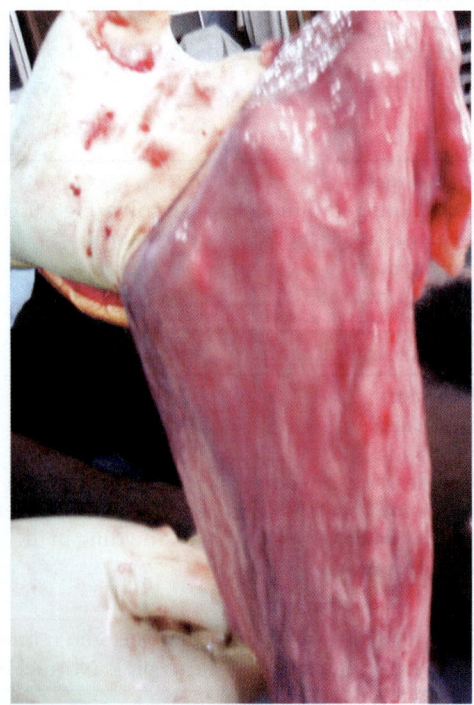

Fig. 20.7: Bright red discoloration of stomach mucosa in CO poisoning

HYDROGEN SULFIDE (H$_2$S)	SULFUR DIOXIDE (SO$_2$)	PHOSGENE (COCl$_2$)
Metal sulfide + sulfuric acid → salt + H$_2$S. It is the product of decomposition of organic material containing sulfur[1]	It is prepared by burning sulfur in oxygen/air	The **choking gas** is prepared if CCl$_4$ is exposed to hot air (i.e. oxidation) or by mixing chlorine gas with carbon monoxide
Properties Colorless, rotten egg smell	**Properties** Colorless, pungent	**Properties** Colorless, phosgene smell
Source: Sewer, cess pool, well-decomposed body	**Source:** Laboratory, industrial, pollution	**Source:** Laboratory, industrial
Uses: Production of sulfuric acid, manufacture of pesticides, and in laboratories for analytical chemistry	**Uses:** Refrigerant and bleaching agent	**Uses:** Production of isocyanates, used in refrigeration, as a chemical weapon
Action: It binds with iron in the mitochondrial cytochrome enzymes to form a complex, thereby blocking oxygen from binding and stopping cellular respiration.[10]	**Action:** Respiratory irritant	**Action:** Prevent diffusion of gas at alveolar membrane
Fatal dose: 1000 ppm **Fatal period:** Min to hrs	**Fatal dose:** 1000 ppm **Fatal period:** Min to hrs	**Fatal dose:** 1000 ppm **Fatal period:** Min to hrs
Clinical features • Lacrimation, photophobia headache, dyspnea, dizziness, confusion, giddiness, weakness, and cramps • This is followed by: – Convulsion, collapse, and coma	**Clinical features** • Lacrimation, photophobia + sneezing, coughing, dyspnea, suffocation, constriction in chest • This is followed by: – Laryngeal spasm and convulsion, collapse, and coma	**Clinical features** • Lacrimation, photophobia + sneezing, coughing, dyspnea, suffocation, constriction in chest. • This is followed by: – Marked restlessness, rapid respiration, cyanosis, convulsion, collapse, and coma
Treatment • Quick removal from source. • Artificial respiration and oxygen inhalation • Supportive: Respiratory stimulant, antibiotic cover	**Treatment[1]** • Quick removal from source. • Artificial respiration and oxygen inhalation • Supportive: Bronchodilators, antibiotic cover	**Treatment** • Quick removal from source. • Artificial respiration and oxygen inhalation • Supportive: Antibiotic cover
PM findings • Suggestive of asphyxia present • PM staining: Greenish color[11] • Organs: Congested, petechial hemorrhage present. Brain may have black discoloration with pulmonary edema[11] • Blood: Dark brown fluid blood, with high level of thiosulfate[11]	**PM findings** • Suggestive of asphyxia present • PM staining: Bluish color • Organs: Congested, petechial hemorrhage present • Blood: Dark red fluid blood	**PM findings** • Suggestive of asphyxia present • PM staining: Bluish color • Organs: Congested, petechial hemorrhage present • Blood: Dark red fluid blood
ML aspects • Suicidal: Not known • Homicidal: Not known • Accidental: While cleaning of unused wells and underground sewerage. Also in unconfined space while dumping of sludge from water purification.[12]	**ML aspects** • Suicidal: Rare • Homicidal: Rare • Accidental: Rare	**ML aspects** • Suicidal: Unknown • Homicidal: Unknown • Accidental: Leakage of gas

HYDROCYANIC ACID

Synonyms: Cyanogen, prussic acid, cyanide.

Properties

Also known as 'Vegetable acid' since it is present in certain fruits kernels. It is very potent, extremely lethal and most rapidly fatal.

Chemically: HCN colourless gas with bitter almond smell. But can be kept in liquid form in cold temperature and under pressure.

Salts: K/Na cyanide are dirty white powder.

Sources: Laboratories, industries and kernels of **almonds**, apple, apricot, cherry, plumb, peach, etc. (Figs 20.8 to 20.10).

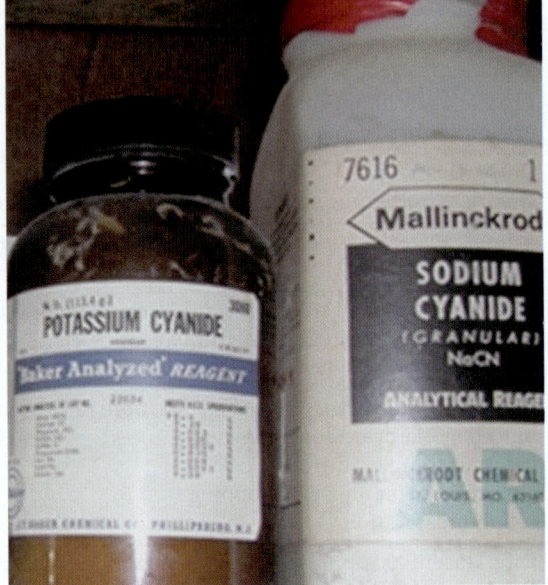

Fig. 20.10: Potassium and sodium cyanide

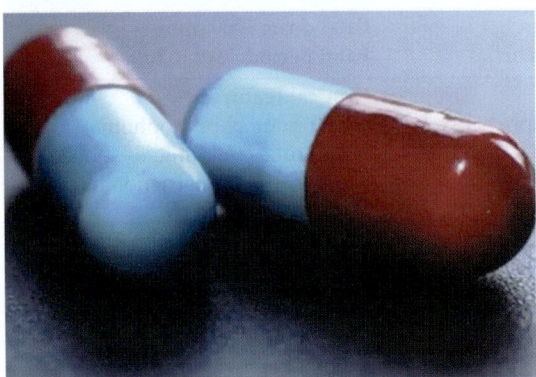

Fig. 20.8: Cyanide capsules (powder)

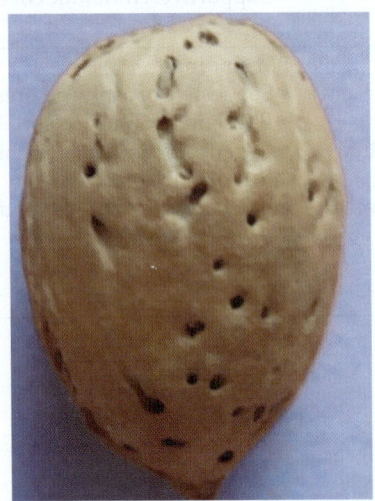

Fig. 20.9: Bitter almond

Uses[1,5]

1. For hardening of metal, metal/gold plating.
2. For purifying metallic ores.
3. In synthetic rubber and plastic industries.
4. In photography and for fumigation.
5. In manufacturing insecticides

Action

It is a protoplasmic poison that acts by **inhibiting the enzymes cytochrome oxidase**[13,14] by chelating the metallic moiety of enzyme, thus reducing oxygen utilization in the tissue resulting in histotoxic hypoxia.[5] Thus it kills person by bulbar paralysis.[1]

Absorption, Fate, Excretion

Cyanide is absorbed quickly through MM of GIT as well as RT and skin (in gases form). It is metabolised to thiocyanate (non-toxic) and is excreted through urine and expired air.

Fatal Dose/Fatal Periods (in Brackets)

HCN gas: 100–2000 ppm   (Immediate)
HCN liquid: 50 ml   (2–5 min)
HCN salts: 200 mg   (30 min)

Clinical Manifestation

The action depends on (i) form of poison [acid/salt], (ii) absence of gastric HCl, (iii) presence of food, (iv) concentration, (v) route of absorption.

- **In gaseous form and in higher concentration:** There is sudden unconsciousness followed by violent breathing, convulsion, and death.
- **When ingested in low dose:** Bitter burning sensation in mouth and feeling of constriction in chest, increase salivation, nausea, vomiting, abdominal pain.
- Fine froth at mouth and nostrils and strong bitter almond smell in expired air.
- There may be low BP, pulse, respiration with absence of reflex.
- This is followed by headache, confusion, vertigo, dizziness, dyspnoea, delirium, convulsion, collapse, coma and cardiac arrest.
- With cyanosis, pink colouration of skin, which does not improved with oxygen therapy.

Treatment

There is hardly any time for treatment (Fig. 20.11).
1. 0.2 ml Amyl Nitrite (3–6 amp) sublingual,[15] to be stopped if BP <80.
2. 3% Na Nitrite (10 ml IV) or (IV Methylene blue or Cobalt acetate/EDTA). Or Hydroxycobalamin slow IV
   [convert Hb → Meth-Hb]
3. 25% Na Thiosulphate (50 ml IV).
   [convert cyanogen → Na Thiocyanate]

4. Artificial respiration and O_2 supply.
5. Stomach wash with activated charcoal[9] or with mixture of 6% $NaCO_3$ + 15.3% Ferrous Sulphate and 3% Citric acid in water[1] or with 0.1% $KMnO_4$ or with 5–10% sodium Thiosulphate solution.

Principles of Treatment of Cyanide[14]

1. To avoid cyanogen-cytochrome combination.
2. To convert Hb to Meth-Hb (by means of Nitrite, Methylene blue[5,16] 50 ml of 1% aqueous solution slow IV, Cobalt acetate[17] 20 ml IV; Hydroxycobalamin[13,15] 5 gm IV.
3. To convert free cyanides to harmless complexes (by Na Thiosulphate, Vitamin B_{12}, Dicobalt EDTA).

PM Findings

- Cyanosis
- S/o Asphyxia
- Pinkish lividity, cherry red blood due to formation of cyanmethaemoglobin[5]
- Froth from mouth/nostril with bitter almond smell, corrosion of stomach mucosa.

Viscera Preservation

- Routine viscera
- Lungs
- Brain
- Preserved in saturated solution of NaCl

ML Aspects

1. **Suicide:** Quite common by goldsmith. Terrorists usually carry cyanide capsule

---

Hemoglobin
   $\downarrow \leftarrow$ Na Nitrite (10 ml of 3% solution IV)

Methemoglobin (has more affinity to cyanide)
   +

Cyanide (of cyanogen-cytochrome complex $\leftarrow$ Cytochrome oxidase + cyanide)
   $\downarrow$

Cyano-MetHB (and release cytochrome oxidase for tissue oxygenation)
   $\downarrow \leftarrow$ Na Thiosulfate (50 ml of 25% sol IV)

Methemoglobin + Na Thiocyanate (which is harmless and excreted in urine)

Fig. 20.11: Treatment of cyanide

to commit suicide rather than to be caught and subjected to torture/confession.[1]

2. **Homicidal:** Rare.

3. **Accidental:** From laboratory/industries. [Bhopal gas tragedy, i.e. MIC.], or from inhalation of fumes from burning polymer product that use nitrile in their production[18]

4. **Cattle poison:** Rare

5. **Judicial execution:** It is carried out in cyanide gas chamber in US.[5]

METHYL ISOCYANATE (MIC)

Properties: Colorless liquid with a sharp odor, which becomes gaseous at 39°C.

It is an extremely reactive chemically and needs to be stored carefully.

Uses

1. In the manufacture of pesticide carbaryl carbamate.

2. Manufacture of polyurethane articles (plastics, foam, adhesives, etc.).

Action

Powerful respiratory irritant.

Clinical Features

1. Inhalation of gas produces immediate lacrimation, photophobia, cough, dyspnea, chest pain, hemoptysis, pulmonary edema, vomiting, convulsion, and coma.

2. Dermal exposure results in erythema and vesiculation.

Treatment

1. Washing of skin and eyes with saline.

2. Oxygen inhalation.

3. Bronchodilators and corticosteroids.

4. Antidote: Sodium thiosulfate.

5. Supportive.

PM Findings

- Suggestive of asphyxia
- **Lungs/brain:** Congested, edematous.
- **Visceral organs:** Congested.

ML Aspect

MIC was involved in one of the most terrible gas disaster which occurred in Bhopal, Madhya Pradesh **(Bhopal Gas Tragedy, 1984)**. There was a leakage of methyl isocyanate from union carbide plant.[19] MIC is required in the manufacture of carbaryl (carbamate). This deadly chemical was stored in huge, double walled stainless steel tanks, one of which burst on the night of Dec 2, 1984, releasing more than 24,000 kg of MIC gas into the atmosphere killing thousands in their sleep and incapacitating several thousands more.

PHOSPHINE (WATER + CALCIUM CARBIDE)

It is a war gas, being prepared by boiling white phosphorus with a solution of KOH or NaOH. It can be easily prepared by moistening calcium phosphide.

- It is a respiratory track irritant and has acetylene like odor.
- **Fatal dose:** 20 ppm.
- It is released from zinc phosphide and metal phosphide.
- It is used as a fumigant to control insects and rodents in foodgrains and fields.

Treatment

1. Quick removal from the source

2. Artificial respiration and O_2 inhalation

3. Supportive

SEWER GAS

Hydrogen sulphide, carbon dioxide and methane gases are formed in sewers and called sewer gas.[4]

IMPORTANT QUESTIONS

1. **Short notes of MIC tragedy.**

2. **Describe action, clinical features, treatment, autopsy findings and medicolegal significance of carbon monoxide poisoning.**

3. **Enumerate the poison which imparts characteristic color of PM lividity. Add a note on Bhopal gas tragedy.**

4. What is the differential diagnosis of death in person while cleaning unused well and sewerage? Describe clinical features, treatment and postmortem findings of any one of them.

5. Describe action, clinical manifestation, management and medicolegal aspect of cyanide poisoning.

SPECIFIC LEARNING OBJECTIVES

After reading this chapter, the reader should be able to:

- **Enumerate different asphyxiant poisons**
- **Classify asphyxiant agents**
- **Enumerate causes of asphyxia due to poisons with examples**
- **Enlist different uses of carbon monoxide and carbon dioxide**
- **Explain clinical manifestation, treatment, postmortem findings and medicolegal aspects of CO/CO$_2$**
- **Delineate the mechanism of action of cyanide and enumerate uses of cyanogen**
- **Explain clinical manifestation, treatment, postmortem findings and medicolegal aspects of cyanide poisoning**
- **Explain methyl isocyanate poisoning and understand the basis of Bhopal gas tragedy**
- **Enlist different gases formed in sewers**

References

1. Nandy A. Principles of Forensic Medicine. 2nd edn, Reprint. New Central Book Agency (P) Ltd: Calcutta. 2004:551–62.

2. Ivan Blumenthal. Carbon monoxide poisoning. J Royal Soc Med. 2001; 94(6): 270–2.

3. Langford NJ. Carbon dioxide poisoning. Toxicol Rev. 2005;24(4):229–35.

4. Bardale R. Principles of Forensic Medicine and Toxicology. 1st edn, Jaypee Brothers Medical Publishers (P) Ltd: New Delhi. 2011: 541–5.

5. Dikshit PC. Textbook of Forensic Medicine and Toxicology. 2nd edn, PEEPEE Publisher and Distributors (P) Ltd. New Delhi. 2014: 560–82.

6. Ganong WF. Review of Medical Physiology. Norwalk Ct: Appleton & Lange, 1995.

7. Touger M, Gallagher EJ, Tyrell J. Relationship between venous and arterial carboxyhemoglobin levels in patients with suspected carbon monoxide poisoning. Ann Emerg Med. 1995 Apr; 25(4):481–3.

8. Cobb N, Etzel RA. Unintentional carbon monoxide-related deaths in the United States, 1979 through 1988. JAMA. 1991; 266(5):659–63.

9. Pillay VV. Textbook of Forensic Medicine and Toxicology. 17th edn, Paras Medical Publisher: Hyderabad. 2016: 640–54.

10. Singh A, Sharma BR. Hydrogen sulphide poisoning: A case report of quadruple fatalities. JPAFMAT. 2008; 8(1): 38–40.

11. Ago M, Ago K, Ogata M. Two fatalities by hydrogen sulphide poisoning: Variation of pathological and toxicological findings. Leg Med (Tokyo). 2008 May;10(3):148–52.

12. Nogué S, Pou R, Fernández J, Sanz-Gallén P. Fatal hydrogen sulphide poisoning in unconfined spaces. *Occupational Medicine*, 2011; 61(3):212–4. https://doi.org/101093/occmed/kqr021

13. Graham DL, Laman D, Theodore J, Robin ED. Acute cyanide poisoning complicated by lactic acidosis and pulmonary edema. Arch Intern Med. 1977 Aug;137(8):1051–5.

14. Tripathi KD. Essential of Medical Pharmacology. 7th edn, Jaypee Brothers Medical Publishers (P) Ltd: New Delhi. 2014:545.

15. Reddy KSN, Murthy OP. The Essential of Forensic Medicine and Toxicology. 32nd edn, Om Sai Graphics: Hyderabad. 2013:583–7.

16. Hanzlik, PJ. Methylene blue as an antidote for cyanide poisoning. JAMA. 1933; 100 (5): 357.

17. Nagler J, Provoost RA, Parizel G (1978). "Hydrogen cyanide poisoning: Treatment with cobalt EDTA". Journal of Occupational Medicine. 20 (6): 414–6.

18. McKenna, Sean Thomas, Hull Terence Richard. The fire toxicity of polyurethane foams. Fire Science Reviews. 2016; 5 (1). doi:10.1186/s40038-016-0012-3.

19. Varma DR, Mulay S. Methyl Isocyanate: The Bhopal gas. In: Handbook of toxicology of chemical warfare agents. 2nd ed, USA: Academic Press. 2015: 287–99.

Drug Dependence and Abuse

Drug abuse is an international problem, which affects almost every country in the world; India is no exception. Illicit drug abuse not only affects the health of the individual but also undermines the political, social and cultural foundation of all countries. With a turnover of around $500 billion, it is the third largest business in the world, next to petroleum and arms trade.[1] According to a UN report, 1 million heroin addicts are registered in India, and unofficially, there are as many as 5 millions.[2] In India, cannabis, heroin, opium, and hashish followed by amphetamines are the most commonly used drugs in India after alcohol and tobacco.[3] A National Survey (2004) on the extent, pattern, and trends of drug abuse in India found that opiates are primary drug abused and 49% of respondent's families had a history of drug abuse.[4]

Drug abuse: It is defined as self-administration of drug for non-medical reasons, which may impair an individual's ability to function effectively, result in social, physical or emotional harm.[5] It is an improper and excessive use of therapeutic medicine even in the absence of addiction

Drug addiction (WHO 1950):[6] It is a state of periodic or chronic intoxication produced by the repeated consumption of a drug	**Drug Habit:** It is a condition resulting from repeated consumptions of drug, which does not cause much harm to the society
It is characterized by a. Tendency to increase the dose b. Harmful effects to the individual and to the society c. It causes both **psychological and physical dependence** d. An overpowering desire to continue the drug or to obtain it by any means	*It is characterized by* a. Tendency to take the drugs with or without increase the dose b. Harmful effect mainly to the individual c. It causes only **psychological dependence** and not physical dependence d. Desire to repeat/continue the drug as and when convenient.

Drug dependence: WHO (1964)[7] has recommended the term drug dependence to **replace the terms** "Drug addiction and drug habit". It has been defined as a state, psychological or physical, in which a person has the compulsion to take a drug on a continuous or periodic basis either to experience its pleasurable effects or to avoid the discomfort.[5]

Physical dependence: It is a biological phenomenon, which depends on the type, dose, and duration of drug used irrespective of personality factor. If the drug is abruptly stopped, withdrawal syndrome will occur.	**Psychological dependence:** It is a compulsive need for a drug in order to maintain state of well-being

CLASSIFICATION OF DRUGS USED FOR ABUSE

I. Depending upon physical or psychological dependence

a. **Drug of addiction:** Drugs that cause both psychological and physical dependence:

- Alcohols
- Narcotic analgesic: Opium, methadon, morphine, heroin, codeine, pethidine
- Depressant (downers):
  Tranquilizers: Diazepam, chlordiazepoxide
  Hypnotics: Barbiturate, paraldehyde, chloral hydrate, hydrocarbon, meprobamate
- Methaqualone

b. **Drug habit:** Drugs which cause only psychological dependence:

- Tobacco
- Cannabis preparations: Ganja, charas, majun, bhang.
- Stimulants (uppers): Amphetamine, caffeine, ephedrine, methyl phenidate (ritalin)
- Volatile anesthetic solvents: Toluene, known as 'glue sniffing'
- Hallucinogens: Lysergic acid diethylamide (LSD), phencyclidine, mescaline

II. Depending upon their effects:

a. **Hard drugs**—narcotics

b. **Soft drugs**—Barbiturates, diazepam, amphetamine, LSD, pentazocaine.

Drug is any substance used in the diagnosis, treatment, investigation, and prevention and modification of disease. It is used to sustain or to prolong life or to get relief. But, it may have physiological and psychological effects on human beings and other animals. However, as actions and powers are misused in all fields, the drugs are not spared. The drug may be misused for following purpose:

1. To terminate their life.
2. To get relief from all stress.
3. To remain undisturbed and pass peaceful time.
4. To be out of touch from reality.
5. To be in an imaginary state of mental happiness and well-being.

The drugs made its path from the doctor's or chemist room to these vulnerable people of the society. Thus, the drugs user may be:[8]

a. **Occasional users:** Depending on the custom and cultural background of the society who accepted the use of alcohol and some preparation of cannabis. However, use of tobacco is almost accepted in all societies.

b. **Heavy users:** They are addicted or dependent on some drugs and cannot do anything without the same.

BRIEF DESCRIPTION OF DRUGS USED FOR ABUSE

1. Opium: It is extracted from unripe fruit of the plant *Papaver somniferum*. It is obtained by giving incisions on the unripe fruit producing milky exude which on exposed to air becomes dark brown opium "AFIM".

Opium is also called 'Black Gold' because of its color and price in international market.

Types of opioid drugs[9]	
Natural	Morphine, codeine, thebaine
Semisynthetic	Heroin, oxymorphone, nalorphine
Synthetic	Pethidine, methadon, fentanyl, tramadol

Opioid drugs are known by many names:

- Heroin—smack, dope, Lady Jane, brown sugar.
- Fentanyl—China white.

2. Cocaine: Cocaine is extracted from the leaves of a *Erythroxylum coca*, which grows in the mountains of South America, Indonesia, and India. It is then purified to the cocaine hydrochloride, which is white crystalline powder.

Street names of cocaine are:[10, 11] Coke, snow, cadillac, white lady, etc.

- Cocaine + ethanol—it is called liquid lady.
- Cocaine + heroin—it is called speedball or crank.
- Newer type of cocaine is known as crack.

3. Cannabis: *Cannabis sativa/indica* grows all over India, but its cultivation and marketing is under strict legislation and control under government.

Active principle: Tetrahydrocannabinol

Preparation of cannabis[11, 12]	
Bhang (siddi)	Consist of dried leaves or stem
Ganja	Consist of flowering tops of female plant
Charas 'Hashish'	Resinous extract from flowering tops and leaves
Majun	Sweet preparation of bhang after **treating with sugar, flour, milk**
Marihuana (marijuana)	Extract from American hemp plant. Ganja smoked in pipe.
Reefers	Cigarettes preparation of ganja/marijuana

Street names: Marijuana, Mary Jane, pot, weed, grass.

4. Alcohol

Arrack: It refers to country made liquor usually distilled from rice/sugar or jaggery, cashew nut, coco palm, and mohua flowers. In India, adulterant like chloral hydrate (knockout drops) or methanol or datura/bhang may be added in order to enhance its effect.

Street names of country liquor: Khopdi, lattha, sura, gudamba, feni, etc.

5. Tobacco: It is obtained from the leaves of *Nicotiana tabacum.*

Active principle: Nicotine—present in leaf.

The dried leaves of tobacco are used in the form of smoke/snuff or chewing with lime or alone. Individual begins with tobacco and alcohol, progress later to cannabis and may eventually to opium/heroin. Hence, it is considered as **"Gateway" to drug abuse.**

6. Sedatives

Barbiturates	Drug for seizure, anesthesia, e.g. gardenal, luminal, veronal
Benzodiazepines	Drug for seizure/sedation/anxiolytics, e.g. calmpose, valium, restyl, libruim

Chloral hydrate (not used now)	Knock out agent, mixed in alcohol for a greater kick

7. Hallucinogens

Hallucinogens	Street names[10]
Lysergic acid diethylamide	The drug is popular among its uses as 'blue pill'. Acid, microdot, purple haze, white lightening, etc.
Phencyclidine [phenyl-cyclohexyl-piperidine (PCP)]	Angel dust, PCP, Angel's mist, peace pill, hog, rocket fuel, etc. Angel dust: Smoking PCP + marijuana. Wack: PCP + formaldehyde + cockroach repellent. Spacebar: PCP + crack (never cocaine).
Mescaline	Extracted from the dried tops of a cactus plant *Lophophora williamsii*

8. Designer drugs are synthetic variations of well-known controlled drugs with similar pharmacological effects but different molecular structures. This makes them immune from the control of the drug enforcement agency. It is abused by athletes to excel their performance.[13] These are also abused by youngsters for rave parties. The most commonly types of synthetic analog drugs available in the illicit drug market includes:

Derivatives	Street name of designer drug
Amphetamine	Ecstasy/adams/XTC. Love drugs; speed/ice; eve
Fentanyl derivatives	China white. Alpha-methyl fentanyl—3000 times as potent as morphine (detected by RI assay)
Flunitrazepam	**Rohypnol 'Roofies':** Reported as being one of the commonest drugs in school and college campuses. It is often combined with alcohol, marijuana or cocaine. It is commonly used for **'Date rape'**

9. Inhalants: The abuse of these drugs is called *'solvent abuse'* because most of these are used as solvents.

Etiology of drug abuse: Factors related to drug dependence are as follows:

Factor	Cause
1. Personal factor	• Psychological status of a person
	• Period of stress/strain, curiosity, adventure and experimentation in young age; and is common in males
	• Individual tolerance and threshold to different odds of life[8]
2. Social/economic and environmental factors[8]	• Family status/environment/liability/responsibility/attachment/happenings and stress events in family
	• Neglected childhood, separated parents
	• Failure in love/exams/achievement/career
	• Social and mental status of friends/associates
	• Environment in school, college, hostel, surrounding
	• Residential and working environment
	• Emotional trends, habits, likeliness and mental makeup
3. Drug factor	• Self-medication, over medication, wrong medication
	• Easy availability of drug
	• Prescription abuse
	• Tolerance to drug

Routes of administration of drugs for abuse	
Routes	*Examples*
1. Oral	Alcohol, cannabis preparation (bhang, ganja, majun), mandrax, LSD, amphetamine (ecstasy), barbiturates, diazepam, cough syrup
Usually they are mixed with something (alcohol) or sometimes one or two drugs may be combined together for a greater kick	
2. Parental	Accessible sites are preferred
a. Subcutaneous (SC)	Opium, heroin—over thigh/forearm
Drug using SC route is known as 'skin popping'[11] and a person who uses this route is called a 'skin popper'.	
b. Intravenous (IV)	Opium drugs
Drug using IV route is known as 'mainlining'[11] and a person who uses this route is called a 'mainliner'	
c. Intra-arterial	Opium drugs in radial/femoral artery, cocaine injection in venous plexuses
Drug using intra-arterial route is known as 'pinkie'	
3. Inhalation	
Snorting/sniffing	Cocaine—when a powder is inhaled (snuff)[11]
Glue sniffing	Toluene, xylene, benzene—when volatile solvent is inhaled
Chasers	Heroin—when foils containing heroin are burnt and the fumes are inhaled
4. Smoking	Ganja, marijuana, tobacco and crack

Commonly used are hydrocarbons, which are classified as:[14]

Aliphatic	Diesel oil, gasoline, kerosene turpentine, naphtha
Aromatic	Benzene, toluene, xylene
Halogenated	Carbon tetrachloride (CCl_4), tetrachloroethane (TCE), organochlorines

10. Others

Mandrax	(Methaqualone + diphenhydramine): It is very popular in India. Many factories manufacturing 'Mandrax' were unearthed by Gujarat and Maharashtra Police and shut down
Cough syrup	It is a newer type of addiction, common in those who have given up alcohol

INVESTIGATION OF DRUG RELATED OR DRUG ABUSE DEATHS

In drug related deaths, the crime scene investigation (CSI) and circumstances leading to death (history of case) is very important, as the toxicological report alone cannot be used to determine the cause of death. Thus, investigation of drug abuse death involves following steps.

I. Crime Scene Investigation

1. Usually the death/circumstances of drug abuse usually occur in isolated place. So, such place/spot should be searched for presence of drugs, needles, syringe, container, etc. and source of heat.
2. Plastic bags, glue tubes or aerosol cans, etc. along with soiled clothes with solvent may indicate death related to 'solvent abuse'.
3. Clothes and body of the deceased should be searched for drugs and apparatus/accessories. Sometimes it may be hidden in between the buttocks, under the breast, etc.
4. Surrounding area should also be searched for home made local remedies used in an attempt to revive, e.g. injecting saliva, milk or water into the arm, back of hands or buttock.

5. Photograph of the crime scene should be taken.

II. History

The drug users may have negative thought, so the past history of drug abuse and police record is very important. The information from friends, relatives and witness as to the behavior of the victim should also be sought.

III. Autopsy Findings

In drug abuse case, the autopsy should be concentrated on external findings and collection of required samples for toxicological analysis.

a. External Examination

1. **In most of the cases, there is no specific autopsy findings:** There may be only wasting or signs of self neglect, i.e. unhygienic condition of abuser.
2. **Burns/stain around mouth or on the tips of finger and long fingernails:** May be seen in cocaine abusers. **Blood tinged froth** oozing from mouth/nostril **with characteristics odor.**
3. **In IV addicts (mainliner):** Typical linear needle track scars appear as 'Railroad tracks'[15] are seen in cubital fossa, forearm and dorsal aspect of hands. They are also seen in area of scalp, neck, sublingual areas, shoulder, inguinal region, penis, vagina, popliteal area, ankle or foot.

In intradermal or subcutaneous drug users—skin popper: There are **typical depressed circular and geographical atrophic scar,** ulceration, infected abscess, etc. at injection site. Healing by fibrosis may produce hyperpigmented macules, circumscribed scars like that of smallpox vaccination scars.

In nasal inhalation (snorting/sniffing): there may be irritation, congestion and atrophy of nasal mucosa; and in some cases perforation of nasal septum, especially in cocaine and heroin abusers.

In solvent abusers (glue sniffing): The face may be red, erythematous pimples or actual excoriations from the irritant action of the solvent. The lesions may become infected, scratched or crusted.

4. **Recent injection sites:** May show zones of inflammation surrounding the puncture site. Incision through skin may reveal a prominent perivenous hemorrhage.

5. **'Soot tattooing':** These are the punctate areas of black discoloration seen along the track of needle due to the deposition of carbonaceous material, as the needle being sterilized over flame. Such tattooing is also called **'turkey skin'**.[11]

6. **Tattoos:** May be seen over the areas of needle marks, which are used **to conceal the injection marks.**

b. Internal Examination

Internal findings are not prominent at autopsy:

1. Examination of needle scars reveals **perivenous fibrosis in IV** addicts, and subcutaneous scarring and acute/chronic abscess in the skin popper.

2. Streaks of carbon may be seen in subcutaneous tissue, which are deposited by heated needle tips.

3. Foreign material such as cotton, piece of cloth, talc, starch, etc. are seen in subcutaneous tissues with surrounding foreign body giant cell reaction on microscopy.

4. Peripheral veins may show old or recent thrombosis, phlebitis in mainliners.

5. Lungs are heavy, congested and edematous, especially in heroin addicts called **'Heroin Lung'**.[16] In mainliners, crystals lodge in pulmonary capillaries and lungs show large quantities of talc, starch and cellulose in the foreign body granulomatous reaction. There is froth in the trachea/bronchi and pleura show petechial hemorrhage.

6. **Stomach** may show undissolved **tablets/pills**. The entire length of GIT should be searched for evidence of an attempt to hide/smuggled drugs.

7. There may be enlarged lymph nodes near porta hepatis. Liver may be slightly enlarged and may show evidence of cirrhosis. This is especially seen in opioid abusers.

8. Pericardial, pleural and peritoneal effusion may be seen; and heart may show valvular disease.

9. Brain may show edema and focal necrosis of globus pallidus and hippocampus due to hypoxia.

IV. Toxicological Analysis

Following samples are preserved for toxicological analysis in drugs related deaths:

1. Routine viscera (V1 + V2) along with gallbladder.

2. **Blood:** Usually venous blood from peripheral sites (femoral vein), kept in fluoride preservative.

3. **Tissue from injection site:** In cases of parenteral users.

4. **Urine:** Usually in opium, datura, cannabis, alcohol, amphetamine, cocaine.

5. **Nasal swabs:** In cases of nasal inhalation of drugs.

6. Any soiling with adhesives or solvent stain.

7. In cases of death due to volatile substances:

   i. **Blood in a glass tube** filled to the top with an aluminium foil lined cap.

   ii. **Whole lungs** with main bronchus and pulmonary vessels, which are to be ligated, should be kept **in a nylon bag** (and not in polythene bags which are permeable to volatiles) and securely tied.

   iii. **Brain half** in opium, barbiturate, diazepam, solvent abuse, cocaine, etc.

CAUSES OF DEATH

I. Mostly due to drug overdose/toxicity

Drug toxicity	Effects
Ethyl alcohol	Alcoholic intoxication
Methyl alcohol	Metabolic acidosis, renal failure
Heroin	Due to combination with alcohol or cocaine
Cocaine	Cardiac arrhythmia, convulsion.

Phencyclidine	Hypothermia, intracranial hemorrhage, cardiac failure
LSD	Traumatic death due to fall from height because the person under influence of LSD think that he can fly and thus project himself out of window
Body packer syndrome	It is due to rupture of packet containing smuggled drugs in the body used as body packer

II. Due to the complication of drug administration/unsterile injection or adulteration:

Infection/septicemia, endocarditis, hepatitis, tetanus, AIDS, with acute muscle neurosis, myoglobinuria and renal failure.

III. Suicidal tendency from drug overdose/

withdrawal, particularly amphetamines, barbiturate, diazepam, alcohol, etc.

IV. Accidental deaths due to electrocutions,

head injury, drowning, aspiration of food, etc.

MEDICOLEGAL ASPECT

In spite of stringent legislation, the drug trade is increasing day by day and often lead to varieties of criminal offences.

1. **Body packing:** For smuggling drugs, person swallows a small packet containing drugs.
2. **Drug abuse and crime**

Drug	Crime
Cannabis	Run amok
Heroin	Assault, mugging to extort money for purchase of drug.
Alcohol	Sexual assaults/rape, etc.
Exchange of drugs for weapons	Narco terrorism
Drug addicts parent	Battered baby syndrome
Morphine	Infanticide

3. **Drugs abuse and suicide:** Barbiturate/ diazepam are commonly used for suicide.
4. **Drugs abuse and accidents**

Drug	Accidents
Alcohol	Vehicular accident if under influence/ industrial hazards
Aphrodisiacs drugs—viagra, cocaine	Accidental death due to excessive dose
Barbiturates	Automatism

5. Drugs abuse and insanity

Drug	Insanity
LSD	Hallucinogens
Datura	Deliriant, stupefying
Cocaine, morphine	Maniacs
Alcohol withdrawal	Delirium tremens

EFFECTIVE DEALING OF THE PROBLEM OF DRUG ABUSE

Following measures are important while dealing with the problem of drug abuse:

1. **Mass education:** Only mass education will not solve problem.
2. **Treatment at de-addiction centres:** Active treatment of victims of drug abuse should be carried out in such centres. Treatment of mild cases should be made at home if the family atmosphere is beneficial and not adverse to the patient.
3. **Stringent legislation:** Strict implementation of the provisions in the law regarding drug trafficking or peddling.
4. **Encouragement for de-addiction:** Effort should be taken to identify the abusers and potential abusers, the factor influencing the abuse and **effective methods to stop drug trafficking/peddling.**
5. **Laboratories for drug testing:** There should be adequate numbers of laboratories for the drug abuser.
6. **Rehabilitation and counselling:** There should be meaningful rehabilitation programmes for de-addicted persons. There should also be counselling for such person.

It must be remembered that drugs are blessed discoveries for the safety and well-being of members of the society and not to cause any harm to any of its members.

IMPORTANT QUESTIONS

1. Define drug abuse and drug dependence. Write difference between drug addiction and drug habit. Describe etiology and route of administration for drug abuse.
2. Write classification of drugs used for abuse. Describe about investigation of drug abuse deaths.
3. Describe the measures to be taken for handling the problem of drug abuse. Add a note on its medicolegal aspect.

SPECIFIC LEARNING OBJECTIVES

After reading this chapter, the reader should be able to:

- Define different terms: Drug addiction, drug habit, drug dependence, drug abuse, physical dependence, psychological dependence
- Enumerate drugs of addiction and drug habit with their street names
- Recognize various routes of administration of drugs for abuse and their causes
- Brief outline for investigation in drug abuse deaths
- Explain medicolegal aspect of drug abuse deaths
- Recognize different measures to deal with problem of drug abuse

References

1. Sharma B, Arora A, Singh K, Singh H, Kaur P. Drug abuse: Uncovering the burden in rural Punjab. J Family Med Prim Care. 2017;6(3):558–62.
2. Miller WR, Sanchez VC. Motivating young adults for treatment and lifestyle change. In: Howard G, editor. Issues in Alcohol Use and Misuse in Young Adults. Notre Dame: University of Notre Dame Press; 1993. pp. 55–82.
3. Nadeem A, Rubeena B, Agarwal VK, Piyush K. Substance abuse in India. Pravara Med Rev. 2009;4:4–6.
4. Ray R. The Extent, Pattern and Trends of Drug Abuse in India: National Survey. Ministry of Social Justice and Empowerment, Government of India and United Nations Office on Drugs and Crime, Regional Office for South Asia. 2004.
5. Park K. Park's Textbook of Preventive and Social Medicine. Bhanot Publisher: New Delhi. 23rd edn, 2015:831–9.
6. Expert Committee on drugs liable to produce Addiction. Report on the 2nd session, WHO Tech. Rep. Ser. 1950:21.
7. Expert Committee on Addiction—producing drugs. Fifteenth report. WHO Tech. Rep. Ser. 1964:273.
8. Nandy A. Principles of Forensic Medicine. New Central Book Agency (P) Ltd: Calcutta, 2nd edn Reprint, 2004:517–43/565–72.
9. Tripathi KD. Opioid Analgesic and antagonists. In: Essential of Medical Pharmacology. Jaypee Brothers Medical Publishers (P) Ltd: New Delhi, 7th edn, 2014:469–85.
10. Pillay VV. Textbook of Forensic Medicine and Toxicology. 17th edn, Paras Medical Publisher: Hyderabad. 2016:618–33.
11. Dikshit PC. Textbook of Forensic Medicine and Toxicology. 2nd edn, PEEPEE Publisher and Distributors (P) Ltd. New Delhi. 2014:528–35/556.
12. Tripathi KD. Antipsychotic and antimanic drugs. In: Essential of Medical Pharmacology. 7th edn, Jaypee Brothers Medical Publishers (P) Ltd: New Delhi. 2014:435–53.
13. Westfall DP, Westfall TC. "Miscellaneous Sympathomimetic Agonists". In Brunton LL, Chabner BA, Knollmann BC. Goodman & Gilman's Pharmacological Basis of Therapeutics (12th ed.). New York, USA: McGraw-Hill. 2010:297–9.
14. Reddy KSN, Murthy OP. The Essential of Forensic Medicine and Toxicology. 32nd edn, Om Sai Graphics: Hyderabad. 2013:537–53.
15. Karmarkar RN. Forensic Medicine and Toxicology: Theory, Oral and Practical. Academic Publishers: Kolkata. 5th edn, 2015:126
16. Wang ML, Lin JL, Liaw SJ, Bullard MJ. Heroin lung: report of two cases. J. Formos Med Assoc. 1994;93(2):170–2.

Food Poisoning

Definition: These are the illnesses resulting from ingestion of food containing bacterial or non-bacterial products. WHO defines food poisoning as diseases usually either infectious or toxic in nature, caused by agents that enter the body through ingestion of contaminated food.[1] However, the term is restricted for the acute gastroenteritis due to bacterial infection of food or drink leading to diarrhea (increase fluid frequency of bowel movement), dysentery (presence of blood and mucus in stool with tenesmus), vomiting and abdominal pain. Food poisoning is due to following causes:

1. Food contaminated with bacteria (bacterial food poisoning), virus (norovirus, rotavirus, hepatitis A/E), parasites (*Taenia solium/saginata, Ascaris lumbricoides* and protozoa like *Entamoeba histolytica, Giardia lamblia*).[1,2]
2. Poisonous food of vegetable origin.
3. Poisonous food of animal origin.
4. Food contaminated with chemicals.

BACTERIAL FOOD POISONING

It is commonly seen in summer season or rainy season and usually occurs in isolated/small outbreaks. The poisoning spreads by consumption of infected food. It is of two types:[2,3]

  a. Infection type
  b. Toxin type

a. Infection type: It occurs due to ingestion of viable microorganism that multiplies in the gastrointestinal tract producing gastroenteritis. It is mainly due to Salmonella group of organism and *E. coli*[1,2] (Table 22.1).

Treatment

1. Fluid replacement therapy
2. Antibiotics

b. Toxin type: In this type, toxin is either produced/present in the contaminated food (exotoxin) or produce after ingestion of contaminated food (enterotoxin) (Table 22.2).

1. Exotoxin Variety (Botulism)

It results from consumption of preformed botulinum toxin (exotoxin) in the preserved food due to infection by *Cl. botulinum*. The toxins bind to the presynaptic nerve terminal at the neuromuscular junction and cholinergic autonomic sites. This prevents the release of acetylcholine and blocks neurotransmission.[2]

2. Enterotoxin Variety

In this food poisoning, the toxins are produced after consumption of the contaminated canned or tinned foods by bacteria. It is due to contamination with Staphylococcus, *Bacillus cereus, Clostridium perfringens*, Shigella and cholera. It acts by producing enterotoxin after consumption of food.

Treatment of bacterial food poisoning:[3,4]

1. Replacement of fluids and electrolyte losses. ORT followed by IV rehydration.
2. Antibiotics.

Table 22.1: Infection type of bacterial food poisoning

Infection type	Source	Incubation period	Clinical features	Diagnosis
Salmonella infection	Beef, poultry products, eggs, dairy products	12 to 48 hours	Main feature is watery diarrhea (foul smelling mixed with blood or mucus), fever and muscle weakness	Widal test, stool culture, isolation of bacteria in suspected food
Escherichia coli (normal flora of intestinal tract of human)	Contaminated food like salad, cheese, meat, water, raw vegetables, apple juice, etc.	1–3 days	(Copious outpouring of fluids from gastrointestinal tract) severe vomiting and diarrhea resulting in dehydration, abdominal cramps, fever and bloody diarrhea	Stool culture, clinical features
Campylobacter jejuni	Water, milk and meat	2–10 days	Watery or bloody diarrhea along with fever, abdominal pain and headache	Stool/blood culture with special media at 43°C, dark field microscopy

Table 22.2: Toxin type of bacterial food poisoning

Toxin type	Source	Incubation period	Clinical features	Diagnosis
Cl. botulinum	Under processed sausages, potted meat, tinned fish, canned vegetables and fruits, etc.	A few hrs to 36 hours	Initial signs and symptoms include blurred vision, mydriasis, ptosis, dysphagia, and dysarthria, dysphonia, and muscle weakness. After 24–48 hours, neuromuscular manifestations progress to symmetric descending paralysis and respiratory failure	• Stool culture, isolation of bacteria in suspected food • Tensilon test—to differentiate it from myasthenia gravis (*see* Table 3.1)
Staphylococcus	Contaminated meat, milk, dairy products, potato, eggs, salad, etc.	2–12 hours	SEB produces nonspecific systemic illness that is characterized by fever, chills, headache, nausea, vomiting, dyspnea, chest pain, myalgia, and a nonproductive cough	Stool culture
Bacillus cereus	Consumption of fried rice, dried fruits, powdered milk, etc. produce toxicity	HL: 8–16 hours HS: 3–6 hours	Two types of toxins: 1. One is heat labile (HL) large molecular protein which produces diarrhea as the main symptom 2. Other toxin is heat stable (HS), low molecular weight peptide which produces severe vomiting	Stool culture, culture of contaminated food
Clostridium perfringens	Consumption of contaminated food particularly canned food, meat, etc.	8–16 hours	Poisoning is characterized by sudden onset of profuse diarrhea and occasionally vomiting	Stool culture
Shigella	Potato, raw milk, eggs, vegetables, lettuce, salad, fruits, etc.	12–96 hours	Patient presents with sudden onset of diarrhea, often with blood and pus in stool, cramps, tenesmus, and lethargy	Stool culture
Cholera	Contaminated water	12–72 hours	The syndrome is characterized by sudden onset of nausea and vomiting and profuse diarrhea with classic rice water stools	• Hanging drop preparation of stool-motile bacteria • Stool culture

3. Supportive care is the mainstay of treatment—clearing of airways, ventilation.
4. Botulinum antitoxin:[3] 10 ml vial by slow IV in 1:10 dilution in normal saline.
5. Guanidine: 15–40 mg/kg/day orally.[3]

FOOD POISONING FROM VEGETABLE ORIGIN

It occurs due to direct toxin effect of the plant or due to the decomposition/contamination. Food poisoning from vegetable origin occurs due to:[5, 6]

a. *Lathyrus sativus*	Due to neurotoxin BOAA present in seeds (kesari dal)
b. Food substance	
Argemone oil	It is mixed with mustard oil
Badly stored groundnut seeds	Contaminated with *Aspergillus flavus* produce aflatoxin causing hepatic damage
Badly stored wheat, rye, oat, barley, etc.	Allows growth of fungus *Claviceps purpurae* leads to ergot poisoning
Potato	Produces solanin (green color)
Cotton seeds	It has gossypol which makes lysine unavailable to the body
Cabbage	It has sulfur containing compound which inhibits thyroxine secretion
Soybean	It has trypsin inhibitor which makes protein unavailable to the body
Poisonous berries	*Atropa belladonna*
c. Food allergy	Particularly with tomato, bean (gavar), milk
d. Mushroom	*Amanita muscaria/phalloides*

Lathyrus sativus

Common name: Kesari, lakhori/tiwra daal.

The seed of this plant is a staple food for low income groups in some areas of central India. The plant is not poisonous and the leaves are used as green vegetables. They have 4–6 cm long beans containing seeds similar to tur daal (Figs 22.1 and 22.2). The toxic principle is present in the seeds. However, the seeds are used in making different food preparations.

Toxic principle: It contains a neurotoxin known as BOAA (beta oxalyl amino alanine)

as a free amino acid in seeds cotyledon which has an affinity for pyramidal systems. Consumption of *Lathyrus sativus* seeds in quantities more than 30% of the total diet for more than 6 months have been known to cause **paralysis (neurolathyrism)**.

Clinical features: The onset of symptoms due to the BOAA is acute, subacute or gradual.

- There is an agonizing pain in calf muscles with paralysis of limbs.
- While working in the field, there may be weakness in the leg with difficulty in sitting.
- Soon the patient becomes unable to walk without help of a stick; the legs tremble and drag along with difficulty.
- Later, the patient has spastic gait characterized by a walk on tiptoes with scissor-like crossing of legs.
- This is followed by paraplegia but there is no atrophy/degeneration or loss of tone of muscle.

Treatment

1. No specific treatment.
2. Exclude pulses from diet.
3. Physiotherapy for muscular and neurological involvement[3]

Argemone mexicana

Common name: Sial Kanta (Bengal), Pila Datura/Bharam Dandi (Maharashtra) and Darvdi (Gujarat), Mexican poppy.[4]

Mustard oil is widely used for cooking purpose in certain parts of India which is more often adulterated with oil of *Argemone mexicana*. This plant grows all over the India.

All parts of the plant are poisonous but maximum concentration is in the seeds. It has sessile, spiny, thistle-like leaves. The flowers are yellow with prickly oblong/elliptic capsular fruit of size 2–4 cm long containing seeds (Fig. 22.3). The seeds are dark brown in color and granular in shape but smaller in size than mustard seeds (Figs 22.4 and 22.5).

Active principle: It contains alkaloids—*berberine and protopine* and sanguinarine and dihydro-sanguinarine in seeds. The oil of Argemone seeds causes **epidemic dropsy**.

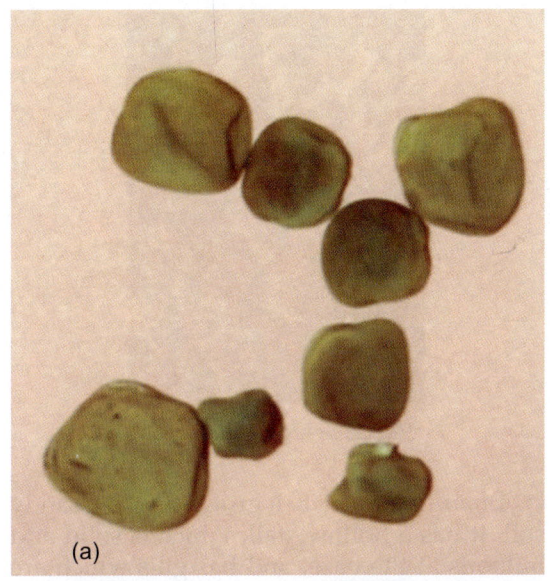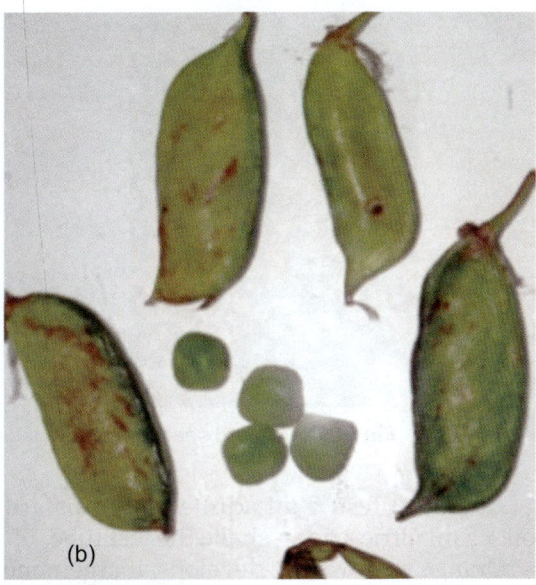

Fig. 22.1a and b: Beans and seeds of *Lathyrus sativus*

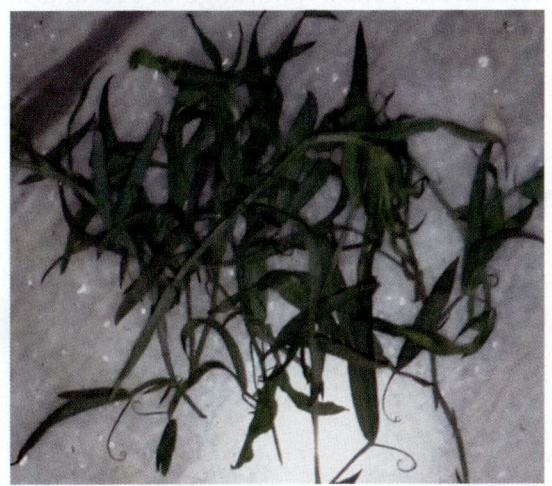
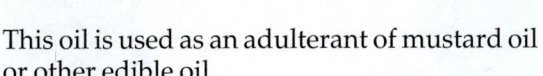

Fig. 22.2: *Lathyrus sativus*

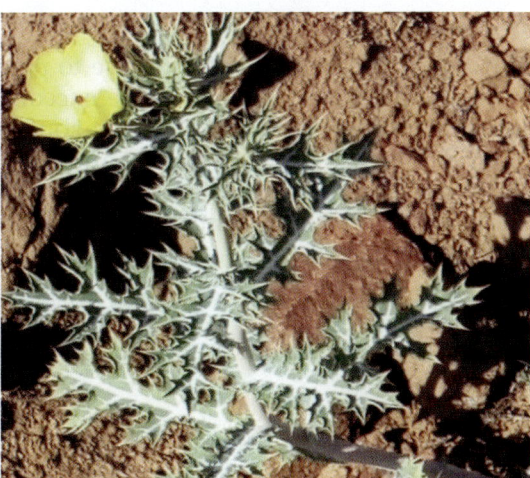

Fig. 22.3: *Argemone mexicana*

This oil is used as an adulterant of mustard oil or other edible oil.

Clinical Features

- The symptoms appear slowly with loss of appetite, nausea, dyspepsia, diarrhea.
- There is also edema of legs or even generalized anasarca.
- There is enlargement of liver with breathlessness on slight exertion.

- It also causes glaucoma with dimness of vision and raised intraocular tension.[3]

Treatment

1. Supportive treatment
2. Diuretics
3. Prednisolone
4. Good nutritious diet, vitamins B_1 and B_{12} and mineral in adequate dose will help in early recovery.
5. Avoid consumption of contaminated oil.

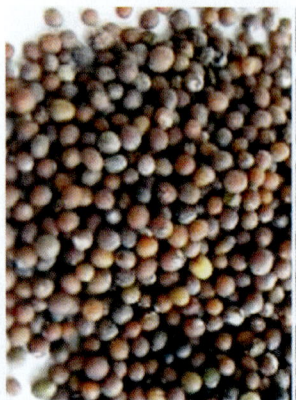

Fig. 22.4: Mustard seeds

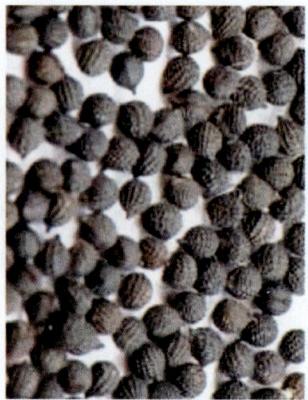

Fig. 22.5: Argemone seeds

Chemical test: 5 ml adulterated mustard oil + 5 ml nitric acid → shake the test tube.

Orange yellow color develops, if argemone is present.

FOOD ALLERGY

It occurs in people who are sensitive to particular food product (usually proteinaceous substance of vegetable and animal source like fish, prawn, egg, milk, etc.) and may show allergic manifestations like rashes, vomiting, diarrhea, asthmatic attack, and circulatory collapse.

Treatment

1. Anti-allergic/anti-histaminic.
2. Symptomatic.
3. Avoid food responsible for allergy.

POISONOUS MUSHROOMS

These are actually the **reproductive portion of the fungus** which grows from an underground mycelium or hyphae constituting the vegetative portion of the fungus. *Some species of the mushrooms are non-poisonous and are used as food. Amanita phalloides/muscaria* are the common varieties of poisonous fungi.

Poisonous mushrooms usually have a bitter, astringent, acid or salt taste. On cut section, brown/green/blue color may be seen on exposure of cut surface. However, it is very difficult to differentiate poisonous mushrooms.

Amanita muscaria: It grows singly in sandy soil. It has a hollow stalk which is solid and bulbous at the base, and has gills which are white. The pileous (top flower-like) varies in color from yellow to orange or red and is covered by warty scales (Fig. 22.6). It contains toxic alkaloids—muscarine, the action of which resembles stimulation of parasympathetic postganglionic nerves.

Amanita phalloides: It is white in color and grows in woody places to a height of 15–20 cm. It has a hollow stalk with a permanent

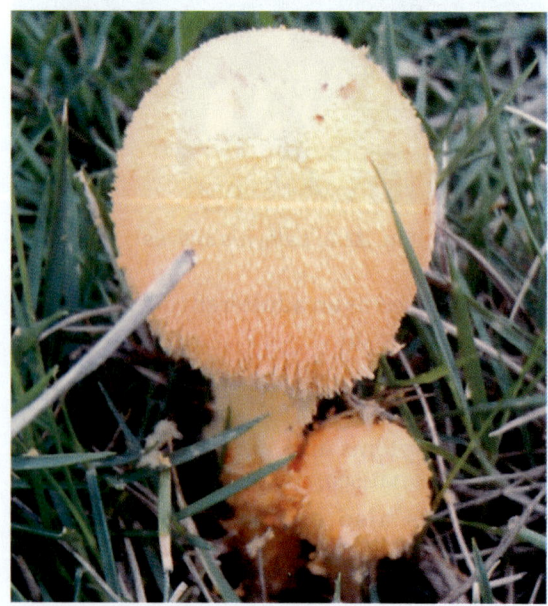

Fig. 22.6: Mushroom: *Amanita muscaria*

Table 22.3: Different species of mushrooms[4]

Species of mushrooms	Common name	Toxin
Amanita muscaria	Fly Agaric	Amatoxin, phallotoxin, virotoxin
Amanita phalloides	Death Cap	Amatoxin, phallotoxin, virotoxin
Amanita pantherina	Panther Cap, False Blusher	Amatoxin, phallotoxin, virotoxin
Amanita virosa	Destroying Angel	Amatoxin, phallotoxin, virotoxin
Clitocybe dealbata	Sweater	Muscarine
Coprinus atramentarius	Inky Cap	Coprine
Galerina autumnalis	Deadly Galerina	Gyrometrin
Gyrometra esculenta	False Morel	Gyrometrin
Psilocybe caerulipes	Blue Foot	Psilocybin, psilocin
Psilocybe semilenceta	Liberty cap, magic mushroom	Psilocybin, psilocin
Lycoperdon	Puffball mushrooms	Amatoxin

bulb at the base. The pileus is usually white, pale yellow or olive; and has gills covered with white spores on its undersurface (Fig. 22.7). It contains polypeptides which are powerful inhibitors of cellular protein synthesis.

Mushroom poisoning: It is usually accidental. It is of three types depending on the toxic principle present in the particular species.[7]

a. Muscarine type (early mushroom poisoning) due to Inocybe and related species. Symptoms characteristic of muscarinic action appear within an hour of eating mushroom. The poisoning is promptly reversed by atropine.

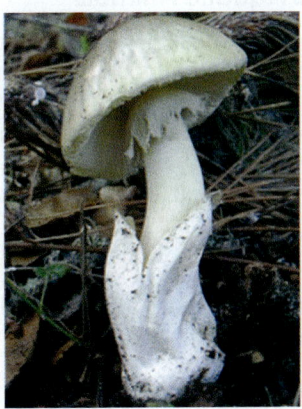

Fig. 22.7: *Amanita phalloides*

b. Hallucinogenic type due to muscimol present in *Amanita muscaria* and related species. It activates amino acid receptors in brain and has hallucinogenic properties. There is no specific treatment and atropine is contraindicated. Another hallucinogenic mushroom is *Psilocybe mexicana*.

c. Phalloidin type (late mushroom poisoning) due to peptide toxin found in *Amanita phalloides* and related species. It inhibits RNA and protein synthesis.

Clinical Features

- The features are due to damage to the GIT mucosa, liver and kidney with neurotic action.[7]
- There is a constriction of the throat, burning pain in stomach with nausea, vomiting, diarrhea followed by cyanosis, slow pulse, laboured respirations, convulsions, sweating, collapsed and death.
- The neurotic manifestations are headache, dizziness, giddiness, delirium, diplopia, constriction of pupils, cramps, twitching of muscle, convulsion, salivation, bradycardia and coma.

Treatment of poisoning with mushrooms:[6]

1. Gastric lavage with $KMnO_4$

2. Activated charcoal

Table 22.4: Types of sea fish poisoning based on the nature of toxin

Type of sea fish	Toxin	Source
Scombroid[6]	Histamine and saurine	Tuna, needle fish, king fish, blue fish
Ciguatera[6]	Ciguatera, maitotoxin, scaritoxin, okadaic toxin, polytoxin	Parrot fish, barracuda, sea bass, red snapper, grouper, king fish
Tetradotoxic[6]	Tetradotoxin	Puffer fish, newts, salamander, blue ring octopus, Ballon fish, Globe fish, toad fish, horseshoe crab eggs
Paralytic shellfish	Saxitoxin, neosaxitoxin	Shellfish like oysters, clans
Neurotoxic shellfish	Brevitoxin	Dinoflagellate, *Ptychodisus brevis*
Amnesic shellfish	Domoic acid	Diatom *Nitzschia pungens*

3. Forced diuresis/hemodialysis
4. Benzyl penicillin
5. Atropine sulfate, particularly in muscarine type.[7,8] It is contraindicated in hallucinogenic type
6. Symptomatic
7. Thiocytic acid—may have some antidotal effect, particularly in phalloidin type.[7]

FOOD POISONING FROM ANIMAL ORIGIN

It is due to the following reasons

a. Decomposed flesh—forms ptomaine which produce manifestation like that of atropine.

b. Venomous fish.

c. Poisonous aquatic animal.

d. Food allergy to fish, prawn, etc.

Ptomaine Poisoning from Decomposed Flesh

Ptomaine is produced by the action of saprophytic microorganism upon nitrogenous material during the decomposition. They also known as **cadaveric alkaloid** when found in dead tissues. And alkaloids secreted during metabolism by **living cells** are called **leucomaines.**

Ptomaine resembles vegetable alkaloids like morphine, codeine, veratrine; mostly non-poisonous except neurine and mydaleine, which are actively poisonous and **produce symptoms resembling those of poisoning by atropine, muscarine and aconite.** But,

by the time ptomaine is formed, the food becomes so unpalatable that it is not likely to be eaten.

Poisonous Fish

Poisoning resulting from fish and other marine creature is known as **ichthyism.** Poisonous fish is divided into three subgroups:

a. Ichthyo-sarcotoxic fish: Contains toxin within its flesh

b. Ichthyo-hemotoxic fish: Contains poisonous blood

c. Ichthyo-otoxic fish: Contains toxin mainly in gonads

Based on nature of toxin, there are six types of sea fish poisoning (Table 22.4).

Poisonous Aquatic Animals[5]

1. California mussel (which eats planktons having deadly toxins): It may cause sensory and motor disturbances like tingling, numbness, muscular weakness and paralysis.

2. Some shells, shrimps and crabs: It may cause chronic arsenic poisoning.

3. Puffer fish: It causes vomiting, retching, lethargy, muscular weakness, fall of BP and respiratory distress.

Treatment

Symptomatic

POISONING FROM INGESTION OF CONTAMINATED FOOD WITH CHEMICALS

a. Contaminated with chemicals, intentionally added flavouring agents to processed food (like MSG), mixing of preservatives or coloring agents to the food, use of hydrocarbon to extract fat from the food.

Monosodium Glutamate (MSG):[4,5,8] It is one of the flavoring agents in foods, especially Chinese food, sausages, canned food, etc. It is fine, white crystalline substance similar to salt and has sweetish saline taste. In large quantities, it causes burning sensation and numbness of face/trunk/ upper limb with flushing, chest pain, headache, nausea, bronchospasm and generalised edema. The symptoms resolve within an hour on their own.

b. Accidentally added or contaminated with pesticides/insecticides or heavy metals.

c. Persistent organic pollutants (POPs):[1] Dioxins and polychlorinated biphenyls are the unwanted by-products of industrial processes and waste incineration that may accumulate in the environment and human body and animal food.

d. Produced as a result of food processing, e.g. smoking of fleshy food.

e. Radio nuclides—polonium—210 (one of the 25 radioactive isotopes of polonium with half-life of 138 days) is the deadly poison that was used to kill the former Russian spy, Alexander Litvinenko, in 2006 in London.[10] He died of acute radiation sickness (ARS).[10] It is administered to victim through food or drink. When swallowed, it becomes concentrated in red blood cells before spreading to liver, kidneys, bone marrow, GIT and the testicles/ovaries.[11] Its radiation causes damage to DNA and lead to cell death and cancer.

Clinical features of polonium poisoning:[11,12] This is characterized by a prodromal phase, in which nausea, vomiting, anorexia, lymphopenia, and sometimes diarrhea develop after exposure. The prodromal phase may be followed by a latent phase during which there is some clinical improvement. Subsequently, bone marrow or cardiovascular/CNS syndromes develop. The triad of early emesis followed by hair loss and bone marrow failure is typical of ARS. The diagnosis of (210) Po poisoning is established by the presence of (210) Po in urine and feces and the exclusion of other possible causes.

Treatment polonium poisoning:[12]

• Good supportive care, gastric lavage
• Prevention of infection
• Blood/platelet transfusion
• Chelation—BAL/penicillamine

Medicolegal importance: Used for homicidal purpose given with food and drinks.

IMPORTANT QUESTIONS

1. **Define food poisoning and enumerate its causes. Describe types, source, clinical features, diagnosis and treatment of bacterial food poisoning.**

2. **Enumerate examples of food poisoning of vegetable source. Describe toxic principle, clinical features and treatment of poisoning with *Lathyrus sativus* or *Argemone mexicana*.**

3. **Describe mushroom poisoning.**

4. **Write brief about poisoning from ingestion of contaminated food with chemicals.**

SPECIFIC LEARNING OBJECTIVES

After reading this chapter, the reader should be able to:

• **Define food poisoning**
• **Enumerate causes of food poisoning**
• **Enlist different types and source of bacterial food poisoning**
• **Explain clinical features and management of bacterial food poisoning**
• **Enumerate examples of food poisoning from vegetable source**
• **Identify active principle of *Lathyrus sativus/ Argemone mexicana***

- **Explain clinical features and treatment of poisoning due to *Lathyrus sativus/Argemone mexicana***
- **Enumerate types of poisonous mushrooms and explain clinical features and treatment of mushroom poisoning**
- **Enumerate different causes of poisoning from ingestion of contaminated food with chemicals and explain monosodium glutamate and polonium**

References

1. WHO. Food safety and foodborne illness. Fact Sheet.WHO, 2007. Available at www.who.int/mediacentre/factsheets/fs237/en/Assessed on 18 Aug 2019.
2. Kapil A (ed). Diarrhea and Food poisoning. In: Ananthanarayan and Paniker's Textbook of Microbiology. 9th edn. Universities Press India Private Limited: Hyderabad. 2016:676–8.
3. Dikshit PC. Textbook of Forensic Medicine and Toxicology. 2nd edn, PEEPEE Publisher and Distributors (P) Ltd. New Delhi. 2014:601–8.
4. Pillay VV. Textbook of Forensic Medicine and Toxicology. 17th edn, Paras Medical Publisher: Hyderabad. 2016:662–74.
5. Nandy A. Principles of Forensic Medicine. 2nd edn, Reprint. New Central Book Agency (P) Ltd: Calcutta. 2004:563–4.
6. Reddy KSN, Murthy OP. The Essential of Forensic Medicine and Toxicology. 32nd edn, Om Sai Graphics: Hyderabad. 2013:603–8.
7. Tripathi KD. Cholinergic system and drugs. In: Essential of Medical Pharmacology. 7th edn, Jaypee Brothers Medical Publishers (P) Ltd: New Delhi. 2014:99–112.
8. Sharma HL, Sharma KK. Drugs affecting parasympathetic nervous system. In: Sharma and Sharma's Principles of Pharmacology. 3rd edn, Paras Medical Publisher: Hyderabad. 2017: 132–58.
9. Monosodium glutamate (MSG): Is it harmful?-Mayo Clinic. Available on: https://www.mayoclinic.org›monosodium-glutamate›faq-20058196. Assessed on 1/09/2019.
10. Markus MacGill. Polonium-210: Why is Po-210 so dangerous? Newsletter: Medical News Today. https://www.medicalnewstoday.com/articles/58088.php. Assessed on 8/Jun/2019.
11. Jefferson RD, Goans RE, Blain PG, Thomas SH. Diagnosis and treatment of polonium poisoning. Clin Toxicol (phila). 2009; 47: 379–92. doi: 10.1080/15563650902956431.
12. Harrison J, Leggett R, Lloyd D, Phipps A, Scott B. Polonium-210 as a poison. J Radiol Prot. 2007 Mar;27(1):17–40.

War Gases:
Chemical and Biological

The term 'War gases' includes **any chemical** (gaseous, liquid or solid) **or biological agents** which is used to cause destruction or damage mostly in times of war but does not include explosives. Deliberate use of such harmful agents results in a huge loss of human lives as well as an adverse impact on the social and economic status of the country.[1] **Warfare agents are the agents used to kill, injure or incapacitate the enemies mostly during war**. However, in civil conditions, these gases are used to disperse the unruly mob. When chemical substance is used, it is called 'chemical warfare', and when biological agent is used, it is called 'biological warfare'.

Chemical warfare: It is the warfare in which there is offensive use of chemical substance having toxic properties to kill, injure or incapacitate the enemies. A chemical used in this warfare is called **chemical weapon agent (CWA)**. About 70 different chemicals have been used or stock piled as CWA during 20th century (in liquid, gas or solid form), which are classified as weapon of mass destruction by the United Nations, and their production and storage was outlawed by the chemical weapon convention of 1993.[2] Some substances are lethal, and some injure or incapacitate people. These agents are dispersed as tiny droplets through chemical shells, spray tanks, bombs and missiles. Harmful effects are caused when the chemical is inhaled, ingested or when it comes in contact with skin or mucous membrane.

There are other chemicals used in military operations that are **not technically considered to be CWA** such as:[3]

1. **Defoliants:** That destroy vegetations. For example, agent orange contained dioxin is known for its long-term cancer effects and for causing genetic damage leading to birth deformities.

2. **Incendiary/explosive chemicals:** Their destructive effects are primarily due to fire or explosive force and not direct chemical action, e.g. Napalm and dynamite

3. **Biological warfare agents:** It includes virus, bacteria, etc.

Classification of warfare agents: According to their primary physiological action

1. Lacrimators: Tear gases
2. Lung irritants: Asphixiant gases
3. Vesicants: Blistering gases
4. Sternutators: Nasal irritant
5. Paralysant: Nerve poison
6. Nerve gases: Acetylcholine like action

Biological warfare: It is the offensive use of living microorganisms to kill, injure or incapacitate the enemies. **Biological weapons (BW)** are defined as microorganisms or their products of metabolism that infect and grow in the target host producing a clinical disease that kills or incapacitates humans or animals. Such microbes may be natural, wild-type strains or may be genetically modified. These include biological toxins and substances that interfere with normal behavior, such as hormones, neuropeptides and cytokines (Table 23.1).

Table 23.1: Clinical manifestation of different warfare agents

Type	Examples	Signs and symptoms	Treatment
1. **Lachrymators or tear gases** (These are the tear gases and cause tearing of eyes)	Chloracetophenone (CAP) Bromobenzyl cyanide (BBC) Ethyliodoacetate (KSK) They are fired in artillery shells or pen guns	The vapors cause intense irritation of the eyes with a copious flow of tears, spasm of the eyelids and temporary blindness. They also cause irritation of air-passages. In long-continued exposure there may be nausea, vomiting and blistering of skin. The effects are transitory	1. Removed the patient to the fresh air 2. Eyes washed with warm normal saline or fresh water or boric acid soda bicarb to the affected skin 3. Application of weak solution of soda bicarb to the affected skin 4. IV aminophylline or salbutamol inhalation
2. **Lung irritants or asphyxiants** (These are the asphyxiants and cause choking of respiratory track)	Chlorine and phosgene chloropicrin and diphosgene. Nitrous oxide, sulfur dioxide, ammonia (choking gases). They can be released from tanks, and gas shells. Phosgene is ten times and chloropicrin four times more toxic than chlorine	The signs and symptoms develop within 2–4 hours of inhalation. Lacrimation, conjunctivitis, coughing, dyspnea with intense air hunger with feeling of pain and tightness of chest. There is headache, vomiting, restlessness, stertorous breathing, cyanosis and collapse Death occurs in 24 to 48 hours due to acute pulmonary edema	1. Eye wash with boric acid 2. Oxygen and adrenaline 3. Antitussives 4. Antibiotics 5. Atropine for pulmonary edema
3. **Vesicant or blistering gases** (These are the agents that cause blisters)	Mustard gas, lewisite (arsenic) sulfur, phosgene, oximes. They are discharged in artillery shells so as to saturate the area of attack	**Mustard gas** (yellow cross)[3] causes irritation of the eyes, nose, throat and respiratory passages. There is lacrimation, conjunctivitis, photophobia with nausea, vomiting and abdominal pain. There is intense itching, redness, vesication, and ulceration especially of the moist areas as it passes through the clothes into the skin. **Lewisite** causes rapid blister with inflammation of mucosa of larynx, trachea and bronchi. It also causes hemolysis, leucopenia and features similar to arsenic poisoning	1. Shift the patient to fresh air 2. Remove all clothing and wash the body with soap and water 3. Irrigation of eyes/nose with cold water/ sodium bicarbonate solution[3] 4. Wash the affected part with soda bicarb solution 5. BAL—in lewisite poisoning[3]

(Contd...)

Table 23.1: Clinical manifestation of different warfare agents (Contd...)

Type	Examples	Signs and symptoms	Treatment
4. Sternutators or nasal irritants (These are the agents that are nasal irritant)	Diphenylchlorarsine (DA), Diphenylaminechlorarsine (DM), and diphenylcyanarsine (DC). DM (sickening gas) is about six times as heavy as air. These are solid, organic compounds of arsenic and are fired in artillery shells	The manifestation is due to inhalation or drinking of contaminated water. The vapors cause intense pain and irritation in the nose and sinuses. There is sneezing, headache, salivation, nausea, vomiting, tightness in the chest and prostration	1. Shift the patient to fresh air 2. Remove all clothing and wash the body with soap and water 3. Irrigation of eyes/nose with cold water/sodium bicarbonate solution
5. Paralysants	Hydrocyanic acid, hydrogen sulfide, carbon monoxide	Already described in respective chapters	Depends on the type of poisons
6. Nerve gases (These are the agents which have acetylcholine-like action. They inhibit the acetylcholinesterase)	GA (Tabun), GB (Sarin), GD (Soman) VE, VM and VX. The vapors are heavier than air, so they tend to sink into valleys, trenches and basements. They are colorless and odorless volatile liquids. They are the most toxic of the known chemical agents	They cause **inhibition of cholinesterase** and produce **features of acetylcholine poisoning** with constriction of pupil, choking, bronchial constriction and photophobia. Exposure to a large amount of vapor will cause loss of consciousness within seconds, followed by convulsions. Muscles become flaccid and breathing stops	Treatment is similar to organophosphates: 1. Decontamination 2. Irrigation of eyes/nose 3. Atropine 4. Oximes 5. Diazepam for convulsion
Chemical crowd/riot control agents[4] used by law-enforcement agencies and the military	Ortho-chlorobenzylidenemalanonitrile (CS, tear gas), CN (Mace), Oleoresin capsaicin (pepper spray, OC) is an extract of hot peppers consisting of capsaicin. These agents are available in varying concentrations and several vehicles, in aerosols or fumes and in particulate form with dispersal device. They are also available in grenades or canisters that can be propelled either by throwing or with a projectile device	**Eyes:** Burning, stinging or pain, conjunctivitis, lacrimation, transient impairment of vision **Nose and mouth:** Burning, stinging or pain, increased secretions **Skin:** Burning, stinging or pain, erythema **Respiratory tract:** Burning and irritation, increase secretions, coughing, tightness in the chest	1. Remove the patient to fresh air 2. Irrigation of eyes/nose with cold water/sodium bicarbonate solution 3. Oxygen inhalation 4. Bronchodilator

Biological warfare agents: *Bacillus anthracis,* smallpox virus, botulinum toxin and ricin are commonly used biological agents followed by bacteria causing plague, cholera, typhus, brucellosis, Salmonella, ebola virus, abrin toxin, etc. Very small amounts of biological agents or toxins can cause mass casualties. The agents are odorless, tasteless and invisible to the naked eye. It is spread through aerosol spray, explosives or food or water contamination.

Precaution while handling the body: The body should be cleaned with **0.5%** hypochlorite or phenol disinfectant and transported to mortuary in an impermeable double bag. Certain bio-agents, such as smallpox, tularemia, viral hemorrhagic fever, ganders, Q fever, can be transmitted to persons performing autopsies. Collect blood, CSF and tissue samples or swabs for isolation of bacteria and virus.

IMPORTANT QUESTION

1. What are chemical and biological warfare agents? Classify warfare agents. Describe any one of them.

SPECIFIC LEARNING OBJECTIVES

After reading this chapter, the reader should be able to:

- **Define war gases, warfare agents**
- **Classify warfare agents with examples**

References

1. Thavaselvam D, Flora SS. Chemical and biological warfare agents. In: Gupta RC (ed). Biomarkers in Toxicology. Academic press. 2014:521–38.
2. Chemical weapon convection, 1993. International committee of Red Cross. Available at: https://www.icrc.org/en/doc/assets/files/other/1993_chemical_weapons.pdf
3. Dikshit PC. Textbook of Forensic Medicine and Toxicology. 2nd edn, PEEPEE Publisher and Distributors (P) Ltd. New Delhi. 2014:583–6.
4. Pillay VV. Textbook of Forensic Medicine and Toxicology. 17th edn, Paras Medical Publisher: Hyderabad. 2016:651.

Appendix

Table 1: Fatal dose, fatal period and antidote of different poisons

Poisons	Fatal dose	Fatal period	Antidotes
Inorganic strong acids	10–20 ml	12–24 hours	CaO, MgO
Oxalic acid	10–15 gm	2–12 hours	Lime, CaO, Ca carbonate
Carbolic acid	10–20 gm	2–12 hours	Magnesium sulfate
Alkalies	Hydroxides: 5–10 gm Carbonate: 15–30 gm	12–24 hours	Weak acid, vinegar, citric acid
Phosphorus	60–120 mg	12 hours to 1 week	Copper sulfate
Iodine	2 gm	24 hours	Starch solution sodium thiosulfate
Arsenic	200 mg	24 hours	Ferric oxide, BAL
Lead/Zinc	20–30 gm	24 hours	Mg/Na sulfate, calcium EDTA
Mercury	0.5–1 gm	2–3 days	Egg albumin, Na formaldehyde Sulfoxylate, penicillamine, BAL
Copper	15–30 gm	2–3 days	Pot ferrocyanide, penicillamine, BAL
Potassium iodate/ $KMnO_4$	12–15 gm	–	Calcium chloride/gluconate
Iron–$FeSO_4$ tablets	10–5 tabs	–	Desferroxamine, deferiprone
Organophosphorus	30 mg to 60 gm	30 min to 3 hours	Atropine, oximes
Organochlorine	30 mg to 5 gm	Within 24 hours	–
Carbamates	–	Uncertain	Atropine
Pyrethroids	–	Uncertain	–
Alum/zinc phosphide	3–5 gm	12–24 hours	–
Abrus precatorius	1–2 seeds	12 hours to 3 days	Anti-abrin
Castor/croton/ semicarpus	6–8 seeds	12 hours to 3 days	–
Poisonous snakes	6–12 mg	Cobra: 20 min Viper: 2–4 days	ASV serum
Opium/morphine	2 gm/100–200 mg	6–12 hours	Naloxone/nalmefene
Ethyl alcohol	150 ml in non-addict	12–24 hours	–
Methyl alcohol	60–120 ml	24–36 hours	Ethyl alcohol, fomepizole
Formaldehyde	30–90 ml	12–24 hours	Sodium bicarbonate
Fuels—kerosene	30 ml	A few hours	Liquid paraffin
Datura/atropine	75–100 seeds; 60 mg	24 hours	Physostigmine/pilocarpine
Cannabis	2–10 gm/kg body wt	12 hours	–
Cocaine	1 gm	2 hours	Amyl nitrite inhalation
Barbiturates	4–5 gm	1–2 days	–
Benzodiazepines	5–10 gm/variable	1–2 days	Flumazenil
Nux vomica/strychnine	1–2 seeds/30–60 mg	30 min to 2 hours	Lorazepam/diazepam
Conium	1 cm of any part	A few hours	–
Curare	30–60 mg	1–2 hours	Neostigmine/physostigmine
Hydrocyanic acid/salts	200 ppm/200 mg	Immediate/30 min	Nitrites followed by Na thiosulfate
Aconite	1 gm root	6 hours	–
Oleander	15 gm root	24–36 hours	–
Paracetamol	10 gm	–	N-acetyl cysteine, methionine
Carbon monoxide	2000 ppm	Min to hours	Oxygen
Nitrobenzene—shoe polish	–	–	Methylene blue

Table 2: Characteristic smell of poison

Typical smell	Poison
Garlicky	Arsenic hydride (Arsine), OP, phosphorus, zinc phosphide, selenium, thallium
Phenolic/sweetish	Carbolic acid
Vinegar	Acetic acid
Fruity, acetone, apple-like	Alcohol
Kerosene/petrol	Petroleum products
Bitter almond	Cyanides
Burnt rope-like	Cannabis
Raw flesh	Opium
Kerosene/turpentine	Insecticidal poisons
Burnt coal gas	Carbon monoxide
Rotten egg	Hydrogen sulfide
Shoe polish	Nitrobenzene
Tobacco	Nicotine
Iodine	Iodine
Mothball	Naphthalene
Formalin	Formaldehyde
Fishy/musty	Aluminium phosphide

Table 3: Characteristic taste of poison

Typical taste	Poison
Sweet	Aconite, carbolic
Bitter	Datura, strychnine
Sour	Acids
Metallic	Metallic irritant

Table 4: Poison acting on enzyme system

1. Metallic irritants
2. Phosphorus
3. Organophosphorus
4. Carbamates
5. Cyanides

Table 5: Poison imparting different colors

1. Urine

Green	Phenol
Red	Lead (coproporphyrin-3), cantharides, phenolphthalein
Orange	Rifampicin, phenothiazines
Blue/greenish blue	Methylene blue
Brown to black	Naphthalene, thymol
Pink	Aniline, eosin, mercury
Yellow	Arsine, dinitrophenol
Liquid gold	Barbiturates

2. Vomitus

Green	$CuSO_4$, copper arsenite, copper acetoarsenite
Blue	Iodine
Brown	Acid, alkali, zinc phosphide
Red	Lead tetraoxide/monoxide, mercury sulfide
Curdy white	Lead
Dark, luminous	Phosphorus

3. Stool

Dark, luminous	Phosphorus
Black	Lead
Colorless, watery	Arsenic

4. Tears

Red	OP (due to porphyrin)

Table 6: Skin manifestation in poisons

Dry skin	Datura
Moist skin/sweating	OP, opium, arsenic, pilocarpine
Flushing	Alcohol, Datura, arsenic, cyanide
Blister/vesicles	Barbiturates, viper bite, CO, semicarpus juice, calotropis, plumbago, croton oil, iodine, arsenic, mustard gas, lewisite gas
Petechiae, purpura, hemorrhagic lesion	Arsenic, phosphorus
Pigmentation	Arsenic
Hair loss	Arsenic, thallium
Hypothermia	Opiates, alcohol, barbiturates, CO
Hyperthermia	Datura, cocaine, strychnine

Table 7: Poison causing eye changes

1. Constriction of pupil	Opium/morphine, OP, carbamate, carbolic, mushroom, cannabis
2. Dilatation of pupil	Datura/atropine, OC, cyanides, cocaine, CO, curare, conium
3. Alternate const/dilatation	Aconite, barbiturate
4. Nystagmus	Alcohol, barbiturate
5. Diplopia	Opium, cannabis, alcohol
6. Lacrimation	Irritant gases, OP, carbamates, pyrethroids
7. Ptosis	Snakebite—cobra, botulism
8. Blindness	Methyl alcohol, chloroquine, arsenic, lead, mercury, tobacco, ergot
9. Photophobia	Irritant gas, iodine, nitric acid fumes

Table 8: Poison causing oral changes

1. Dryness of mouth	Datura, lead, cocaine, opium
2. Excess of salivation	Corrosives, OP, carbamates, pyrethroids, vegetable irritants, aconite, scorpion bite, strychnine
3. Stomatitis/glossitis	Cyanide, calotropis, iodine
4. Discoloration of gums/teeth	Blue-copper, mercury, lead, iron, thallium, silver; fluoride, tetracycline

Table 9: Poison causing GIT manifestation

1. Vomiting	Almost all poisons, copper sulfate is potent emetic
2. Diarrhea	Organic acids, alkalies, arsenic, food poisoning
3. Constipation	Inorganic acids, lead, opium, thallium
4. Gastroenteritis	Almost all local poisons; arsenic, oleander, phosphorus
5. Abdominal pain	Corrosives, irritant, cocaine, iron, oleander, formaldehyde, kerosene
6. Thirst	Corrosives, arsenic, lead, phosphorus, atropine
7. Dysphagia/odynophagia	Corrosives, metallic poison
8. Froth at mouth/nostrils	OP, OC, cyanide, barbiturates, strychnine, opium, CO, $CuSO_4$

Table 10: Poison causing genitourinary system manifestation

1. Oliguria	Corrosives, arsenic, lead, mercury, copper, phosphorus
2. Polyuria	Alcohol, digitalis, mercury
3. Dysuria	Mushrooms, OP, arsenic
4. Hematuria	Organic corrosives, arsenic, mercury, lead, copper, phosphorus
5. Albuminuria	Organic corrosives, arsenic, mercury, lead, copper, phosphorus
6. Hemoglobinuria	Snakebite, acetic acid, arsenic, copper
7. Glycosuria	Morphine, anesthetic agents
8. Porphyrinuria	Lead, mercury

Table 11: Poison causing CVS manifestation

1. Bradycardia	OP, aconite, digitalis
2. Tachycardia	Datura, conium, cannabis, CO, amphetamine
3. Hypotension	OP, aconite, snakebite, arsenic, alcohols
4. Hypertension	Amphetamine, zinc phosphide
5. Arrhythmias	Cyanide, digoxin, quinidine

Table 12: Poison causing RS manifestation

1. Dyspnea	CO, phosphine, irrespirable gases, strychnine, arsine, opium, alcohols
2. Pulmonary edema	OP, OC, snakebite, opium

Table 13: Poison causing CNS manifestation

1. Ataxia	Bromides, carbamazepine, alcohol, sedatives/hypnotic, thallium
2. Coma	Alcohol, CO, opium, organophosphorus
3. Convulsion	Strychnine, cyanides, phosphorus, arsenic, lead, copper, opium, datura, cobra bite, alcohol, OP, aconite, CO
4. Paralysis	Arsenic, lead, curare, conium
5. Paresthesia	Arsenic, lead, conium, alcohol, aconite, cannabis
6. Delirium	Datura, cannabis, cocaine, calotropis
7. Psychosis	Datura, cannabis, cocaine, alcohol

Table 14: Poison causing blood manifestation

1. Anemia	Arsenic, lead, copper
2. Leukocytosis	Snake poisoning
3. Leukopenia	Arsenic, lead, antimony
4. Hemolysis	Sea snakes, viper bite, copper sulfate, lead, arsenic
5. Methemoglobin	Nitrobenzene, methylene blue, copper
6. Basophilic stippling	Lead, antimony, bismuth

Table 15: Poison causing different color of postmortem lividity

Color of lividity	Poisons
Deep blue color	Asphyxiant/aniline
Cherry red	CO poisoning
Pink	Cyanide
Brown	Phosphorus
Black	Opium
Green	Hydrogen sulphide

Table 16: Colour of stomach mucosa in different poisoning

Whitish, bleached	Alkalies
Yellow	Nitric acid
Bluish green	Copper sulphate
Green	Ferrous sulphate
Black	Sulphuric acid
Grey/slate colour	Mercury chloride
Red velvety	Arsenic
Discolour/staining	Coloured salts of arsenic, lead, copper

Table 17: Condition of stomach wall in different poisoning

Thickened and soft	Corrosive, irritant
Hard wall	Formaldehyde
Hard and leather like	Carbolic acid
Red velvety	Arsenic

OP	: Organophosphorus	OC	: Organochlorines
CO	: Carbon monoxide	GIT	: Gastrointestinal tract
CVS	: Cardiovascular system	RS	: Respiratory system
CNS	: Central nervous system		

Multiple Choice Questions

1. **Who is called the Father of Toxicology?**
   - a. Francis Galton
   - b. Edmond Locard
   - c. Imhotep
   - d. Paracelsus

2. **Who is called the Father of Modern Forensic Toxicology?**
   - a. James Marsh
   - b. Carl Scheele
   - c. Mathieu Orfila
   - d. Hans Gross

3. **Characteristic features of both ideal homicidal and ideal suicidal poison include all *except*:**
   - a. Easily available
   - b. Highly toxic
   - c. Completely metabolised
   - d. Easily mixed with food

4. **Usually the concentrated form of poisonous substance is more rapidly absorbed *except*:**
   - a. Oxalic acid
   - b. Acetic acid
   - c. Carbolic acid
   - d. Hydrochloric acid

5. **Demulcent and fatty foods should be avoided in:**
   - a. Phosphorus
   - b. Organochlorine
   - c. Pyrethroids/pyrethrins
   - d. All of these

6. **It can be used for induction of vomiting (emesis) in weak solution:**
   - a. Arsenic oxide
   - b. Mercuric chloride
   - c. Lead tetraoxide
   - d. Copper sulfate

7. **All are contraindicated for both gastric lavage and emesis *except*:**
   - a. Coma
   - b. Convulsion
   - c. Corrosives
   - d. Pregnancy/esophageal varices

8. **In gastric lavage, the first washing is done with:**
   - a. Fresh lukewarm water
   - b. $KMnO_4$ solution
   - c. Activated charcoal
   - d. Antidote of poison

9. **Gastric lavage can be done in injected poisoning with:**
   - a. Curare
   - b. Morphine
   - c. Cocaine
   - d. None of these

10. **All of the following are the chelating agents *except*:**
    - a. Dimercaprol
    - b. EDTA
    - c. Cuprimine
    - d. Desferrioxide

11. **Constriction of pupil is not seen in:**
    - a. Morphine poisoning
    - b. Phenol poisoning
    - c. OP poisoning
    - d. Cocaine poisoning

12. **Rectified spirit is used for preservation of viscera for toxicological analysis in poisoning with:**
    - a. Acetic acid
    - b. Carbolic acid
    - c. Sulfuric acid
    - d. Formalin

13. **The route of administration for BAL in arsenic poisoning is:**
    - a. ID
    - b. SC
    - c. IM
    - d. IV

14. **Universal antidote contains all *except*:**
    - a. Charcoal
    - b. Tannin
    - c. Caffeine
    - d. Magnesium oxide

15. **This drug is used for narcoanalysis:**
    a. Atropin   b. Phenobarbitone
    c. Scopalamine   d. Pethidine

16. **The colour of the tissue on contact with nitric acid turns to yellow due to:**
    a. Xanthoprotein reaction
    b. Carbonisation of organic matter
    c. Conversion of haemoglobin to acid hematin
    d. Yellowish colour of an acid

17. **Vinegar is dilute solution of:**
    a. Oxalic acid
    b. Carbolic acid
    c. Acetic acid
    d. Acid of sugar/Chinese acid

18. **It is commonly called 'caustic soda'.**
    a. Sodium hydroxide
    b. Potassium hydroxide
    c. Calcium hydroxide
    d. Ammonium hydroxide

19. **It does not act on enzyme system.**
    a. Phosphorus   b. OP
    c. Cyanides   d. Aconite

20. **Red colour urine is one of the manifestations seen in poisoning with:**
    a. Arsenic   b. Lead
    c. Mercury   d. Copper

21. **Red velvety appearance of stomach is seen in poisoning with**
    a. Arsenic   b. Lead
    c. Mercury   d. Copper

22. **Garlicky odour is present in all *except*:**
    a. Arsine
    b. Phosphorus
    c. Zinc phosphide/carbamate
    d. Aluminium phosphide

23. **Burnt rope like smell is suggestive of:**
    a. CO   b. CO_2
    c. Cannabis   d. Opium

24. **It is not a 'toxalbumin'.**
    a. Cerberin   b. Abrin
    c. Crotin   d. Snake venom

25. **'Hyderabadi goli' is the ....**
    a. Paste of chilli powder used to push in the rectum for torture and confession
    b. Paste of *Abrus precatorius* and Datura powder used to kill cattle and humans
    c. Sweet meat preparation of bhang
    d. Dark brown or black 'Afim'

26. **It is not a poisonous snake.**
    a. Dhaman   b. Ghonus
    c. Maniyar   d. Nag Raja

27. **The tail of viper is short/tapered and scales are ....**
    a. Not divided
    b. Divided throughout
    c. Divided distally
    d. Divided proximally

28. **This manifestation is not present in colubrine bite.**
    a. Ptosis
    b. Drooling of saliva
    c. Pupils dilated not reacting to light
    d. Staggering gait

29. **Patient with clear evidence of neurotoxicity after snakebite should receive all *except*:**
    a. Pretreat with atropine
    b. Anti-snake venom
    c. Neostigmine
    d. Dopamine

30. **Naloxone is used as an 'antidote' in intoxication with:**
    a. Cannabis   b. Datura
    c. Aconite   d. Opium

31. **In honey bee bite, the site should be washed with solution of ....**
    a. Vinegar
    b. Sodium bicarbonate

c. Tincture iodine
d. Rectified spirit

32. **'Afim' is a derivative of:**
    a. Opium b. Cannabis
    c. Cocaine d. None of these

33. **Beers, an alcoholic beverage, is an example of:**
    a. Spirit b. Liquor
    c. Wines d. All of these

34. **Wines, an alcoholic beverage, is obtained by fermentation of:**
    a. Germinating cereals and un-distilled
    b. Natural sugar in fruits and un-distilled
    c. Juice extracted from palm trees and un-distilled
    d. Cereals, fruits, flower, etc. followed by distillation

35. **Absorption of alcohol is delayed:**
    a. In high concentration of alcohol
    b. In fatty and *proteinaceous* food
    c. In chronic gastritis
    d. When mixed with aerated water

36. **Widmark formula is used to estimate:**
    a. Blood alcohol concentration
    b. Alcohol absorbed in the body
    c. Breath alcohol concentration
    d. All of these

37. **In methyl alcohol intoxication, the treatment includes all *except*:**
    a. Folate therapy b. IV NaHCO$_3$
    c. IV ethanol d. IV fomepizole

38. **All are the features of Datura poisoning *except*:**
    a. Dysphagia b. Dysuria
    c. Diplopia d. Dementia

39. **Tactile hallucination is seen in all these poisoning *except*:**
    a. Datura b. Narcotics
    c. Cocaine d. Amphetamine

40. **Visual and auditory hallucination is particularly seen in poisoning with:**
    a. Datura b. Cannabis
    c. Cocaine d. Alcohol

41. **All are the preparation of cannabis *except*:**
    a. Charas b. Afim
    c. Majun d. Hashish

42. **The smuggler smuggled following contraband drug in body packer (packing) *except*:**
    a. Cocaine/heroin
    b. Amphetamine
    c. Benzodiazepine
    d. Hashish

43. **In barbiturate poisoning, the treatment includes all *except*:**
    a. Maintain respiration/circulation
    b. Forced alkaline diuresis
    c. IV flumazenil
    d. Stomach wash with activated charcoal

44. **All of the following are used in 'Date Rape' *except*:**
    a. Alcohol b. Cocaine
    c. Flunitrazepam d. Amphetamine

45. **'Dope Test' is carried out in athletes for the detection of all drugs *except*:**
    a. Amphetamine b. Diazepam
    c. Cannabis d. Cocaine/heroin

46. **All of the following are potent hallucinogens *except*:**
    a. LSD b. Phencyclidine
    c. Mescaline d. Amphetamine

47. **This alkaloid is not an active/toxic principle of strychnos nux vomica.**
    a. Strychnine b. Brucine
    c. Loganine d. Conine

48. **Strychnine acts on spinal cord by blocking:**
    a. Presynaptic inhibition at anterior horn cell (AHC)

b. Postsynaptic inhibition at AHC

c. Presynaptic inhibition at posterior horn cell (PHC)

d. Postsynaptic inhibition at PHC

49. **Curare is an active principle obtained or derived from:**

a. *Chondrodendron tomentosum*

b. *Conium maculatum*

c. *Cinchona pubescens*

d. *Cytrullus colocynthis*

50. **This poison acts an enzyme system causes histotoxic anoxia.**

a. Cyanide   b. Phosphorus

c. Arsenic   d. Lead

51. **It is commonly called 'Cyanogen'.**

a. Mixture of $O_2 + CO_2$

b. Mixture of $CO_2 + Hb$

c. Carbon monoxide

d. Cyanide

52. **It is commonly called 'Mitha Jaher'.**

a. Arrow poison

b. Aphrodisiac agent

c. Majum

d. Aconite

53. **It is not useful in cyanide poisoning.**

a. Sublingual amyl nitrite

b. IV Na nitrite

c. IV Na thiosulfate

d. IV Na bicarbonate

54. **Quinine is obtained from the bark of:**

a. Cinchonine

b. *Cinchona pubescens*

c. *Conium maculatum*

d. *Cytrullus colocynthis*

55. **It is not an active principle of 'Tobacco'.**

a. Loganine

b. Lobeline

c. Nicotine

d. Nicotianine

56. **This poisonous plant is not found by roadside.**

a. *Cerbera thevetia*

b. Datura

c. *Jatropha curcas*

d. *Calotropris/Ricinus communis*

57. **Mecamylamine is a specific antidote of:**

a. Nicotine   b. Quinine

c. Aconite   d. Strychnine

58. **It is not the natural derivative of opium.**

a. Morphine   b. Pethidine

c. Codeine   d. Thebaine

59. **Reefers is the cigarette preparation of:**

a. Cocaine   b. Afim

c. Ganja   d. Charas

60. **It is considered as 'Gateway to drug abuse'.**

a. Tobacco   b. Ganja

c. Heroin   d. LSD

61. **Drug of abuse using the parental route is called 'skin popping':**

a. Intradermal

b. Subcutaneous

c. Intravenous

d. Intra-arterial

62. **Drug of abuse using intra-arterial route is known as ....**

a. Mainlining   b. Skin popping

c. Chasers   d. Pinkie

63. **Run amok is seen in poisoning with:**

a. Opium   b. Cannabis

c. Cocaine   d. Datura

64. **Blister/vesicle is one of the manifestations seen in:**

a. Barbiturate poisoning

b. Snakebite

c. Both a and b

d. None of these

65. Blister/vesicle formation is seen at the site of contact with juice/oil of all vegetable irritants *except:*
   a. *Ricinus communis*
   b. *Croton tiglium*
   c. *Semicarpus anacardium*
   d. Calotropis

66. In this bacterial food poisoning, the toxin is present/produced in the contaminated food.
   a. *Clostridium botulinum*
   b. Shigella
   c. Salmonella
   d. Cholera

67. It contains beta oxalyl amino alanine (BOAA) causing 'paralysis'.
   a. *Argemone mexicana*
   b. *Lathyrus sativus*
   c. Mushrooms
   d. *Cannabis sativa*

68. Mustard oil adulterated with oil of .... causes epidemic dropsy.
   a. *Argemone mexicana*
   b. *Lathyrus sativus*
   c. Badly stored groundnut
   d. *Jatropha curcas*

69. Leather bottle appearance of stomach is seen in:
   a. Oxalic acid   b. Carbolic acid
   c. Acetic acid   d. Alkalies

70. Basophilic stippling is seen in all *except:*
   a. Arsenic   b. Lead
   c. Antimony   d. Bismuth

71. In carbamate insecticidal poisoning, all of the following are true *except:*
   a. Blood cholinesterase level is decreased
   b. It inhibits the acetylcholine esterase
   c. Clinical features similar to OP poisoning
   d. Pralidoxime (PAM) is given as an antidote

72. Antidote of ethyl alcohol poisoning is:
   a. Methanol   b. Fomepizole
   c. Flumazenil   d. None of these

73. Datura, cocaine and cannabis are the examples of all *except:*
   a. Aphrodisiac agents
   b. Stupefying poison
   c. Cattle poison
   d. Deliriant poison

74. It is an antidote of copper sulfate poisoning.
   a. Ferric oxide
   b. Potassium ferrocyanide
   c. Ferric chloride
   d. Potassium permanganate

75. Cherry red postmortem lividity is seen in poisoning with:
   a. CO   b. CO_2
   c. Cyanide   d. Opium

76. Egg albumin is an example of:
   a. Physical antidote
   b. Chemical antidote
   c. Both a and b
   d. None of these

77. For toxicological analysis, urine is preserved in:
   a. Potassium oxalate
   b. Potassium acetate
   c. Sodium fluoride
   d. Formalin

78. It is an example of both diluents and demulcent.
   a. Oil   b. Ghee
   c. Water   d. Milk

79. All of the following chemical tests are used to detect metallic poison *except:*
   a. Marsh's test
   b. Marquis test
   c. Reinsch test
   d. Gutzeit test

80. Marquis test is used to detect all the following poisons *except:*
    a. Benzodiazepines
    b. Ergot and Abrus
    c. Opium
    d. Cyanide

81. Hyperpigmentation of palm and sole (black foot disease) is seen in:
    a. Arsenic poisoning
    b. Mercury poisoning
    c. Lead poisoning
    d. Copper poisoning

82. Forty-five years male comes in the hospital with hyperkeratosis/rain drop pigmentation of palms, paraesthesia of hands and feet, whitish Mee's lines on nails. The most likely diagnosis is:
    a. Chronic arsenic poisoning
    b. Chronic mercury poisoning
    c. Chronic lead poisoning
    d. Chronic copper poisoning

83. Delayed rigor mortis occurs in poisoning with:
    a. Arsenic   b. Lead
    c. Mercury   d. Copper

84. It is detected even in highly decomposed bodies, charred bodies and burnt ash.
    a. Strychnine   b. Lead
    c. Copper   d. Arsenic

85. Golden yellow hair is seen in poisoning with:
    a. Cadmium   b. Copper
    c. Lead   d. Arsenic

86. All are associated with lead poisoning, *except:*
    a. Coproporphyrin in urine-red colour
    b. Basophilic stippling of red cells
    c. Cutaneous blisters
    d. Deposited in bones and nails

87. A person with anaemia, abdominal colic, constipation, basophilic stippling, blue lines over gums, wrist drop and encephalopathy are the characteristic features of poisoning with:
    a. Arsenic   b. Lead
    c. Mercury   d. Thallium

88. Acrodynia, Hatter's shakes, pink disease, erethism and brownish spot in the lens are seen in poisoning with:
    a. Arsenic   b. Lead
    c. Mercury   d. Copper

89. Mercury is a nephrotoxic agent acts on:
    a. Proximal convoluted tubules
    b. Distal convoluted tubules
    c. Loop of Henle
    d. Collecting ducts

90. Clapton's line over gums and Kayser Fleischer ring in cornea with low serum ceruloplasmin level are characteristic of poisoning with:
    a. Arsenic   b. Lead
    c. Mercury   d. Copper

91. Chemical antidote for copper is:
    a. Ferric oxide
    b. Potassium ferrocyanide
    c. Potassium permanganate
    d. None of these

92. All are the features of organophosphorus poisoning *except*
    a. Dilated pupil   b. Lacrimation
    c. Sweating   d. Bradycardia

93. Which of these statements is false about snakebite?
    a. Cobra venom is neurotoxic
    b. Deranged blood coagulation in viper bite
    c. Ptosis, staggering gait with loss of speech/deglutition in cobra bite
    d. Neostigmine has a role in krait bite

94. False about snake envenomation:
    a. Tourniquet should be applied proximal to the bite
    b. Affected limb should be splinted

c. Wound should be immediately cauterized

d. Washing the wound with antiseptic

95. Neostigmine is used in the treatment of all *except:*

a. Datura poisoning

b. Cobra bite

c. Mushrooms

d. Myasthenia gravis

96. In cyanide poisoning, the death is due to:

a. Anoxic anoxia by inhibiting succinyl oxidase

b. Cytotoxic anoxia by inhibiting cytochrome oxidase

c. Histotoxic anoxia by inhibiting cytochrome oxidase

d. Inhibition of DNA and protein synthesis

97. A young lady committed suicide by consuming 50 tablets of paracetamol. What is the drug of choice?

a. Gastric lavage

b. Alkaline diuresis

c. Dialysis

d. N-acetyl cysteine

98. The most common cause of parasuicide is:

a. Hanging

b. Cutting wrist

c. Consumption of drug

d. Jumping from height

99. Antidote of ethylene glycol is:

a. Flumazenil

b. Fomepizole

c. Ferric chloride

d. Potassium chlorate

100. Hemodialysis is used in all poisoning *except:*

a. Barbiturates

b. Cocaine

c. Cannabis

d. Kerosene

101. *Argemone maxicana* **contains all toxic principles** *except:*

a. Protopine

b. Loganine

c. Berberine

d. Dihydrosanguinarine

102. St. Anthony's fire refer to poisoning by:

a. Ergot alkaloids   b. Aflatoxin

c. Spanish fly   d. Phosphorus

103. Atropine is an antidote in all poisoning cases *except:*

a. Organophosphorus

b. Carbamates

c. Cyanide

d. Mushroom

104. Atropine is used in the treatment of all poisoning cases *except:*

a. Mushroom

b. Aconite

c. Curare

d. Cannabis/cocaine

105. The drug of choice for mushroom poisoning is:

a. Adrenaline   b. Atropine

c. Physostigmine d. None of these

106. It is used to produce artificial bruises:

a. Abrus   b. Ricinus

c. Calotropis   d. Semicarpus

107. These are the postmortem findings in cyanide poisoning *except:*

a. Characteristics bitter almond taste

b. Pinkish or cherry red lividity

c. Pale organs

d. Erosion and hemorrhages in mucosa of stomach

108. All are true for carbolic acid poisoning *except:*

a. Greenish brown urine

b. Tough and leathery stomach wall

c. Dilated pupil

d. Ochronosis

109. **Brown colored urine is seen in poisoning with:**
    a. Sulfuric acid
    b. Nitric acid
    c. Hydrochloric acid
    d. Carbolic acid

110. **This statement is not correct about chemical burns due to strong acids.**
    a. Trickle marks are present with absence of singeing of hair
    b. Ulcerated patches and coagulation necrosis present
    c. Blister over burnt area is common
    d. Red line of demarcation is not present

111. **It is also known as knock out drops, or dry wine or Mickey finn.**
    a. Barbiturates   b. LSD
    c. Mescaline   d. Chloral hydrate

112. **It is commonly known as ecstasy.**
    a. LSD   b. Mescaline
    c. Phencyclidine   d. Amphetamine

113. **All are true about methanol poisoning** *except:*
    a. It is metabolized to formaldehyde and formic acid
    b. It causes snow field vision/blindness
    c. Fomepizole is an aldehyde dehydrogenase inhibitor
    d. Critical level of methanol is 1.25 ml/kg body weight

114. **It is not correct about barbiturate poisoning.**
    a. Coma   b. Blister
    c. Hypothermia   d. Hypertension

115. **It is an antidote of benzodiazepine.**
    a. Naltrexone   b. Naloxone
    c. Flumezenil   d. Fomepizole

116. **Opium is derived from which part of the plant?**
    a. Root
    b. Leaf

117. **Black tongue is present in abuse of:**
    a. Tobacco smoking
    b. Cocaine
    c. Heroin
    d. Afim

118. **Poisonous snake 'Krait' belongs to:**
    a. Colubridae   b. Elapidae
    c. Viperidae   d. Crotalide

119. **All of the following causes 'Priapism'** *except:*
    a. Spanish fly
    b. Scorpion bite
    c. Honey bee bite
    d. Viper bite

120. **All are the characteristic features of poisonous snakes** *except:*
    a. Presence of fangs
    b. Belly scales are complete
    c. Usually large head
    d. Abruptly tapering (compressed) tail

121. **In snakebite poisoning, antivenom is usually started by giving a dose of:**
    a. 20 vials   b. 10 vials
    c. 5 vials   d. 2 vials

122. **Lee Jones test is used for:**
    a. Arsenic   b. Lead
    c. Cocaine   d. Cyanide

123. **Urine is preserved for toxicological analysis in all the following preservatives** *except:*
    a. Saturated solution of common salt
    b. Hydrochloric acid
    c. Thymol
    d. Sodium fluoride

124. **Bluish green color of postmortem lividity is seen in poisoning with:**
    a. CO   b. CO_2
    c. H_2S d. Cyanide

c. Poppy seeds
d. Unripe poppy capsule

125. **Brown hypostasis is seen in poisoning with:**
    a. Cannabis
    b. Aniline
    c. Phosphorus
    d. Organophosphorus

126. **Red-brown postmortem lividity is seen in poisoning with:**
    a. Cannabis   b. Nitrites
    c. Opium   d. Barbiturates

127. **All are the composition of sewer gas except:**
    a. CO_2 b. H_2S
    c. Phosgene   d. Methane

128. **Acrid (pear) smell is seen in:**
    a. Cocaine
    b. Cannabis
    c. Ether
    d. Paraldehyde/chloral hydrate

129. **All are the examples of 'Tear gas' except:**
    a. Diphenyl chlorarsine
    b. CAP: Chloracetophenone
    c. BBC: Bromobenzyl cyanide
    d. Ethyl iodoacetate acetate

130. **All are the examples of 'Blistering gas' except:**
    a. Mustard gas   b. Chlorine gas
    c. Lewisite   d. Phosgene

Keys for MCQs

1. d	2. c	3. c	4. a	5. d	6. d
7. d	8. a	9. b	10. d	11. d	12. c
13. c	14. c	15. c	16. a	17. c	18. a
19. d	20. b	21. a	22. c	23. c	24. a
25. a	26. a	27. b	28. c	29. d	30. d
31. b	32. a	33. b	34. b	35. b	36. b
37. c	38. d	39. a	40. a	41. b	42. c
43. c	44. d	45. b	46. d	47. d	48. b
49. a	50. a	51. d	52. d	53. d	54. b
55. a	56. c	57. a	58. b	59. c	60. a
61. b	62. d	63. b	64. c	65. a	66. a
67. b	68. a	69. b	70. a	71. d	72. d
73. c	74. b	75. a	76. c	77. c	78. d
79. b	80. d	81. a	82. a	83. a	84. d
85. d	86. c	87. b	88. c	89. a	90. d
91. b	92. a	93. d	94. c	95. c	96. c
97. d	98. c	99. b	100. d	101. b	102. a
103. c	104. d	105. b	106. d	107. c	108. c
109. b	110. c	111. d	112. d	113. c	114. d
115. c	116. d	117. b	118. b	119. c	120. c
121. b	122. d	123. a	124. c	125. c	126. b
127. c	128. d	129. a	130. b		

Index